The Clinical Handling of Dental Materials

Second Edition

Bernard G.N. Smith, BDS, PhD, MSc(Mich), FDSRCS(Eng)
Paul S. Wright, BDS(Hons), PhD, FDSRCS (Eng)
David Brown, MSc, PhD, CEng, MIM

With contributions by

Keith G. Isaacson, MOrth, FDSRCS (Eng)
Richard M. Palmer, BDS, PhD, FDSRCS (Eng)
Tom R. Pitt Ford, BDS, PhD, FDSRCPS (Glasgow)

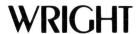

Wright
An imprint of Butterworth-Heinemann Ltd
Linacre House, Jordan Hill, Oxford OX2 8DP

℞ A member of the Reed Elsevier plc group

OXFORD LONDON BOSTON
MUNICH NEW DELHI SINGAPORE SYDNEY
TOKYO TORONTO WELLINGTON

First published 1986
Second edition 1994
Paperback edition 1995

British Library Cataloguing in Publication Data
A catalogue record for this book is available from the British Library

ISBN 0 7236 1023 1

Library of Congress Cataloguing in Publication Data
A catalogue record for this book is available from the Library of Congress

Filmset by Bath Typesetting Ltd, Bath
Printed in Scotland by Cambus Litho Ltd, Glasgow

Contents

Authors and contributors

The Authors

BERNARD G.N. SMITH
BDS, PhD, MSc(Mich), FDSRCS(Eng)

Professor and Head of the Department of Conservative Dental Surgery,
United Medical and Dental Schools of Guy's and St. Thomas's Hospitals (UMDS),
Guy's Hospital, London.
Formerly of the Royal Dental Hospital, School of Dental Surgery and The London Hospital Medical College Dental School.
Examiner for the Universities of London, Birmingham, Sheffield and Malta and The Royal College of Surgeons of England.

PAUL S. WRIGHT
BDS(Hons), PhD, FDSRCS(Eng)

Senior Lecturer and Consultant,
Department of Prosthetic Dentistry,
The London Hospital Medical College Dental School,
Turner Street, London.
Examiner for the University of London and The Royal College of Surgeons of England.

DAVID BROWN
MSc, PhD, CEng, MIM

Head of the Department and Senior Lecturer in Dental Materials Science,
UMDS, Guy's Hospital, London.
Formerly Lecturer in Dental Materials Science in the Turner Dental School, University of Manchester, and Visiting Lecturer in Dental Materials at the College of Medicine in the University of Lagos, Nigeria and the College of Health Sciences in the University of Nairobi, Kenya..
Examiner for the Universities of London, Cork, Manchester and Nairobi.

The Contributors

RICHARD M. PALMER, BDS, PhD,
FDSRCS(Eng)
Senior Lecturer and Consultant
Department of Periodontology and Preventive Dentistry,
UMDS, Guy's Hospital, London.

KEITH G. ISAACSON, MOrth, FDSRCS(Eng)
Consultant Orthodontist
Royal Berkshire Hospital.

TOM R. PITT FORD, BDS, PhD,
FDSRCPS(Glasgow)
Senior Lecturer and Consultant
Department of Conservative Dental Surgery,
UMDS, Guy's Hospital, London.

Preface

This book is primarily for postgraduate clinicians, although much of it is of interest to undergraduate students as well. This represents a shift in emphasis from the first edition in which an attempt was made to address the needs of both undergraduates and postgraduates equally. With the rapid development of new materials and their use in different applications, together with the expansion of postgraduate education, the decision has been made to concentrate more on the needs of the postgraduate student in this second edition. New sections have been added to all chapters in the book, some by additional contributors. Colour illustrations and sections on further reading have also been added.

The book approaches the science of dental materials from the clinician's viewpoint. Materials are discussed in relation to clinical procedures, concentrating on properties which affect both their handling at the chairside and their subsequent behaviour in service. Armed with this information, clinicians should be able to select an appropriate material for any application.

Part One sets the scene for an understanding of materials and Part Two follows a sequence of clinical procedures, starting with the examination of the patient. Since materials are discussed in the context of each procedure, some, which are used in several applications in different ways, for example self-activated acrylic resins, appear in a number of chapters.

In Part Two a series of numerical references, in parentheses after the headings, directs the reader to further details of the materials, composition and properties which are set out in Part Three. Parts Three and Four are for reference and it is not envisaged that they will be read from beginning to end.

Part Four lists the more common materials available by trade name. This list will of course become out of date fairly quickly, but once the principles described elsewhere in the book are understood the place of any new material in the general scheme of things should be clear.

Acknowledgements

We are grateful to our three new contributors, Keith Isaacson, Richard Palmer and Tom Pitt Ford who have written new sections for this second edition on orthodontics, periodontology and oral surgery and endodontics respectively. We also thank several colleagues who have lent illustrations. They are acknowledged individually in the relevant captions.

We are also grateful to Martyn Sherriff for coordinating our word processing.

Cover illustrations

We would like to thank Tim Watson for permission to use the two confocal micrographs which illustrate the book cover. *Left* A high resolution optical section made with a confocal microscope through the interface between composite resin, bonding agent and dentine, the so-called hybrid layer. The adhesive has been specifically labelled with a dye and is approximately 30 μm wide. *Right* A confocal microscope image of the enamel margin produced after a 1 mm diameter, fine diamond bur has finished cutting. The 7 μm diameter, horseshoe-shaped enamel prisms can be seen within the bulk of the tooth and the diamond grit of the bur can be seen.

Abbreviations

μm	micron (1 micron $= 10^{-6}$ metres; 1 mm $=$ 1000 microns)
ADA	American Dental Association
BHN	Brinell Hardness Number
bis-GMA	a dimethacrylate resin derived from the reaction between bis-phenol A and glycidyl methacrylate
BPDM	biphenyl dimethacrylate
BS	British Standard
CAD/CAM	computer-aided design/computer-aided manufacture
CPITN	Community Periodontal Index of Treatment Needs
E	elastic modulus (Young's modulus)
EDTA	ethylene diamine tetra-acetic acid
EGDMA	ethylene glycol dimethacrylate
EPT	electronic pulp tester
FG	friction grip (burs)
g	gram
g/cc^3	grams per cubic centimetre (density)
GHM	commercial name for occlusal shimstock foil
GN/m^2	giga-newtons per square metre. Giga $= 10^9$. Encountered when elastic modulus of rigid solid is quoted. Also known as GPa
GP	gutta percha
GPa	giga-pascal; equivalent to GN/m^2
HEMA	hydroxyethyl methacrylate (also poly[HEMA])
HTV	high temperature vulcanization
ISO	International Organization for Standardization
K$_{1C}$	the characteristic energy needed to propagate a crack through a solid. It is a measure of the fracture toughness of a material
kHz	kiloHertz (1 kHz $=$ 1000 cycles per second)
LC	light cured (resin)
MDP	10-methacryloxydecyl dihydrogen phosphate
mm	millimetre (1000 mm $=$ 1 metre)
MN/m^2	mega-newtons per square metre. Mega $= 10^6$. Encountered when the tensile, compressive or adhesive bond strength are quoted. Also known as MPa
MOD	mesial-occlusal-distal (a 3 surface cavity or restoration)
MPa	mega-pascal; equivalent to MN/m^2
NPG-GMA	N-phenyl glycine – glycidyl methacrylate
NTG-GMA	N-tolyl glycine – glycidyl methacrylate
p.p.m.	parts per million
pH	measure of the acidity or alkalinity [neutral $= 7, 1\text{-}6 =$ acidic, 8-14 $=$ alkaline]. It is the logarithm of the reciprocal of the hydrogen ion concentration in moles per litre of solution.

PMDM	pyromellitic acid dimethacrylate
PTFE	poly(tetrafluoro-ethylene)
PVC/PAN	poly(vinyl chloride)/polyacrylonitrile
r.p.m.	revolutions per minute
RTV	room-temperature vulcanization
TBB-O	tri-N-butyl borane oxide
TEG-DMA	triethylene glycol dimethacrylate
Tg	glass transition temperature
TLV	threshold limit value of a toxic substance (e.g. mercury in air)
USP	United States Pharmacopoeia
UV	ultra-violet radiation
VLC	visible light cured (resin)
W/(m.K)	watts per metre degree Kelvin. This is a measure of the thermal conductivity which is measured under steady state conditions. Such conditions do not occur in the mouth and a more realistic property is thermal diffusivity. This is an indication of heat flow under transient conditions. It is defined as the thermal conductivity divided by the product of the thermal capacity and the density of the material.
WHO	World Health Organization
YS	yield strength
4-META	4- methacryloxyethyl trimellitate anhydride

Part One

An introduction to the general properties of dental materials

The limitations of dental materials

Limitations on the practitioner's use of any dental material are controlled by the inevitable interrelation of the three factors outlined below – chemistry, handling characteristics and performance in service – together with considerations of cost.

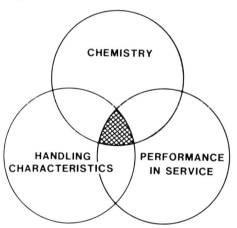

The factors that limit the use of dental materials.

Chemistry

The chemistry of a material covers its composition and also those factors which enable it to be formed or shaped. The material may become a restoration or appliance, or may be used and then discarded in the sequence of making a restoration or appliance.

All the basic structural materials of the universe can be categorized as ceramics, metals, polymers or composites.

Ceramics

Ceramics are the most abundant structural materials in the earth's crust and are either simple or complex combinations of the metallic and non-metallic elements of the periodic table. They are characteristically hard and abrasive. Examples of simple ceramics found in use in dental materials include alumina (aluminium oxide), silica (silicon dioxide) and tungsten carbide. Examples of complex ceramics include potassium, aluminium silicate (potash feldspar), hydrated aluminium silicate (kaolin) and tetra-silicic fluor-mica.

Although they all have high melting points, mixtures of both simple and complex ceramics will react together at high temperatures to form the viscous liquids we know as glasses and porcelains. Whilst at low temperatures these materials appear to have the properties normally associated with solids, they are in fact not true solids but very viscous, supercooled liquids.

Metals

Metals are rarely found in the natural state, the exceptions being gold and platinum and occasionally copper, silver and mercury. More usually they are found combined with non-metals such as oxygen and sulphur as oxides and sulphides respectively, or as carbonates, nitrates, sulphates, nitrites or phosphates when combined with two non-metallic elements. These compounds are solids, but metals are also found in solution in the sea as chlorides, bromides and other compounds. Still others are found as complex mixtures of oxides in clays and soils. In most cases the metal has to be won from the ore by some sort of energy-consuming process, such as high temperature reduction or the electrolysis of a fused salt. In all cases, even when found in the natural state, metals have to be separated from the rocks in which they lie, whence they are refined and purified.

Pure metals are generally very soft and can be easily bent and shaped and many can be rolled to produce thin sheets or drawn through dies to produce wires. Examples of pure metals used as dental materials include aluminium (temporary crowns), copper (bands and electroplating electrodes), gold (cohesive foil), lead (foil behind X-ray films), platinum (matrix foil for the build-up of porcelain), silver (endodontic points and electroplating electrodes), tin (separating foil and electroplating electrodes) and titanium (endodontic points). In each case they are used because of the ease with which they can be permanently bent or shaped. However, this weakness is not acceptable in structural or engineering components and metals are frequently combined with one another or with non-metallic elements such as carbon or nitrogen to produce alloys. Alloys used in dentistry range from the simple, two component nickel–titanium to the complex, six component gold–platinum–palladium–copper–silver–zinc alloys.

Polymers

Polymers of all sorts are now synthesized by humans from the simple organic compounds found in fossil fuels such as gas, oil and coal. However, natural polymers in the form of cellulose (wood pulp and cotton), nucleic acids and collagen have existed in nature much longer and are the structural building blocks of all living things.

Apart from the polymeric nature of the soft dental tissues and certain components of the hard tissues, examples of natural polymers found in dental materials include agar-agar, alginates, several resins and gums extracted from trees, and a whole range of animal, vegetable and mineral waxes. Examples of synthetic polymers used in dental materials include acrylics, urethanes and silicones. Generally these materials have low melting points, are fairly soft and are not particularly stiff.

Composites

Composites are combinations of any of the basic ceramic, metallic and polymeric materials, as shown below. Their properties tend to be somewhere

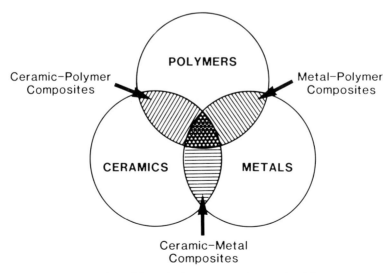

Composites derived from the basic structural materials of the universe.

between those of their basic constituents and they are used when performance in service or the handling characteristics can be improved.

An example of a ceramic–metallic composite used in dentistry is the tungsten carbide (ceramic)–cobalt (metal) tip used on both scaling instruments and burs. The ceramic–polymer composites used as restorative materials in dentistry are generally just known as composites, and metal–polymer composites are sometimes employed as die materials in the dental laboratory. Enamel and dentine are both magnificent examples of natural ceramic–polymer composites.

Handling characteristics

The handling characteristics of any dental material are of vital importance and frequently they control absolutely the selection of a material for a particular application. No matter how excellent its other properties may be, the material is not acceptable if it cannot be readily controlled to produce what the practitioner wants in the time available.

Shelf life

As all dental materials spend much of their time prior to being used sitting in some cupboard or on a shelf, the first essential requirement is a good shelf-life. During this out-of-use period the material must not 'go off' – that is, its constituents must not separate or evaporate, nor must they react together. In fact, anything which causes the material to change its viscosity or which causes it to become a solid when it is presented as a liquid or a paste, or vice versa, is not desirable.

Presentation and mixing

Many dental materials are presented for use as two components which have to be mixed together. Frequently these are a powder and a liquid, as in most dental cements, amalgams or laboratory materials such as plaster, artificial stone and investment. However, others such as composites and impression materials are often presented as two pastes. In these cases the two-component pastes have to be mixed together to produce a single paste

which is then deployed. Whatever its starting components, the fluid paste, once in position is required to undergo a change in its viscosity such that, in the case of the cements, filling materials, model and die materials and investments they become rigid solids, and in the case of the elastic impression materials they become solids capable of considerable elastic distortion.

These changes, which are generally thought of as setting reactions, can be brought about by several mechanisms. In the case of most cements and model dies and investment materials, setting occurs due to the precipitation and interlocking of new compounds. In unfilled resins or filled polymeric systems such as the dental composites, the setting occurs due to polymerization reactions, in which molecules join together to produce chains of high molecular weight. Sometimes the chains themselves can be joined by cross-links, rather like the rungs of a ladder, and such reactions are utilized in both the strengthening of restorative and denture base resins, and in the setting of the elastomeric or rubber-like impression materials. Those materials which undergo neither chemical precipitation nor polymerization reactions change from being mouldable fluids into rigid solids by physical phase changes such as those seen in the solidification of metals and alloys with cooling and in the crystallization of solid wax from the melt. A physical change also occurs when an elastic gel forms from a sol of agar-agar.

Not all materials are handled or shaped whilst fluid. Orthodontic wires and bands, for example, are cut, bent and joined as solids. In such cases the inherent ductility of the metal is utilized. Such plastic deformation is also utilized in the formation of impressions in dental composition, in the shaping of thermoplastic baseplates and in the creation of mouthguards from soft polymers. In the case of these thermoplastics the material is heated to enable plastic deformation to take place readily.

A special forming process is used to create dental porcelain crowns and veneers. The particles of porcelain are packed together as closely as possible using water or other suspension medium. The consolidated particles are then heated in a vacuum and they fuse together in the process known as sintering. The air in the spaces between the particles is drawn to the surface in the vacuum process, and solid porcelain is the result.

Behaviour of materials at the chairside

Two-component materials   Because many dental materials used at the chairside are shaped as fluids and then harden by one of the reactions outlined above, they are often presented as two components. These require proportioning and then mixing — both processes which should be simple and foolproof. Some materials are more sensitive to the use of the correct ratio of components than others and in such cases variation can affect fluidity of the mix and/or the rate at which the material hardens. It may even ultimately influence the performance of the material in service.

Whether a two-component system is presented as a powder and a liquid or as two pastes or as a paste and a liquid, the result on mixing is a paste into which air has inevitably been incorporated. Thus the set material is always porous, and although the minute air-filled cavities within it are not interconnected, the porosity represents regions of structural weakness.

Placing materials in the mouth   Premixed or freshly mixed materials which are being used at the chairside need to be transferred from the mixing pad into the patient's mouth using an appropriate instrument or carrier. It is most desirable that the material should not escape from the carrier until it has reached its intended destination. The ideal material would not in fact show any flow until a force was applied to it. The way in which fluids, including pastes, behave under loads is included in the science of rheology, and a material which appears to get thinner and flows more readily when stressed is termed pseudoplastic. In dentistry we are fortunate that either by accident or by design many restorative and impression materials behave in this way. Those that do not are either applied using a brush (in which case the material is retained on the bristles by surface tension) or they are viscous enough to be controlled by suitable manipulation of the carrier in the same way that honey, for example, can be retained on a knife.

If the material is pseudoplastic then when it is inserted into the mouth and loaded it will readily flow around and into those areas where it is required. Once it is inserted and the load is removed, the ideal material stays in place. In the mouth this is generally assisted by the increase in

viscosity which occurs during the setting stage. However, during insertion the material may be experiencing conditions which may either help or hinder its ability to flow and ultimately its ability to set. These include the increase in temperature from room to open-mouth conditions, and exposure to the inherent high humidity and possibly even oral fluids. At some point most materials are obliged to come into contact with other materials and there may be some chemical interaction, which might affect the properties of either. It is clearly important that good compatibility should exist between such materials. In those whose setting is brought about by light-activated polymerization their exposure to normal lighting levels around the chair may start their setting reaction and their viscosity will increase as a result. This could make their handling more difficult.

Wettability   On contact with the oral tissues materials need to 'wet' the surfaces. When a material flows in contact with either the hard or soft oral tissues the effects of surface tension, which manifest themselves as 'wettability', are of consequence. The adaptation of a filling material to the cavity or the flow of an impression material to give a good detail of the tissues is related to this behaviour. In addition, although the retention of any material to another can be brought about by several processes, assuming that one is a fluid and the other is a solid, the ability of the fluid to wet the solid provides the first contribution towards the forming of a bond between them. This involves the weak physical attraction known as the van der Waals forces. True chemical adhesion can then develop subject to a chemical reaction taking place between the components of the surface (adherend) and the material placed in contact with it (adhesive) which has to wet the surface. If the adhesive has good fluidity it will flow into all the nooks and crannies of the surface, which is never microscopically smooth, and once the fluid becomes a solid those parts of the adhesive which are in the surface pits and scratches (surface asperities) contribute a mechanical component to any bond which forms. Many so-called adhesives rely on this mechanical component almost entirely.

Setting behaviour   The change from being a fluid into a rigid or elastic solid, and the rate at which this change takes place is the next consideration in the handling of any chairside material. The mechanisms by which such a change can take place have been indicated above, and these reactions can be influenced by the conditions within the mouth. Many materials set more readily when the temperature is raised and in some cases the set is accelerated by the high humidity. Those materials which polymerize as a result of light activation need exposure to light of the appropriate wavelength and once they are *in situ* this will only come from a high-intensity activating lamp via a suitable light guide.

Assessment of set   Assessing whether or not the material has completely set in relation to the conditions within the mouth is never the easiest task, and most practitioners tend, in the absence of experience with any particular material, to expect that it will take longer than the manufacturer indicates or, in the case of the light-activated polymers, that it will require a longer exposure to the light source. During their setting reactions many materials evolve heat, that is they undergo exothermic reactions. In general, the amount of heat produced within the small volume of material normally used within the mouth is not enough to cause any problems, particularly with modern materials. However, this is always a property which should be stated for any material which is to set in contact with freshly cut dentine or with the mucosa.

Behaviour after setting   Once a material has set, its treatment will depend on its application. A restorative material will probably require some degree of finishing, which may involve trimming and polishing and could also require additions. The handling characteristics of such a material are difficult to generalize, except to say that each should be capable of being adjusted or modified without too much difficulty. However, if the set material is an impression there are several more stages in its handling sequence still to follow. These include the removal of the impression from the mouth − a stage at which it is important that it sticks to, or is held mechanically on to, the tray rather than the tissues. If the impression is an elastic one then on its removal it must deform readily as it is withdrawn, and must recover completely. If it is

to be an accurate impression of the tissues it should not tear as it is deformed, and once it has recovered from its elastic distortion it should not undergo any other dimensional changes during the period in which it is stored prior to the preparation of a model or die.

Performance in service

The selection of a material for any particular application is strongly influenced by the practitioner's experience of its handling characteristics, but he or she may also need to consider the performance of the material in long-term service in the mouth. An impression material spends only minutes in the mouth, and its performance during that short period is clearly important, but a material used as a component of a long-term restoration or appliance must be capable of performing efficiently in the dynamic working conditions pertaining in the mouth. These will include variations in temperature, pH, conductivity and bacteriological activity and the complex mechanical stresses generated during both the masticatory and silent periods. In the course of time all these influences combine to produce changes in the surface or substance of the restoration or appliance, and can result in what the practitioner or patient deem to be failure. A consideration of the effect of changing biological, chemical, mechanical and other physical factors of the oral environment upon dental materials is therefore appropriate here.

The performance in service of the natural dental tissues

The performance in service of any restorative material should emulate or supersede that of the enamel, dentine or other tissue which it is called upon to replace. Natural hard dental tissues are reasonably good at the job which modern human beings ask them to carry out, although they do fall short of ideal in some respects. Biologically there is, as yet, nothing to surpass them when they are healthy and the soft tissues and supporting periodontal membrane are also free from disease. No synthetic dental material can yet persuade the periodontal ligaments completely that it is cementum, for although considerable success has been achieved in implantology with transmucosal abutments made of titanium, there is really no substitute for healthy, natural hard tissue when it comes to forming a periosteal seal.

As natural composites, teeth are prone to chemical attack by any substance which can dissolve their organic or inorganic components. In particular, solutions with low pH can readily demineralize the enamel, causing either caries or erosion. Any material employed as a replacement for damaged or lost hard dental tissues should resist all forms of *in vivo* chemical attack. The enamel surface in contact with saliva in a healthy mouth is in a continuous state of ionic exchange, some ions being lost into the saliva whilst others are being absorbed. Under normal conditions the net exchange should be zero, but the excessive intake of acidic foods or the unchecked development of acid-producing plaque can alter the equilibrium of the ionic exchange and excessive and irreplaceable losses can occur.

Mechanically, teeth are rigid and their composite structure and shape endow them with high strength and a good resistance to the propagation of cracks when they are clinically vital and sound. However, when non-vital or when part of their structure is weak or missing, they become brittle and can readily fracture, particularly when subjected to a sudden blow or impact. Enamel and dentine do not deform under the loads to which they are subjected in the mouth such that their dimensions change, that is, they neither creep (as metals can) nor do they flow (as fluids do). They do not appear to suffer from fatigue fractures. However, they are prone to some structural loss due to wear, either from contact with opposing teeth during strong muscular activity or from agents introduced into the mouth such as food, toothbrushes, dentifrices and pipe stems. Any material called upon to replace enamel and dentine should have mechanical properties roughly similar to those of the natural materials. Improvements in some properties are not necessarily good, for example, if the replacement material is harder or rougher than enamel it may cause wear or damage to opposing teeth.

The physical properties of a tooth are produced by its complex composite structure, its internal blood supply and its seating within its mucosa-covered bony housing. Under such conditions the significance of simplistic measurements of the physical properties is questionable; however, two properties of enamel and dentine which should be

copied as closely as possible by any replacement material are the coefficients of thermal conductivity and thermal expansion. The complex combination of colour, translucency, fluorescence and an opacity to X-rays gives the optical properties which the ideal replacement material should possess.

Biocompatibility of dental materials

The reality of materials used as replacements for lost teeth or for restoring them has to take into account a number of other failings from which the natural dentition does not suffer. We have to be concerned about the risk to which both the patient and the staff in the dental surgery and laboratory might be exposed when they come into contact with dental materials. The level of this risk can range from potentially fatal, through harmful and irritant to mere nuisance. At the harmful and irritant levels materials may operate systemically or just on some localized area of the body. It is an essential requirement of all dental materials that their biological interaction should be minimal. Natural dental materials are at home in the wet conditions of the mouth and, except as indicated above, are not prone to dissolution. Any material which purports to act as a replacement should be at least as resistant to dissolution and to the concurrent loss of potentially hazardous solutes into the mouth. In practice several restorative dental materials are prone to the leaching out of various constituents and this effect is occasionally utilized for the controlled release of therapeutic agents which have either a prophylactic or pharmacological action.

Some restorative materials are metallic and almost all metals and metal mixtures (alloys), given the right conditions, show a thermodynamic tendency to form metallic compounds. The environmental conditions of the mouth are ideal for this process and metallic restorations should be alloys with an inherent resistance to corrosion. Such materials either contain large amounts of the noble metals — gold, platinum or palladium — which are fundamentally insensitive to corrosive aqueous environments, or they contain large amounts of elements such as chromium or titanium whose oxides form a thin but highly protective surface film. Natural dental materials, having existed in equilibrium with their aqueous environment since their formation, tend to be unaffected by strongly coloured or flavoured foodstuffs, although the enamel will develop superficial staining quite readily from the habitual use of tobacco. Restorative dental materials, as strangers to the aqueous oral environment, take some time to reach equilibrium, and there may be either an uptake of oral fluids whilst this equilibrium develops or an exchange of oral fluids with soluble components within the restoration or appliance. In the ideal restorative material no absorption or surface staining will occur, but if it does it must not be to the detriment of the mechanical and other physical properties of the material.

A property which is often desirable is that of adhesion. True adhesion involves a chemical reaction between the adherend and the adhesive and should not be confused with mechanical attachment, which has been described above. Once a chemical bond has formed, its stability within its working environment should be maintained. It should not therefore be weakened by the chemical action of anything that enters the mouth.

Mechanical properties of dental materials

The mechanical properties which have to be taken into account when considering a material as a replacement for enamel and dentine or as a component of a dental appliance or restoration are those which affect both its stiffness and its strength. A careful distinction between the two is important.

Stiffness

Stiffness is an indication of how easy it is to bend something without causing it to stay bent or to break. The 'something' has to be defined, as it is clearly always easier to bend long, thin pieces of material than it is short, thick ones. When materials are used they are not just lumps but are shaped by one of the processes described above into a useful object. This may be complete in itself, as is often the case with a dental restoration, or it may be just a component part, as in the case of a machine. Whatever the application it must be designed to resist the anticipated load. Structures may be described as rigid or flexible, although in fact even

the most apparently rigid structure will deform imperceptibly when loaded. The secret of designing structures is to ensure that they do not bend elastically to such a degree that their function as a useful structure is in question. For example, a road bridge over a river, which twisted when vehicles crossed it such that they fell off, would be unacceptable as a road bridge, even though it returned to its original shape once the vehicles had been dumped in the river. In a similar manner, a denture base which was so flexible that it allowed its teeth to be displaced during mastication would be of little use to its owner. The rigidity of any structure is controlled by three major factors – the inherent elastic modulus of the materials from which it is made, the size of the structure and its shape. Varying one of these factors whilst keeping the other two constant can give a wide range of stiffness values for the particular structure.

Yield strength

The concept of stiffness is only relevant up to the point at which the loaded structure starts permanently to deform; that is, once the load which has been elastically deforming it is removed, the structure stays deformed. The point at which this occurs is called, amongst other things, the yield strength. Unless we are trying permanently to shape a material by applying a load, this is the point at which, to all intents and purposes, the structure has failed, even if it has not broken. In many materials catastrophic failure occurs once this point has been reached but in metals a considerable amount of *plastic deformation* (permanent bending) may occur before the structure breaks. Returning to the analogy of the road bridge, even if the vehicles are not thrown into the river by the twisting of an excessively flexible structure, it would be embarrassing if, after the passing of a heavy vehicle, the bridge was discovered to have been permanently distorted such that its centre had become lower than its ends. Structures thus have to be designed not only to be rigid but to resist permanent deformation. Once again, the resistance to this form of distortion is dependent on the inherent strength of the material, its size and its shape. In order to compare different materials and variations in size under a range of loads the concept of *stress* is invoked. This relates the load to the cross-sectional area of the material and it is often quoted in units such as pounds per square inch, kilograms per square centimetre or, in the currently preferred SI unit, newtons per square metre (N/m^2). When a particular structure is loaded, stresses are generated within it and these stresses create deformation of the structure. This deformation is also size dependent and hence the concept of *strain* is invoked. If a material is being pulled in tension it will increase in length; if this increase is divided by the original length we get the strain, which has no units. It is often quoted as a percentage. Most natural and synthetic dental materials have strengths quoted in MN/m^2, where the prefix M indicates that they are meganewtons (10^6).

The *elastic modulus* of a material is a fundamental property and is the theoretical stress which would be needed to strain the material 100%. It is theoretical because most materials permanently deform at stresses well below this. The elastic moduli of most dental materials are quoted in GN/m^2, where the prefix G indicates that they are giganewtons (10^9).

Test methods

A further complication which arises in comparing the strengths of materials is that they are sensitive to the method by which they are tested. Materials can thus be made into structures, albeit simple ones, which are then pulled in tension, pushed in compression or bent in a transverse manner. Such methods of loading are further complicated by the rate at which the load is applied, and many materials are sensitive to the rate of loading. In general, materials are tested to failure and their behaviour under test often suggests the best method of testing them. Many non-metallic materials (such as dental cements, composites and gypsum products) fail catastrophically as soon as they cease to deform elastically. Such materials are brittle and cannot be meaningfully tested by pulling in tension. It is thus necessary to test them either in compression or in a transverse test. In this latter test the material is made into a simple beam which is supported at each end and loaded in the middle until it breaks – rather like breaking a matchstick in the fingers. Metallic materials, on the other hand, are good examples of

those which behave in a *ductile* manner once they cease to deform elastically. In some cases they can undergo considerable plastic deformation and 20–40% is not uncommon in pure metals and soft alloys. However, even metals show sensitivity to the rate at which they are loaded and three time-dependent loading effects are worth noting – creep, impact and fatigue failure.

Creep

Creep is the name given to the slow plastic deformation that occurs when a material is placed under a static or dynamic load which would not produce any detectable permanent distortion when applied over the few minutes that a laboratory test would normally take. The slow deformation is akin to the flow of material, and creep and flow are sometimes used to express the same idea, although the mechanisms which permit these apparently similar phenomena are usually different. Creep is a phenomenon generally associated with solid metals and occurs more rapidly as the metal approaches its melting point. *Flow*, on the other hand, is a time-dependent phenomenon of fluids rather than solids under load. However, it is sometimes difficult to see the exact dividing line between the two states and it is here that confusion can occur.

Impact strength

No such confusion occurs when solids are loaded extremely rapidly. Under these conditions even normally ductile materials can behave in a brittle manner. Such conditions occur when structures are subjected to sudden blows or impacts, and when tested by sudden blows in the laboratory an indication is provided of the impact strength of a particular material. Impact strength is itself an indication of the amount of energy which can be absorbed before a material fails when struck rapidly and, whilst vital teeth have a high impact strength, non-vital ones are apparently easily fractured by sudden blows.

Restorative materials may also be subjected to sudden high loads, as in a blow to a crowned tooth or the classic 'biting on a piece of lead shot whilst eating game'. These forces are resisted to some extent by the elasticity of the periodontal membrane, and in the latter case by the rapid reversal of the contraction of the muscles of mastication by the proprioceptive mechanism. However, despite these physiological restraints, both natural and restorative dental materials are stressed suddenly and fracture can occur. Perhaps the most common example of fracture due to impact of a dental material is seen when a complete denture is dropped, and many thousands of pounds are spent each year in repairs and replacements. The need for an economic, easy-to-process, high impact resistant material for this application is still to be satisfied.

Fatigue failure

Structures which are subjected to stresses which fluctuate in a regular manner are prone to yet another form of time-dependent stressing. This is called *fatigue*, and fatigue failure can occur when a crack, often aggravated by a stress-raising feature such as a notch, grows step-by-step as the structure undergoes cyclic loading. Rotating components in machines are prone to this sort of failure, and the cyclic nature of mastication can also lead to fatigue failure in those restorations and appliances that are capable of considerable elastic distortion on loading. Once again it is usually in large structures such as denture bases where this type of failure can be seen, and under certain conditions the fraenal notch is the stress-raising feature at which the crack starts.

Hardness and wear

One property which humans can judge subjectively is hardness. The fingernail or tapping test is carried out even by those with no scientific training when they are presented with a piece of a material which is new to them. However, hardness is measured much more objectively by pressing something very hard, either a steel ball or a diamond pyramid, into the surface of the material. The size of the hole produced is then measured and related to a scale of hardness. Although hardness is simple to measure, its interpretation is related to the resistance of the material, both to elastic and plastic deformation. Thus in one simple measurement we obtain an indication of the strength of the material and its ability to deform both plastically and elastically.

Such indications are useful guides when comparing materials for particular applications and they also provide some idea of the resistance of any particular material to abrasion. This can be useful when considering the manipulation of the material, particularly with regard to adjustments and finishing procedures. It can also suggest how the material might stand up to those forces which are going to wear it away whilst it is part of an engineering structure, even if that structure is as small as a dental restoration or appliance. As wear infers a loss of structure, a high resistance to wear is a major requirement of any material which is to be used in the mouth. Loss of material by wear not only brings with it a weakening of the structure of which it is part, but the subsequent ingestion of the particles which are worn away may also present a toxic hazard not normally associated with the bulk material.

Fracture toughness

Many of the properties outlined above are related to the energy needed to propagate a crack through the material. Laboratory tests have been devised to measure this *fracture toughness* and they provide a value known as K_{1C}, which is a characteristic for a particular material. In general, cracks in materials with low K_{1C} values require little energy to get them moving and to propagate them. In the mouth such materials would be observed to be friable and bits would readily chip off them during normal masticatory loading. Synthetic dental materials behaving in this way would be observed to wear away faster than natural ones.

Other physical properties

The physical properties of materials used in dentistry are all those generally covered by the scope of physics, namely heat, light, sound, magnetism, electricity, radiation and the properties of matter. This last heading includes all the mechanical properties already discussed and also includes density or specific gravity. This really only becomes an important consideration when using materials which have high densities. Gold is such an element, and in the days when swaged gold upper denture bases were common, retention of such a heavy base was often a problem. Nowadays, as will be considered later, its effect on the economics of restorations is the main concern.

Thermal conductivity

Thermal properties become important as soon as enamel and dentine start to be replaced with synthetic dental materials in an environment where the temperature can range almost instantaneously from 0 to 60°C. Sound enamel and dentine have low coefficients of thermal conductivity (less than 1 watt per metre degree Kelvin — W/(m·K)), and, as they are contained in a moist environment and held within living tissue, they provide good protection to the pulp from thermal trauma. However, if a heat-conducting path is created by the use of a material with a high coefficient of thermal conductivity such as amalgam (over 20 W/(m·K)), then trauma to the pulp is distinctly possible. In this case a protective lining with a low conductivity to heat such as a dental cement is recommended. Denture base acrylic has a coefficient of thermal conductivity of about 0.2 W/(m·K), whereas that for cobalt — chromium is about 70 W/(m·K). Patients' sensitivity to hot or cold food is thus going to be much greater when their palate is covered by a metallic rather than a polymeric base.

Thermal expansion

Thermal expansion and contraction become significant once different materials are used together. The coefficients of thermal expansion of most restorative materials differ considerably from those of enamel and dentine. However, the thermal equilibrium of vital teeth within the mouth is such that, even when very hot or very cold foods are introduced, there is insufficient time for restorations to undergo bulk dimensional changes before the hot or cold food is equilibrated to mouth temperature. The most important area where the differences in the coefficients of thermal expansion need careful consideration is when trying to create and maintain a bond between metal and porcelain in crowns and bridges. The manufacturers of such systems have to arrange by careful control of the constituents that the coefficient of thermal expansion of the porcelain matches closely that of the metal so that, when the

metal — porcelain composite is cooled from a firing temperature of 800–1000°C to room temperature of about 23°C, high interfacial stresses are not created, since these can lead to catastrophic failure of the metal–porcelain bond.

Exotherm

Although not strictly a physical property as such, the exotherm — the amount of heat evolved in the setting reaction — should be mentioned here again because a high exotherm can traumatize the pulp or the soft tissues when the material is used in the mouth. In the laboratory, overheating of materials can also lead to problems, notably the production of gaseous porosity within an acrylic denture base, which can occur when it is heated too rapidly during its curing cycle. In this case a combination of the exotherm and a low thermal conductivity can cause unpolymerized monomer to boil and thus produce trapped bubbles in the deep parts of thick sections of the acrylic.

Optical properties

The optical properties of dental materials are those which affect their perceived appearance. The dental tissues are both translucent (i.e. they transmit light but only by dispersing it, so that no detail is visible) and have a wide range of colours. Colour itself is a complex phenomenon and its perception is closely related to the wavelength (colour, if the light is in the visible range) and the intensity of the light falling on the object in view. White light, for example, can be split into its spectrum of wavelengths from red through orange, yellow, green, blue and indigo to violet. These are the *hues* and their concentration (i.e. whether they are pale or intense) is called the *chroma*, while a third component, *value*, is used to describe the lightness or darkness of a colour. A vital tooth, for example, would have a high value, whereas the same tooth when non-vital would be dark and have a low value. Colour comparisons must often be made in clinical dentistry and these must be made under optimal lighting conditions. Extraneous colour reflections from wall surfaces and furnishings must be avoided and the light used to illuminate the subject must be as close to daylight as possible. Failure to do this can result in restorations with some very peculiar shades, particularly when viewed in light from artificial sources, each of which has its own characteristic distribution of colours within the visible spectrum.

A further problem of our time arises from the exposure of the dentition to various sources of ultraviolet (UV) radiation. Whilst natural sunlight has some UV radiation associated with it, high-intensity artificial lighting, as found in television and film studios and in the special effects lights of discothèques and the like, can contain a high proportion of UV light. Natural teeth fluoresce under UV light; that is, they absorb the UV radiation and emit light in the blue region of the spectrum. If restorative materials do not fluoresce in the same way they appear dark to the observer and this can be unacceptable to the patient.

Several dental materials rely on light of various wavelengths to activate chemical initiators and thus cause the resins which they contain to undergo polymerization, and hence setting occurs. Whilst UV radiation with a wavelength of approximately 365 nm was popular for some years, initiators which are activated by visible blue light with a wavelength of approximately 470 nm are now preferred.

Sound, magnetism and electricity

Although the characteristic clicks of natural and artificial teeth when they are brought into contact with one another can be used to identify problems associated with occlusion, sound is not a property which is of any great consequence in dental materials, and no effort is made to match restorative materials to natural teeth in this respect. Likewise the magnetic properties of enamel and dentine are not those which we have to try and emulate in restorative materials, although modern magnetic materials are being tried as aids to the retention of certain prosthetic appliances and have been suggested for use in orthodontics.

The electrical properties of dental materials are, to a large extent, tied up in the problems associated with galvanic cells. These are electrical current generators consisting of two different metallic materials connected together (possibly by a tissue pathway) and submerged in an electrically conducting aqueous medium or electrolyte (saliva in this case). These electrical currents can be both irritating to the patient and deleterious to at least one of the metallic materials, which is undergoing galvanic corrosion and thus dissolution during the production of the electrical current. Efforts are thus needed to eliminate as far as practicable the close contact of different metallic materials within the mouth, or at least to provide reasonable protection to the pulp in the form of insulating cements and varnishes.

Radiation

The radiation which is of dental interest is that of X-rays, whose diagnostic use is widespread in seeking all sorts of conditions which are difficult or impossible to detect in any other way. To assist in this process, materials intended for use within the mouth should be opaque to X-rays so that their presence and their position can be readily detected, either in normal use or when they are swallowed, inhaled or traumatically displaced.

Although modern dental materials are not permitted to contain substances which themselves emit ionizing radiation, some dental porcelains hitherto contained very small amounts of mildly radioactive salts to promote the fluorescence mentioned above. Modern materials achieve this without the use of this type of fluorescing agent. Clearly the continuous exposure of the dental tissues to even small amounts of ionizing radiation is undesirable and nowadays is unnecessary.

The cost of dental materials

The economics of dental materials are not easy to specify, since the amounts needed for different applications vary and the cost of a sales unit is often negotiable according to the quantity purchased from any particular supply house.

Mention has already been made of the historical significance of density to the weight of a restoration or appliance and the problems associated with its retention. However, in modern dental practice its significance lies not so much in the problems of retention but in the inherent cost. The volume of metal required, say, for a bridge is going to be similar whether it is cast in a gold alloy or a non-precious alloy (Table 1).

However, the density of gold is at least twice

Table 1 The relative mass of alloy needed for a three-unit bridge together with the approximate cost in 1993 for the metal contained in the finished restoration

	Bonding alloy			Casting alloy		
	Density (g/cm^3)	Mass (g)	Cost (£)	Density (g/cm^3)	Mass (g)	Cost (£)
High-gold	19	6.65	70	18	9.0	80
Medium-gold	15	5.25	36	14	7.0	43
Low-gold	12	4.20	15	11	5.5	16
Base metal	9	3.15	2.5	9	4.5	3.5

Data courtesy of Johnson Matthey Dental Materials, Birmingham

that of any non-precious metal used in dentistry and so the weight required for a similar volume of material is going to be at least twice. As gold alloys are, at the time of writing, about 10 times the price of non-precious alloys, the fact that twice the weight is needed to produce a bridge in gold alloy is a double disincentive to use them. There is thus a strong economic movement towards the use of non-precious alloys wherever possible but, as with all materials for use in dentistry, the simple economic equation needs to be modified by factors relating to the chemistry, handling characteristics and performance of the material in service.

Whilst it is an easy exercise to calculate the cost of the materials needed for any particular clinical procedure and thus rank them from the cheapest to the most expensive, the real cost of using them must include the time of the dental surgeon and, where appropriate, that of the dental technician. Hence, although material *A* may be inherently cheaper than *B*, if *A* takes longer to manipulate, or worse still has a greater propensity to fail either during its manipulation or shortly after being supplied to the patient, the time penalty incurred in repeating the procedure, replacing a restoration or remaking an appliance may well outweigh the original saving. Unfortunately, it is only by using a

material under clinical conditions that an individual practitioner is able to assess the reality of such savings.

Further reading

Combe, E. C. (1992) Section I. Basic scientific principles. Section in *Notes on Dental Materials*, 6th edn. Churchill Livingstone, Edinburgh, pp. 5–69

Craig, R. G., O'Brien, W. J. and Powers, J. M. (1992) Properties of materials. Chapter in *Dental Materials. Properties and Manipulation*, 6th edn. Mosby Year Book, St Louis, Missouri, pp. 10–31

Gangler, P., Hoyer, I., Krehan, F., Niemella, S. and Weinart, W. (1990) Biologic testing and clinical trial of a visible-light-curing composite resin restorative materials. *Quintessence International*, **21**, 833–842

McCabe, J. F. (1990) Properties used to characterize materials. Section in *Applied Dental Materials*, 7th edn. Blackwell, Oxford, pp. 4–27

Mjör, I.A. (1990) Current views on the biological testing of restorative materials. *Journal of Oral Rehabilitation*, **17**, 503–507

Svanberg, M., Mjör, I.A. and Orstabik, D. (1990) *Mutans streptococci* in plaque from margins of amalgam, composite and glass-ionomer restorations. *Journal of Dental Research*, **69**, 861–864

Van Noort, R. (Ed.) (1993) Dental materials: 1991 literature review. *Journal of Dentistry*, **18**, 5–30

Part Two
The use of materials in clinical procedures

Chapter 1
Examination and diagnosis

Introduction

Dental materials are most commonly thought of in connection with restorative procedures (in the wider sense) and most texts on the subject concentrate on this area of their use. However, a surprising number of materials are used before treatment commences during the examination, special investigation and diagnostic procedures that occupy the initial stages of treatment planning.

Cross-infection control

During the late 1980s there developed an increasing emphasis on cross-infection control, which has now led to the routine use of gloves, face masks and eye protectors for the operator and dental surgery assistant. In addition, eye protection is used for the patient to protect against mechanical damage as well as infection.

Gloves are most commonly made from natural latex rubber, but poly(vinyl chloride or acetate) may also be used. Allergic reactions occasionally occur on the hands of the wearer, related to the powder used as a release agent or to the accelerator used in the curing of latex gloves, or to the compounds added as antioxidants and to prevent cracking and drying. Plastic (vinyl) gloves produce less allergic contact dermatitis despite the greater potential of the allergens they contain. Some latex gloves are claimed to be hypoallergenic and are powder free.

The use of antiseptic or bland hand creams helps to reduce allergic reactions, skin cracking and skin infection in the event of glove porosity. Washing gloves leads to porosity.

Materials used in the prevention of cross-infection are dealt with in Chapter 2.

Hand instruments (1.1)*

Most hand instruments are made from stainless steel in order to facilitate wet sterilization by autoclave without risk of corrosion. However, stainless steel can be corroded by some disinfectants, for example hypochlorite.

It is fortunate that instruments used in the examination procedure do not need to be sharp, as stainless steel is difficult to sharpen effectively. Sharp probes or explorers are the obvious exception to this and, to facilitate the maintenance of a sharp

*see section 1.1 of Part Three

point on these instruments, the taper from shank to point should be minimal. However, it is no longer recommended that a sharp probe is used to diagnose the initial caries lesion because its sharp point is capable of penetrating a demineralized but otherwise intact enamel surface which may be in the process of being remineralized. Thus if a probe is to be used in diagnosing caries it should be blunt.
*See section 1.1 of Part Three.

The periodontal probe is intentionally blunt and is marked so that it can be used to measure depths of periodontal pockets. For screening and monitoring purposes the CPITN (Community Periodontal Index of Treatment Needs) probe is used. Instead of the usual markings at 1 or 2 mm intervals the CPITN probe has a single 2 mm wide black band extending between 3.5 and 5.5 mm from the tip, which is a tiny (0.5 mm diameter) sphere. Other versions have the addition of two lines at 8.5 mm and 11.5 mm from the tip, but either version can be used to provide information as part of the CPITN system.

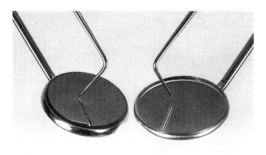

Figure 1.1 Front surface mirror (left) gives a single reflected image but a mirror silvered on the rear surface may give a double image. From Kidd, E.A.M. and Smith B.G.N. (1990) *Pickard's Manual of Operative Dentistry*, Oxford University Press, Oxford, p. 86, with permission of Oxford University Press.

Dental mirrors are provided with the silvering either on the back or front of the glass surface. Front-surface mirrors are superior in providing a clear image uninfluenced by secondary images from the glass surface, but are easy to damage if scratched against other instruments. Clear vision is so important that front-surface mirrors are almost

certainly worth the extra expense involved (Fig. 1.1). It is also possible for patients to purchase quite cheaply front-surface plastic mirrors as an aid to proper oral hygiene procedures.

Cleaning the teeth prior to examination (15.1.3)

A proper examination of the teeth can only be made following removal of plaque and calculus from the tooth surface if this is not already being done by the patient. This is usually referred to as scaling and polishing the teeth. However, strictly speaking, enamel is too hard to be polished in the mouth. The objective of all 'polishing' pastes used in the mouth is to be sufficiently abrasive to remove plaque and stains from the enamel surface without abrading the enamel surface itself. None of the commercially available prophylaxis pastes (15.1.3) will abrade enamel, and they usually contain such mild abrasives as pumice, calcite, quartz, talc or zirconium silicate (15.1.3). These abrasives will, however, abrade dentine and cementum, so that care is necessary where gingival recession has occurred. The technique of air-polishing which utilizes an air-driven stream of sodium bicarbonate as the abrasive, will similarly not damage enamel but will abrade dentine, cementum, some restorative materials and soft tissues.

Disclosing agents1
(plaque indicators; 15.1.4)

It is often appropriate to illustrate the presence of plaque by the use of disclosing agents prior to removal, both as an education for the patient and in the recording of plaque indices. Disclosing agents are available as tablets or liquids and usually contain the dye erythrosin, which is also used in food colouring, and which stains plaque red. Other colours are available and a disclosing solution which contained a dye which was only visible under ultraviolet light used to be used, but this was unnecessarily complex and ultraviolet lights are no longer used at the chairside to cure composite materials.

Disclosing tablets dissolve in saliva and the

resultant solution is spread around the mouth and teeth. This is convenient for home use but is not always totally effective, so in the surgery disclosing solutions are often used on a cotton bud to reach selected tooth surfaces reliably.

Diagnostic aids

Caries indicators

Caries indicator dyes are available but these are not intended for use in the initial diagnosis of caries. Their value is in identifying in the base of partially prepared cavities dentine which is demineralized by the carious process and infected, therefore warranting removal prior to the placement of a restoration. Conversely, non-infected dentine, which will remineralize with appropriate treatment, does not stain. These indicators should not be used on their own, but in conjunction with conventional visual and tactile identification of softened dentine.

Commercially produced caries prediction kits are available to measure salivary buffering power and counts of salivary *Streptococcus mutans* and *lactobacilli*. The best predictive value obtainable using combinations of these variables is 75%.

Occlusal indicators (4.5.2)

Identification of normal and abnormal occlusal contacts between natural and artificial teeth is essential in the diagnosis of occlusal disturbances and in the diagnosis of pain related to appliances. Articulating papers, typewriter ribbons, wax and Chinagraph pencil, occlusion test foils based on mylar films, liquid paints and powder aerosols have all been used to mark such occlusal contacts. The requirements of such materials are that they should be thin enough so that only actual contacts and not near contacts are marked; that the material should reliably mark contacts between teeth no matter what the material (either natural or artificial) of the contacting surfaces, using a reasonable occlusal force; and that the material should not be so thick that it disturbs the normal occlusal relationship. None of the available methods works well when there is a layer of saliva covering the teeth and therefore the teeth should always be dried prior to testing.

Some articulating papers and occlusal indicator waxes are clearly so thick as to cause erroneous marking of near contacts, disturbance of occlusal relationship and displacement of appliances supported by soft tissue. Conversely, GHM foils include 8 μm double sided foils and 12 μm single sided foils. Such thin foils need special forceps (Miller) or tweezers to hold and control them. Foils of various colours may be used for differentiating between contacts in intercuspal and retruded contact positions and in eccentric excursions.

One type of articulating paper successfully overcomes these disadvantages by having marking dyes of different colours on the upper and lower surfaces. Following the marking of the surfaces with the paper between the teeth the paper is removed and the teeth brought into direct contact. Only where the two colours (usually red and blue) are superimposed is actual contact occurring (Fig. 1.2).

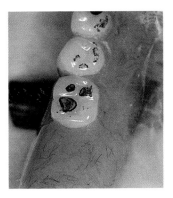

Figure 1.2 Superimposition of the red and blue markings from 'Radar' articulating paper giving dark purple markings on acrylic teeth where actual contact with the lower teeth has occurred.

Testing for contact between individual teeth can also be carried out using GHM 8 @m shimstock foil which does not mark the teeth but tests contact by resistance to withdrawal from between the teeth. This is a plastic material with a silvery appearance which makes it easy to see in the mouth (Fig. 1.3).

Advocates of the use of occlusal indicator waxes claim that only where the wax is fully penetrated is actual contact occurring (Fig. 1.4). However, difficulty may be experienced in identifying the areas of penetration before marking through the penetration on to the tooth with a Chinagraph pencil, and a possible deflection of the occlusal relationship by the force necessary to penetrate the wax may occur. Care should be taken when used with soft tissue-supported appliances since the displaceability of the supporting tissues may prevent penetration of the wax. With experience this method may be successfully used with natural teeth and tooth-supported appliances.

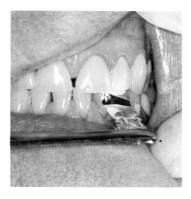

Figure 1.3 GHM 8 μm 'shimstock' foil tests contact by resistance to withdrawal from between the teeth.

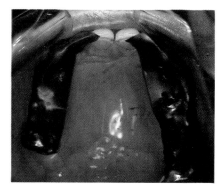

Figure 1.4 Use of occlusal indicator wax in a patient wearing a mocosa supported acrylic partial denture showing heavy contacts on three of the abutment teeth and on one of the artificial teeth. This latter contact had caused trauma to the underlying denture bearing mucosa.

All the thinner test foils and typewriter ribbon (as well as some of the thicker papers) often fail to mark polished gold, porcelain, tooth and acrylic even when dry. Sand-blasting or other abrasive treatment will make the recording of marks more reliable, but acrylic resin and porcelain are unsuitable for abrasive treatment and it should not be used on enamel.

Liquid paints consist of a pigment or powder in a volatile solvent which rapidly evaporates leaving the pigment to mark the contact between the teeth. Aerosol powders are used either alone or as an intermediate coating and like the liquids can be used on the tooth to be adjusted or the opposing tooth. However the powder rubs off the teeth very easily and many dentists find it difficult to control.

Pressure indicators (13.7)

These are used to identify areas of heavy contact (or pressure) between appliances (or restorations) and oral tissues. In the case of teeth, the heavy contact will usually stop the appliance or restoration from seating correctly, the objective of the pressure indicator being to assist in fitting the appliance. With soft tissues the heavy contact may not initially prevent seating of the appliance, but may result in discomfort or pain after a period of wear. Pressure will also result in some distortion of the soft tissues concerned, which makes subsequent alteration of the appliance rather difficult. Ideally, the appliance should be removed from the mouth for 24–48 hours to allow healing and recovery of the distortion before the use of a pressure indicator to identify the area where the appliance should be adjusted. Realistically, a small adjustment may need to be followed by a further adjustment as the distortion of the soft tissue recovers. This, accompanied by the adaptability of the living tissues, should result in a satisfactory and comfortable fit.

A number of different materials have been used as pressure indicators, some of which are specifically designed for that purpose. The material used must form a thin layer adherent to the appliance to be tested, which will not stick to the oral tissue involved and yet is sufficiently fluid to be displaced away in the area of pressure. This kind of differential adhesion is assisted by drying the appliance while the tissues remain wet with saliva.

For fitting cobalt–chromium or gold castings to teeth, an accurate fit is required and therefore a very thin layer of indicator material is desirable. Powder aerosols and liquid paints are readily adherent to the metal casting, are easy to apply and record only actual contacts reliably. Care must be taken to differentiate between passing contacts and contacts occurring when the appliance is fully seated, and the pigment must be carefully cleaned from cast restorations before cementation. However, cleaning is reasonably easy as the pigments are either water-soluble or an organic solvent is supplied.

When testing for heavy contacts between appliances and soft tissues, slightly different properties are required. The material must have a low viscosity, otherwise the soft tissue rather than the test material will be displaced. For this reason pressure indicator waxes are not very satisfactory and only indicate areas of very high pressure. They are therefore best reserved for localizing small areas of pressure causing identified local soreness. Low-viscosity creams are messy, and being oil-based are difficult to clean from the appliance. There is also a tendency for these materials to adhere to the oral mucosa even when wet with saliva, but with experience good results can be obtained and only reasonable manual force is needed to demonstrate areas of localized pressure (Fig. 1.5). Simple versions of this type of material can be easily made from zinc oxide powder and glycerine, which has the advantage of being easily removed with water, or by mixing equal parts of petroleum jelly and the white zinc oxide paste used in impression pastes. Occlusal force should not be used, as this could superimpose occlusal errors on to fit-surface errors, confusing the disclosed pattern of pressure.

A cleaner and more effective alternative is provided by low-viscosity silicone rubber wash impression materials used with minimal pressure (Fig. 1.6; 5.2.5; 13.7). These adhere well to the dry appliance and do not adhere to the oral mucosa. They are, however, more time-consuming and expensive, especially if repeated applications are necessary, as time has to be allowed for the material to set. They are very easy to clean from the appliance since it is not necessary to use an adhesive. They are most useful where the whole fitting surface of the appliance requires testing for heavy contacts, while testing of smaller areas is probably best achieved with pressure indicator pastes.

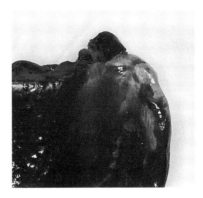

Figure 1.61 Low-viscosity silicone rubber wash impression material used to identify areas of contact between the fit surface of a denture and the denture-bearing mucosa.

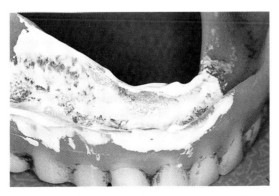

Figure 1.5 Disclosing cream demonstrating areas of contact between the fit surface of a denture and the denture-bearing mucosa.

Testing the vitality of teeth

Teeth are defined as vital when they have an intact blood supply. This can only be tested directly without damage by using expensive laser Doppler equipment, and so instead the sensory nerve supply is tested. The nerve supply may be tested using the response of the teeth to heat, cold or a small electric current. Heat is applied using a stick of gutta-percha (4.7.2), heated until it is soft and just beginning to burn, allowed to cool for a few seconds, and placed on the tooth. Cold may be applied using a small pledget of cotton wool on to which is sprayed ethyl chloride, which readily evaporates resulting in cooling and the formation of ice crystals on the cotton wool. Conveniently shaped pieces of solid ice may also be used.

These methods are rather crude and can be painful as there is little control of the temperature used. It is therefore preferable to use an electric pulp tester (EPT) which is precisely controlled. An electric current is applied to the tooth from the EPT via an electrode. To transfer the current from the electrode to the tooth effectively a good conductor of electricity must be used, either in paste form (e.g. prophylaxis paste) or as a special conductive rubber tip on the electrode.

The stimulus is increased slowly from zero and the electrode withdrawn from the tooth as soon as the patient responds, before pain is felt. Although the EPT does not give a reliable quantitative measure of vitality, it can detect hypersensitive pulps and those with a reduced response, particularly if comparisons are made with similar teeth elsewhere in the mouth.

Radiographic materials (18)

Radiographic film is packaged in sizes convenient for the structures to be imaged. Intraoral films are supplied in sealed paper or plastic envelopes measuring 4.5 x 3.2 cm, packaged between black paper and protected on one side (away from the X-ray source) by a thin sheet of lead foil, which has the dual function of preventing scattered X-rays from fogging the film and preventing the X-rays passing beyond the film into other oral tissues. This size of film will normally cover three teeth comfortably, while smaller sizes are also available for access to difficult areas and for the smaller mouth of a child.

Occlusal films are similarly packaged in 7.7 x 5.8 cm envelopes, which will conveniently cover the occlusal surface of all the teeth in one arch with some surrounding area. Extraoral films range from sizes suitable for producing images of the whole head, through the panoramic radiograph (rotational tomograph) which covers all of both jaws, to the half-jaw size usually used for lateral oblique films. Extraoral films may be supplied prepackaged but are often loaded by the operator (in a dark room) into reusable metal cassettes. In both cases intensifying screens are usually used to reduce the radiation necessary for exposure of the film. Intensifying screens consist of a suitable base coated with a phosphor material which emits light when irradiated. Materials used include calcium tungstate, and rare-earth phosphors containing elements from the lanthanide series.

Most films are provided separate from their developer, but rapid development films are provided which include developer and fixer in an attached package. This system allows rapid development for use in diagnosis or root canal therapy, but the resultant films are not usually suitable for long-term storage.

Radiopacity of dental materials

All metals are strongly radiopaque, thus giving good images on radiographic film. Temporary restorations, cavity lining materials and gutta-percha root filling materials containing barium or calcium salts are usually visible on radiographs, although this depends on their thickness and the amount of masking by the tooth enamel or metallic restorations. Polymeric materials are generally radiolucent and this is a disadvantage of both composite restorations and polymeric denture base materials. Methods of improving the radiopacity of these materials are discussed in Chapters 3 and 7.

Study casts or models (6.1)

Articulated study casts of the upper and lower jaws are often valuable aids for treatment planning and patient education. Where complex restorations or appliances are to be provided they become essential. Since these are usually cast in dental stone they should be handled with care as the surface may be easily abraded or chipped.

Impression trays for study casts

These may be of metal or of polymer. The former have the advantage of being rigid, robust enough to withstand cleaning procedures and tolerant of high temperatures, therefore enabling them to be easily sterilized. Thus they may be reused almost indefinitely. Conversely, polymer trays are less rigid, less easily cleaned and are distorted by heat. They are not therefore autoclavable and should be disposed of after a single use. Both types may be perforated or have undercuts incorporated around the periphery (rimlock) to aid the retention of impression material within them. A variety of shapes and sizes is available, designed for the full arch or part of it, with teeth or without.

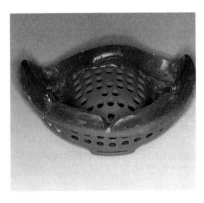

Figure 1.7 Modelling or baseplace wax used to make moderate extension to a tock tray. Properly cooled and in thick section this material is acceptably rigid.

Modification of the peripheral extension may be carried out using pink modelling wax (Fig. 1.7; 7.1.1) or composition (5.1.2). The latter is more rigid but more time-consuming to apply; soft wax is insufficiently rigid or stable for any but the smallest extensions. Where some teeth are missing a large void exists within the tray and this is best filled by modifying the tray using either silicone rubber putty (Fig. 1.8; 5.2.5) or composition. An impression of the edentulous area in one of these materials is taken, it is removed from the mouth and set material trimmed from around the standing teeth with a sharp knife prior to completing the impression of the teeth (see below). The impression material used for the teeth is allowed to flow over the silicone rubber or composition, as this gives better surface detail and because it is usually difficult to reseat the modified tray in the mouth in exactly the same position. If an impression of the teeth only is required, the palate of the tray can be left uncovered with impression material, or even removed to improve patient comfort. Stock impression trays

and study casts for the edentulous patient are discussed in Chapter 7.

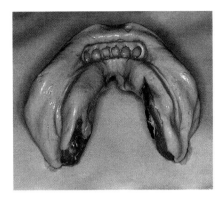

Figure 1.8 Teeth are missing in both lower posterior segments. The large void that exists within the tray is filled by modifying the tray using silicone rubber putty. The impression is completed using alginate which is allowed to flow over the silicone rubber to give better surface detail.

Impression materials for study casts (5.2)

An elastic impression material is necessary to record the undercuts around natural teeth, and because of its low cost and convenience, irreversible hydrocolloid (alginate; 5.2.2) is almost invariably used for study casts. The shelf-life is good, provided it is kept dry and not stored at elevated temperatures. Alginate has a pleasant taste and odour and good compatibility with oral tissues, the only identified hazards being associated with lead-containing alginate which have now been withdrawn from use, and from inhalation of the silica filler, which represents nearly three-quarters of the unmixed alginate. Modern alginate tends to be dust-free. Different commercially available alginates have different viscosities and different working and setting times, so a material may be selected to suit individual preferences. In addition, selection of the temperature of the water used in mixing facilitates further control, for example, the colder the water the longer the working and setting times.

Careful handling is important to achieve the best results. The most common difficulties are due to poor extension and fit of the impression tray, defects due to inadequate material available to fill the space, lack of adhesion of the alginate to the tray, and poor dimensional stability on storage of the set impression. Lack of extension should not occur if the tray is properly modified to carry the impression material to every part of the mouth. Filling defects occur because of the use of a spaced tray which is poorly adapted to the shape of the mouth. The use of wax, silicone putty or composition to modify the fit surface of the tray can overcome this problem or alternatively parts of the mouth can be filled with alginate manually before the tray is seated. The latter technique is particularly useful in the case of a high palatal vault.

It is important to achieve a good impression of the occlusal surfaces of the teeth, free of air bubbles, so that the study casts can be properly articulated. A simple way of doing this is to wipe the alginate into the occlusal fissures with a finger before seating the tray (Fig. 1.9).

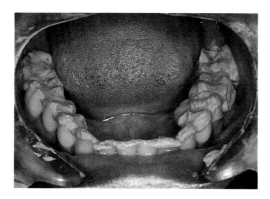

Figure 1.9 Alginate wiped into occlusal fissures prior to seating the loaded tray to prevent air being trapped in the depth of the fissures.

Lack of adhesion to the tray is overcome by the use of a perforated or rimlock tray plus the use of an adhesive. The adhesive, dissolved in a volatile solvent, is painted or sprayed on to the tray (5.2.2). It should be applied sparingly because, if too great a thickness is applied, it acts as a lubricant and actually reduces the retention of the impression in the tray. Unfortunately it is very messy and if excess adhesive is allowed to contact the gloves,

fingers or working surface it remains sticky and collects dust and debris. Contaminated gloves should be discarded. There is an organic solvent available for cleaning the adhesive from work surfaces and trays, but cleaning the adhesive off reusable trays is time-consuming.

Poor dimensional stability of a set impression on storage is related to its high water content. Syneresis and evaporation will occur if the impression is allowed to dry while water can be absorbed or imbibed if the impression is immersed: both processes cause dimensional changes. Ideally, the impression should be cast immediately, but if storage is unavoidable it should be covered with a damp cloth or tissue and sealed in a plastic bag or other airtight container to maintain 100% humidity. This difficulty has been highlighted by the need to improve cross infection control related to impressions in general.

To be on the safe side, all impressions should be regarded as infected. Impressions should be washed in running water to remove all visible signs of contamination before being sent to the dental laboratory. Rinsing, or better still an air/water spray in a closed cabinet (not the three-in-one syringe at the chairside), removes many of the microbes together with the harbouring media (plaque, blood and saliva).

The single use of disposable impression trays is now strongly recommended, and bearing in mind the difficulty of disinfection, technicians should wear gloves when handling these impressions and pouring casts.

Neither alginate nor composition impression materials are compatible with disinfection solutions when immersed for the recommended time (see Chapter 5) and, while silicone putty is, problems with mixing and handling may be experienced because contact with most latex gloves inhibits the polymerization. Ways of overcoming this without placing personnel at risk must be devised.

One manufacturer has added a quaternary ammonium salt to the alginate powder. This product has been shown to have some bactericidal properties, but these salts are usually ineffective against viruses. Another suggestion is the use of solutions of disinfectants instead of plain water in preparing the impression material. Materials which may be used to disinfect impressions are described in Chapter 2.

Occlusal registration materials (4.5.1)

Study casts are articulated using a variety of occlusal records depending on the type of articulator chosen. Occlusal registration rims may sometimes be required in the partially edentulous mouth (see Chapter 7) but, conversely, accurate intercuspation of the natural teeth may sometimes eliminate the need for any additional occlusal record. Both contact and precontact records may be necessary, depending on the amount of detail of analysis of the occlusion that is clinically required. Because of the problem of ensuring accuracy of these records, more than one record is often taken to improve confidence with reproducibility. Occlusal registration materials are discussed in detail in Chapters 5 and 7.

Diagnostic occlusal appliances

In the diagnosis of disorders attributed to the occlusion, appliances to disocclude the natural teeth may be used. These appliances may cover all the teeth in one of the arches, or alternatively provide for occlusal contacts in one area of the mouth only, thus separating the natural teeth in the other areas, for example, an anterior or incisal bite plane or occlusal pivots.

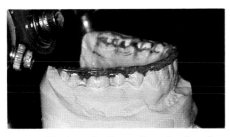

Figure 1.10 Hard acrylic diagnostic occlusal appliance fitted on the cast.

These appliances are constructed on the study casts, either in hard acrylic (Fig. 1.10; 12.1) as used in partial and complete dentures or in a soft thermoplastic polymer (15.4.3). Hard appliances are processed in the laboratory and the disadvantages of this material are discussed in Chapter 7. In these appliances the polymerization shrinkage of acrylic makes fitting the appliance to the complex occlusal surface often difficult and time-consuming.

Of the soft materials, the polyethylene is softer and more flexible than the polypropylene and a variety of thicknesses of both materials is available. Appliances are formed in the laboratory on the study casts using an air pressure process. In this the polyethylene or polypropylene in sheet form is softened by heat and then blow-formed on the cast using air pressure. Controlling the thickness of the appliance is difficult as the material tends to be stretched thinnest over the most prominent parts of the cast, often the cusp tips. However, the soft flexible appliance can easily be adjusted, using scissors or acrylic burs; it fits readily into all areas of the mouth (including undercut areas, which provide retention of the appliance), and it is comfortable to wear.

Further reading

Baragona P. M. and Cohen H. V. (1991) Long-term orthopedic appliance therapy. *Dental Clinics of North America*, **35**, 109–121

Bergman B. (1989) Disinfection of prosthodontic impression materials: a literature review. *International Journal of Prosthodontics*, **2**, 537–542

Field E. A. and King C. M. (1990) Skin problems associated with routine wearing of protective gloves in dental practice. *British Dental Journal*, **169**: 281–285

Martin M. V. (1991) *Infection control in the dental environment*. Martin Dunitz, London

Wilson R. F. and Ashley F. P. (1989) Identification of caries risk in schoolchildren: salivary buffering capacity and bacterial counts, sugar intake and caries experience as predictors of 2-year and 3-year caries increment. *British Dental Journal*, **166**, 99–102

Chapter 2
Prevention and stabilization

Introduction

There are many excellent texts dealing with the prevention of dental disease and so only those preventive materials which are used by the dental worker in the surgery will be described. For this reason important topics such as dietary factors are excluded. However, dentists are so often asked for advice concerning toothbrushes, toothpastes and other tooth-cleaning aids that some information on these materials has been included. Materials used in the prevention of cross-infection have also been included under this heading.

Materials used in the prevention of cross-infection

Disinfectants do not kill the most virulent organisms and should be used only for those items which cannot be sterilized by more effective methods. The use of chemical agents is restricted by many factors, including variable effects on microorganisms, reduced efficiency in the presence of organic matter, deterioration on storage and potential toxicity. Disinfectants deteriorate with use due to evaporation or dilution by adding wet items. They are therefore mainly used for cleaning work surfaces and equipment. The following agents are commonly used:

Sodium hypochlorite or sodium dichloroisocyanurate

Fresh aqueous solutions of either of these are recommended for general surface disinfection, including surfaces contaminated with blood spillage in a concentration equivalent to 10 000 parts per million (p.p.m.) available chlorine (about $1:10$ dilution of household bleach, although household bleach varies in concentration). The World Health Organization recommendation is to use this concentration for 1 hour. Hypochlorite has the disadvantages of being corrosive to metals and bleaching fabrics.

Alkaline glutaraldehyde

For non-corrosive disinfection freshly activated 2% alkaline glutaraldehyde may be used. Immersion for a minimum of 3 hours is recommended but this solution must be handled with great care as it has irritant and sensitizing properties. The recommended maximum safe exposure level is 0.2 p.p.m.

Isopropanol

Immersion in 70% isopropanol or industrial methylated spirits for a minimum of 1 hour is the last resort for materials which are incompatible with the above disinfectants.

Descriptions of methods of disinfecting impressions are given in Chapters 1, 5 and 7.

Materials used in the prevention of dental disease

Tooth-cleaning materials

Toothbrushes (15.1.1)

To be effective, toothbrushes need to have straight and rather stiff (medium or hard) bristles. All toothbrushes are manufactured with straight bristles but they become bent and worn in use and so need to be replaced fairly frequently. Nylon bristles are better than natural bristles as they remain straight and stiff for longer and dry out quicker between uses. A small brush-head is desirable to simplify manoeuvring the brush around all of the surfaces of the teeth. Numerous closely packed small diameter bristles are probably more effective than fewer larger diameter bristles. A typical toothbrush might have a head which is 18 mm long and 8 mm wide with 32 tufts. Each tuft has 40 filaments 11 mm long and 0.21 mm in diameter.

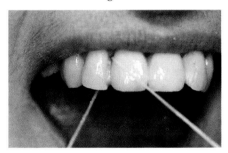

Figure 2.1 Super-floss is particularly good for cleaning beneath bridge pontics.

Dental floss

Dental floss is a thread of synthetic fibres and is supplied either waxed or unwaxed. The unwaxed version may be more effective at collecting plaque but it tends to fray rather easily. Waxed floss is therefore more popular. A wider version of this is dental tape which is more expensive but easier to handle. It may also be more effective if larger interdental spaces are present.

Another variation is Super-floss, which has a stiffened end and a furry section in the middle. This is also good for larger spaces but is particularly good for cleaning beneath bridge pontics (Fig. 2.1).

Toothpaste (15.1.2)

Toothpastes are not necessary for the removal of dental plaque. They do, however, contain abrasives such as calcium carbonate, calcium pyrophosphate, sodium metaphosphate and alumina which may assist in the removal of stains. These abrasives would need to be used for an unusual amount of time to abrade enamel significantly, but they may abrade the softer cementum and dentine when the root of the tooth is exposed. They will also significantly abrade acrylic when toothpaste is used to clean appliances (Fig. 2.2). Tooth powders and some toothpastes (often designated for use by smokers) have more coarse abrasives and these will abrade enamel if used regularly. Most toothpaste now contains fluoride which it is an important aid in the prevention of dental decay (see later). Other additives include the detergent sodium lauryl sulphate and the antimicrobial triclosan, both of which are said to inhibit plaque proliferation; chlorhexidine which has a chemical effect in inhibiting plaque bacteria; and pyrophosphate, which it is claimed is a calculus control agent. Chlorhexidine also causes staining of the teeth if used regularly, although this can be removed by brushing with a conventional toothpaste. Tooth-pastes which contain desensitizing agents will be described later.

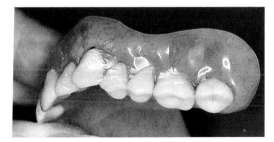

Figure 2.2 Abrasion of acrylic teeth caused by overzealous brushing with toothpaste.

Mouthwashes

Antiseptic mouthwashes have little effect on plaque, with the notable exception of those containing chlorhexidine. Like toothpastes containing this chemical, these cause staining and in addition cause an alteration in the normal oral bacterial populations. They should not therefore be used on a continuous basis. Other mouthwashes may also cause irritation of the oral mucosa if used excessively, especially those that are alcohol-based. Prebrushing rinses have become available recently, but published evidence for their value has been contentious. Fluoride mouth rinses, which are another method of topical application of fluoride to the teeth, are described later.

Denture (or other appliance) cleansers (13.5)

Apart from a brush and soap, toothpaste or other paste cleaner, three main types of denture cleanser are available: oxygenating cleansers, dilute sodium hypochlorite and dilute mineral acids.

Oxygenating cleansers are supplied as a powder or tablet containing alkaline percarbonate or peroxide and an alkaline detergent such as trisodium phosphate (13.5.2). The oxygen bubbles released are supposed to loosen the deposits on the denture so as they may be washed away. This process is only effective on lightly held deposits and more adherent deposits tend only to be bleached, thus giving the appearance of cleanliness, while the bubbling of the solution is visually encouraging. Unfortunately, prolonged use tends to bleach the denture base acrylic and the artificial teeth and may also be harmful to some types of soft lining material. The instructions for this type of cleanser usually prescribe the use of warm water. Unfortunately, this is somewhat imprecise and hot water can significantly increase the bleaching effect (Fig. 2.3).

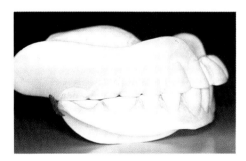

Figure 2.3 Bleaching of acrylic following regular immersion in an oxygenating denture cleanser dissolved in hot water.

Dilute sodium hypochlorite cleansers also cause bleaching of the deposits and the denture, but may in addition dissolve some of the organic components of the plaque (13.5.3). They have a tendency to cause corrosion of stainless steel and cobalt–chromium alloys (although an anticorrosive agent is usually added to the solution) and they may leave an odour on the denture.

Dilute mineral acids such as hydrochloric acid are effective at removing calculus deposits and some staining, but they may also corrode some alloys (13.5.4).

In every case these cleansers should be used with the assistance of a brush, and preferably a disclosing agent, which is then the most effective part of the cleaning regime.

Improving the resistance of teeth to dental caries

Fluoride agents are the most effective method of increasing the resistance of the tooth enamel to dental decay. Water fluoridation (optimum ratio 1 part fluoride per million parts water) or systemic fluoride in the form of drops or tablets produces dramatic reduction in caries levels. The intermittent topical application of fluoride to the teeth by dentists or others provides some benefit, but not as much as more frequent application by the patient in the form of mouthwashes and toothpaste. The occlusal fissures of those teeth which are especially susceptible to dental decay and least benefited by fluoride preparations may be sealed by the dentist with fissure sealants or sealant restorations (preventive resin restorations; 15.3).

Topically applied fluoride (15.2)

Fluoride may be applied topically to the teeth by means of toothpastes, mouthwashes, solutions, gels or varnishes. Fluoride toothpastes contain stannous fluoride, sodium fluoride, sodium monofluorophosphate or amine fluoride which have all been shown to have anticariogenic properties. A low concentration of approximately 0.1% of fluoride is used, because otherwise there may be a danger of children eating a toxic quantity of toothpaste.

Fluoride mouthwashes contain either sodium fluoride in concentration of 0.05–0.2%, or acidulated phosphate fluoride in concentration of 0.02–0.2%. Both mouthwashes have been found to have an anticariogenic effect which is best achieved if the mouthwash is used daily. The use of the mouthwash should be supervised in children or confined to older individuals who can be relied upon not to swallow significant quantities of the mouthwash. However, if carefully controlled, the lower-concentration fluoride mouthwashes containing acidulated phosphate fluoride can also be used to supply the daily dose of systemic fluoride by swallowing the mouthwash.

The lethal toxic dose of fluoride is now considered by the National Poisons Centre to be 14–28 mg/kg bodyweight. This means that if a 5-year-old child of 20 kg swallows two-thirds of a 500 ml bottle of 0.2% sodium fluoride rinse, this could be lethal. Only 32 ml of a 2% concentrate could be lethal and 2.2 ml would be enough to cause acute symptoms.

Solutions of sodium or stannous fluoride are now less commonly used for topical application of fluoride to the teeth. This is because the need to dry the teeth and apply the solution for up to 4 minutes makes the technique difficult and time-consuming. Conversely, the use of fluoride gels is simple and the whole mouth can be treated at one time (15.2.4). This is achieved by the use of trays or applicators which may be formed in the mouth or on a study cast. Wax, foam rubber, alginate impressions and soft, blow-formed polymer slips have all been used to apply the fluoride gels, but it is important to obtain a close fit of the tray. Because the gels flow under pressure, a close fitting tray will force the gel on to every surface of the tooth, including the approximal surfaces. The gel also adheres to the teeth better than a solution thereby prolonging the effects of the gel and improving the effectiveness of host protection. Acidulated fluoride phosphate is usually used in fluoride gels because this has been shown to be more effective in reducing caries.

The most effective way of retaining the fluoride in close apposition to the enamel is by using a fluoride varnish applied to the dried teeth (2.2). Although some success in caries reduction has been achieved, the use of these varnishes is still considered experimental.

Fissure sealants (15.3)

Numerous different synthetic resins have been used in the attempt to seal caries-susceptible occlusal fissures. The two most successful are based on either bis-GMA resins or glass-ionomer cements.

Bis-GMA resins are also used in modern anterior restorative materials which either use chemicals or visible light as a means of activating the setting reaction. Resins may be tinted and both filled (ceramic fillers) and unfilled versions are available; the current preference is for the use of a filled resin. Combination of a posterior composite resin (see Chapter 3) to restore small occlusal cavities with a similar unfilled resin to seal the remainder of the fissure system is also used and is known as a sealant or preventive resin restoration. In clinical handling the most critical features are the maintenance of a totally dry operating field and the production of an etched enamel surface which provides mechanical retention for the fissure sealant. Contamination of the etched enamel surface with saliva prior to placing the sealant will invariably cause failure of the bond, so the most reliable technique involves the use of total isolation of the tooth using a rubber dam. With these techniques a high level of retention of the fissure sealant can be obtained and even if the bulk of the fissure sealant is lost, the retention of tags of fissure sealant in the etched enamel may well render it that much more resistant to caries than the adjacent sound enamel surface (Fig. 2.4).

Glass-ionomer cements bond chemically to the enamel surface rather than by acid-etch retention. The enamel surface is cleaned by polishing and by applying poly(acrylic acid). Glass-ionomer cement used as a fissure sealant has the advantage of containing fluoride, which may further prevent caries.

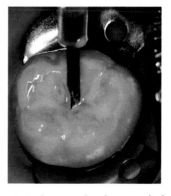

Figure 2.4 Resin fissure sealant being applied with a brush.

Remineralization of carious enamel

The initial phases of dental decay cannot be simply represented as the demineralization of the enamel surface. Rather, there is an intermittent progress with both demineralization and remineralization occurring, and external factors such as changes in diet and oral hygiene practices may alter the balance between the two processes, either leading to advancing or arrested dental caries. Clinically the availability of a topically applied remineralization agent would be attractive, even though the elimination of demineralization agents from the mouth is a more logical approach.

An example of such a mineralizing agent is of a saturated solution of dicalcium phosphate dihydrate in a phosphate buffer at pH 4.5, which is mixed immediately before use with an equal part of phosphate buffer, pH 9.0, containing 2000 parts per litre of fluoride in the form of the sodium salt.

However, despite successful clinical trials, this agent is not yet commercially available. Meanwhile, it has been clearly shown that part of the effect of fluoride mouthwashes and toothpastes is the enhancement of natural remineralization of initial carious lesions from the saliva by favouring the precipitation of well-crystallized apatite in the enamel surface.

Saliva

Natural saliva

From the preceding section it is clear that an adequate amount of salivary flow is essential in the host's resistance to dental caries. It is also of vital importance in the comfortable and successful mastication and swallowing of food and the comfortable wearing of dental appliances. Where salivary flow is reduced, salivary stimulants or artificial salivary substitutes have been proposed. Salivary stimulants are most satisfactory in the form of a pastille which requires chewing, as chewing also acts as a stimulant. The active ingredient is usually acidic in nature as this is well known to provoke salivation. Unfortunately, this acidity can cause erosion of the teeth and there is a need for non-acidic forms to be developed. In the meantime

patients may be advised to chew and suck pastilles or chewing gum produced for diabetics. These contain sorbitol rather than sugar; they also have an acceptable pH. Chewing gum specifically marketed to assist in the prevention of caries probably has its greatest effect by stimulating saliva.

Artificial saliva

No fully satisfactory artificial saliva has yet been formulated. Both carboxymethyl cellulose and hydroxypropylmethyl cellulose in aqueous solutions are in common use and are used as a mouthwash as frequently as required. Neither of these materials has the viscoelastic properties of natural saliva and both require frequent use to maintain a moist oral environment. A possible alternative is high molecular weight polyethylene oxide. Although a 2% aqueous solution of polyethylene oxide has similar viscoelastic properties to natural saliva, the sticky, stringing and viscous liquid is difficult to handle and transport to the mouth.

Many artificial saliva solutions, for example, those used after radiotherapy to the jaws (which damages the salivary glands and reduces saliva flow), contain acid. These should be avoided in dentate patients if possible. Typical formulae for acid-containing and acid-free artificial saliva solutions are:

Acid solution (pH = approximately 2)

Citric acid	25 g
Chloroform spirit	60 ml
Concentrated anise water	10 ml
Methyl cellulose	20 g
Water to 1 litre	

Non-acid solution (pH = approximately 6)

Calcium chloride	0.5 g
Magnesium chloride	0.25 g
Potassium chloride	1.25 g
Sodium chloride	1.75 g
Di-potassium hydrogen orthophosphate	2.0 g
Potassium di-hydrogen orthophosphate	0.65 g
Sodium fluoride	0.01 g
Lemon spirit	16 ml
Sorbitol (70% solution)	85 ml
Methyl cellulose	100 g
Methyl hydroxy-benzoate	4 g
Water to 2 litres	

Whilst the above solutions can be made up by a pharmacist, commercial mouth lubricants in the form of sprays are available. Glandosane has a pH of approximately 5 and contains hydroxymethyl cellulose together with calcium, phosphate, sodium, potassium and magnesium ions. Saliva Orthana has a pH of 7 and is now available containing sodium fluoride. Unusually, instead of methyl cellulose, it contains mucin extracted from the gastric mucosa of the pig to provide the appropriate viscosity.

Prevention of tooth wear

Attrition, erosion and abrasion of natural teeth are largely controlled by alteration of dietary factors or control of oral habits. Occasionally occlusal protection using appliances covering the occlusal surfaces may be indicated, particularly for wear at night in cases of bruxism. The hard acrylic diagnostic occlusal appliances described in Chapter 1 can be used for this purpose but the polyethylene and polypropylene appliances are not suitable as they rapidly become penetrated by occlusal wear in such patients. If the appliance does not wear through in a few days or weeks, either the patient is not wearing the appliance or he or she is not a nocturnal bruxist and the aetiology of the tooth wear is erosion rather than attrition.

Prevention of traumatic damage to teeth (15.4)

Mouthguards are becoming more popular in all contact sports. Traditionally boxers have worn mouthguards to counteract the direct blow to the mouth but all other contact sports, notably rugby and hockey, also have a significant incidence of traumatic injury to the teeth.

Mouthguards act by cushioning the blow to the teeth and by splinting several teeth together by distributing the force of the blow harmlessly around the arch. For this to happen effectively the appliance should fit the teeth accurately and should be neither too flexible nor too rigid. A rigid appliance may itself fracture or, if even a slight inaccuracy in fit occurs may, selectively load individual teeth. Too

flexible an appliance will not effectively distribute the load around the arch. Numerous materials or combinations of materials have been suggested for their manufacture and both professionally constructed and user-formed appliances are available. Thermoplastic materials may be readily adapted to the teeth within the mouth after softening in hot water, are cheap, and are readily available from sports shops. They do not, however, fit the teeth accurately and are often too flexible. Rigid, loosely fitting appliances, rather like stock impression trays may be modified in the mouth with self-curing silicone rubbers (5.2.5). These provide an accurate fit with a happy compromise between overall rigidity and energy-absorbing softness at the tooth–appliance interface. They may, however, be too bulky for comfortable use and the silicone rubber is inclined to absorb oral fluids and become unpleasant after a limited period of use.

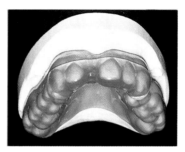

Figure 2.5 Blow-formed polyethylene thermo-formed to a stone cast to provide a mouthguard. A 3 mm sheet is used and a double thickness is applied over the anterior teeth. Note that the loss of some anterior teeth previously will give extra motivation to wear a mouthguard.

Professionally constructed appliances have been made from rigid acrylic, blow-formed polyethylene or polypropylene sheets and silicone rubber or plasticized acrylic materials. Acrylic is difficult to construct so as to fit accurately because of the polymerization shrinkage but does provide the most durable type of appliance. Silicone rubber (13.2.2) and plasticized acrylic resins (13.2.1) are probably too flexible to be effective, are often bulky and again suffer from oral degradation in a limited period. Most nearly ideal and also very simple to construct are the blow-formed appliances (15.4.3). Provided the sheet of material from which they are formed is adequately thick (3–6 mm depending on the sport), these provide an accurately fitting, durable appliance that is neither too rigid nor too flexible. Although an impression and stone cast are required for their construction, thereby necessitating professional help, they are reasonably cheap to provide and are comfortable and unobtrusive to wear (Fig. 2.5).

Stabilizing materials

These are materials used to stabilize the disease process, thus preventing progression of the disease until elective and more permanent treatment can be completed.

Obtundent materials

Desensitizing materials

Sensitivity of teeth to cold, heat and tactile stimuli may occur as a result of exposure of dentine at the cervical margin or occlusal surface of the tooth, even in the absence of any pathological changes in the tooth or its pulp. Restorations in the area of the exposed dentine may resolve the sensitivity but this is unsatisfactory because the tooth–restoration junction may favour the collection of plaque and predispose to further pathology. The use of lasers to desensitize teeth has also been described, but this treatment is not generally available and its effectiveness is not established. Consequently, attempts are made to reduce the sensitivity by the application of chemical obtundents or by blocking the dentinal tubules with polymeric materials.

Such materials may be found in toothpastes formulated for sensitive teeth or in materials to be applied by the dentist (2.2; 4.9). Several types of desensitizing toothpastes (15.1.2) are available, all of which have been found to be clinically effective in some cases. They may contain 10% strontium chloride hexahydrate, 0.76% sodium monofluorophosphate, 2% sodium citrate or 5% potassium nitrate as the active agent. The use of 1.3% formaldehyde has been questioned following the receipt of reports by the Committee on the Safety of Medicines of adverse reactions in the form of a burning sensation in the mouth, followed by

redness and thickening of the mucosa and in some, ulceration and sloughing. The condition was completely reversible on discontinuing the use of the toothpaste.

Materials for professional application include fluoride pastes, varnishes and a silicone polymer. The fluoride pastes are applied to the exposed dentine with a burnishing action – often a painful procedure which, together with the lack of evidence of effectiveness, has led to the use of this material being largely discontinued. Varnishes (2.2) may or may not contain fluoride and are usually based on a solution of a polymer in a highly volatile solvent, for example, copal-ether varnish. They do not adhere well to the moist dentine so that their effect is probably short-lived and storage is a problem – any leakage in the container leads to rapid evaporation of the solvent and hardening of the varnish, while leakage of the varnish around the lid of the container may effectively seal the container forever. The most favoured material at present is a liquid siloxane ester (4.9) which polymerizes in the presence of moisture to form a retentive thin polymeric film over the exposed dentine. It is applied on a cotton wool pledget and several layers may be applied to improve the durability of the film. How long the film is retained is uncertain but the material is clinically successful.

Pulp capping materials (2.1.11.1)

In stabilizing carious cavities it may be necessary to approach the pulp closely in the removal of the carious dentine. In such cases the pulp may already have pulpal inflammation and a clinical decision has to be taken as to whether to commence endodontic therapy or to treat this by pulp capping. Two types of materials are available for pulp capping – calcium hydroxide or antibiotic–steroid preparations.

Calcium hydroxide (2.1.11), being alkaline, has a bacteriostatic action and appears to promote dentine formation and possibly cementum formation. Calcium hydroxide powder may be mixed with sterile distilled water, or one of the proprietary materials which sets to a soft consistency may be used.

In some cases of acute pulpitis with an actual exposure of the pulp which is bleeding, materials containing antibiotics and steroids (e.g. Ledermix) may be used for 24–48 hours in order to suppress the inflammation and therefore the symptoms, kill the organisms and allow the pulp to recover. The material should, however, be entirely removed after as short a period as possible and replaced with calcium hydroxide; otherwise, as long-term studies have shown, the pulp eventually becomes necrotic.

It is very difficult to make the clinical decision between three groups of pulpitic teeth. Group 1 has a pulpitis which will recover with a calcium hydroxide dressing; group 2 will not recover with calcium hydroxide but may possibly recover with Ledermix; group 3 will not recover whatever treatment is applied. Although some pulps undoubtedly fall into group 2, there are no clear indications of which these are beforehand, so many dentists have abandoned this use for Ledermix and treat all pulps as if they fall into groups 1 or 3.

Pulp-dressing materials

In addition to root canal sealers (Chapter 4), chemically active agents are used in the pulp chamber or in the root canal for a number of purposes. These include devitalizing the tooth chemically when it is difficult to remove a vital pulp mechanically, because of problems with access, difficulty with anaesthesia, or lack of time, and materials used to treat an inflamed pulp in the hope that it will remain vital.

In the early days of endodontics, pastes containing arsenic were used and were apparently very effective at devitalizing pulp. Still in use is a traditional material, carbolized resin, which is a paste containing phenol. This material is effective in suppressing symptoms and producing a pulp which is easy to remove mechanically at a subsequent visit. It is simply applied to the bleeding exposure and sealed over. The seal must be entirely reliable as the material is irritant if it leaks back into the mouth.

Some dentists use materials containing antibiotics and steroids with the intention of devitalizing pulp (e.g. Ledermix). This material was originally designed to *maintain* the vitality of pulp, and in some cases does so for some years (see above). However, pulp so treated seems inevitably to become necrotic, the only advantage being the suppression of the symptoms while the pulp dies a natural death. In other words the material has failed

in its intended purpose but its side-effect has had a satisfactory result.

In deciduous teeth, materials used to dress or treat inflamed or necrotic pulp must not damage the permanent successor. They should be resorbable so that the material does not remain when the deciduous root resorbs. They should also be effective as a one-visit treatment. Formocresol and iodoform pastes have traditionally been used and are effective.

Root canal dressing materials

Stabilization of individual teeth may involve placing materials into non-vital root canals, to prevent spread of infection to the periapical tissues which might cause abscess formation. Sometimes the tooth needs to be stabilized in this way for weeks or months while other treatment is carried out, while the periodontal prognosis is established or if the patient is unavailable for treatment. Both antiseptic and antibiotic preparations have been used in the short and long term. The reason for the decline in their use is discussed earlier and in Chapter 4. For long term stabilization there is a preference for chemical antiseptic agents rather than antibiotic preparations. However, despite the disadvantages of the long-term use of low doses of antibiotics, the use of antibiotic–steroid preparations as a dressing for a non-vital root canal is common, presumably because it has the advantage of reliably suppressing symptoms of pulp death until such time as root canal therapy may be commenced. Its use in this way is deprecated.

Commercially available, non-setting calcium hydroxide preparations, which can be injected directly into the root canal are the preferred dressing materials. Alternatively, calcium hydroxide powder mixed with sterile distilled water may also be used as root canal dressing material. These materials remain effective for a long time and are easily removed to permit conventional endodontic therapy at a later date.

Temporary restorations

Stabilizing the crown of a tooth until it can be restored often requires a temporary restoration.

This may be either intracoronal or extracoronal, depending on the degree of tooth destruction. Extracoronal temporary restorations are discussed in Chapter 5.

Choice of temporary restorative material

The choice of a temporary restoration material is based in part on how closely the material matches the ideal properties listed below. Possible materials are discussed in an order which demonstrates that the larger the cavity, the better the materials need to be. The choice of material depends not only on the size of the cavity, but also on its form, the period during which the temporary restoration is required to remain in place and the eventual restoration which is planned to replace it.

Intracoronal temporary restorations

These are usually cements and are retained in the cavity either by its undercut form or by adhesion. The ideal properties of a cement for a temporary restoration include:

1. Easy and rapid mixing.
2. Easy to place in the cavity and shape with hand instruments.
3. Rapid set to ensure stability before the patient leaves the chair.
4. Good strength, especially when used in larger cavities.
5. High abrasion resistance and low oral solubility to maintain tooth contact and occlusal relationships.
6. Adhesion to dentine and/or enamel.
7. Easy to remove to facilitate placement of permanent restoration.
8. Non-irritant to pulp and other oral soft tissues. Ideally the base of the temporary restoration may be left as a lining material when the permanent restoration is placed.
9. No taste or odour (or at least a pleasant one).
10. Acceptable colour for use in the anterior teeth.
11. Cheap and readily available.

Zinc oxide–eugenol cement (2.1.1)

Unmodified zinc oxide–eugenol cement has been used as a temporary restoration for many years. It is easy to mix, place and shape, and is cheap. The set of the unmodified material is very slow, which can lead to the temporary restoration being distorted by masticatory forces before it is fully set. It is now seldom used.

Accelerated zinc oxide–eugenol cement (2.1.2) is the obvious development from the basic material and this has clear advantages in ensuring stability of the temporary restoration. Neither the basic material nor the accelerated versions are very strong and therefore they cannot be used in large cavities without the danger of breakage. Reinforced (2.1.4) or resin-bonded (2.1.3) versions of the accelerated material are available and are more satisfactory for the larger cavities, but in all cases zinc oxide–eugenol materials exhibit poor abrasion resistance and rather high oral solubility and should not be left in place for long periods of time, because loss of tooth contacts may lead to drifting of adjacent teeth or over-eruption of the occluding teeth. Ready-mixed zinc oxide-containing cements for temporary restorations are available in tubes and pots and these perform as well as the materials mixed at the chairside and are therefore popular, despite the higher cost.

All zinc oxide–eugenol materials are non-irritant to the pulp and may have an obtundent effect on the slightly inflamed pulp, maintaining vitality and reducing the likelihood of pain. Part of the temporary dressing may consequently be left under a permanent restoration as a lining. They have a rather strong taste of oil of cloves (eugenol) and when set are too white and opaque to be ideal for visible teeth. Zinc oxide–eugenol should not be left in a tooth which is to be restored with composite as it affects the curing of the composite.

Zinc phosphate cement (2.1.6)

This is also based on zinc oxide but mixed with a 50% aqueous solution of phosphoric acid. The chief advantages as a temporary restoration are strength, which is more than double that of accelerated zinc oxide–eugenol, superior abrasion resistance and lower oral solubility. It may therefore be used in larger cavities and will provide a stable temporary dressing for a longer period. The chief disadvantage is the low pH in the early stages of setting which can irritate the pulp unless a lining of a more bland material is placed over deeper parts of the cavity. As it is harder it is also more difficult to remove. It is easy to use, cheap and has no taste once set, but the appearance is again unsatisfactory and has now been largely superseded for temporary restorations by the zinc polycarboxylate and glass-ionomer cements.

Zinc polycarboxylate cement (2.1.9)

Both zinc oxide–eugenol and zinc phosphate cements require undercuts to retain them in place and where the cavity is large this may seriously weaken the structure of the crown of the tooth. Indeed it is unjustifiably destructive to remove sound tooth structure for this purpose. In poly-carboxylate cement the phosphoric acid is replaced by poly(acrylic acid) which is less irritant to the pulp and forms a cement which is adherent to clean dry enamel. The strength, abrasion resistance and oral solubility are similar to zinc phosphate and it may therefore be used in larger cavities without the need to weaken the crown by providing undercuts. Unfortunately, adhesion is not totally reliable when used as a temporary dressing and the extra cost reduces its attractiveness.

Glass-ionomer cement (3.4.2)

This is essentially a permanent restorative material and has better properties than a temporary cement. However, the significant advantages of its adhesion and tooth colour make it a very useful long-term temporary restorative material. Like polycarboxylate cements it is not irritant to the pulp and can be applied directly to cut or fractured dentine and enamel for optimum adhesive results. The major disadvantages in using glass-ionomer cement as a temporary material are the time required to place it, the difficulty in removal without damaging sound tooth substance and the cost of the material. Glass-ionomer cement is covered in greater detail in Chapter 3.

Acrylic or other resin inlays (4.6; 4.7)

Another alternative for the non-undercut cavity, especially if undercuts are contraindicated because the cavity is eventually to be restored with an inlay, is an inlay made from poly(methyl methacrylate) or preferably one of the higher acrylics. The strength and abrasion resistance of the resins used are not ideal, but are considerably better than the cements described above. Strength is poor in thin section so such sections should be avoided, while the relatively poor abrasion resistance limits their use to periods of a few months or less depending on the level of the occlusal forces, otherwise occlusal wear may allow tooth movements.

Temporary inlays are usually formed in the mouth and matrix bands may be used to ensure a good fit at the cervical margins of Class II cavities. The occlusion may be roughly shaped when moulding the inlay and finally adjusted using occlusal marking material on the cured inlay.

Methyl methacrylate (acrylic) has been largely superseded by materials which have a lower exotherm during setting, are less irritant to soft tissues and are more elastic immediately prior to the final set (4.6).

Powder–liquid and two- and three-paste systems are available. When a powder–liquid system is being used, the proportions of powder (polymer) and liquid (monomer) are judged by partly filling a dappens dish or paper cup (not a plastic cup which will melt) with the monomer, adding polymer to excess, tapping the pot on the work surface to assist saturation of the liquid with the powder, discarding the excess polymer and finally adding one drop of monomer. Very little stirring of the mixture is necessary or desirable as this incorporates air which produces a weaker, cured material. In curing the acrylic passes through a mouldable plastic stage, to a rubbery stage and finally a hard set. The material is placed and moulded in the cavity in the plastic stage, and then removed and replaced several times during the rubbery stage before being allowed to cure on the bench or in hot water; the latter speeds the curing cycle considerably. In this way there is no danger of the inlay becoming fixed in the cavity by unnoticed undercuts, or because of the polymerization shrinkage locking the inlay around retained cusps or other cavity features. The removal and replacement of the inlay also help to dissipate the heat produced by the exothermic setting reaction.

The cured inlay is trimmed to extend exactly to the margins of the cavity, so as to contact adjacent teeth and occlude with opposing teeth, before being cemented with a temporary cement (see Chapter 5). The retention of the inlay and the protection of the pulp rely in part on the properties of the temporary cement but, since these are usually based on zinc oxide cements the latter is less of a problem than the former. Temporary acrylic inlays have the additional advantage of being tooth coloured.

Temporary splints

In traumatic loosening of anterior teeth, particularly in children, a temporary splint will stabilize the traumatized, mobile tooth and allow healing. Although the tooth may subsequently lose its vitality and even undergo root resorption, the temporary splinting is usually effective in reducing traumatic mobility. Permanent splints are discussed in Chapter 6.

Temporary prosthetic materials

Patients often present with prosthetic problems which require the eventual provision of a new or replacement denture. However, it is usually necessary to provide one or more forms of preparatory treatment. This may be restorative treatment in the partially edentulous mouth, treatment to resolve inflammatory changes in the oral mucosa or surgical preparation of the denture-supporting tissues. In such cases provision of a temporary appliance or modification of an existing appliance will allow comfortable wear and provide some therapeutic benefit.

Temporary appliances may be simple mucosa-supported acrylic dentures, which will later be replaced by more technically demanding tooth-supported cobalt–chromium alloy dentures, in which case an account of the materials used and their handling may be found in Chapter 7. The provision of emergency prostheses and the modification of existing dentures are described later.

However, it should be noted that patients often try to find their own solutions to denture problems. Consequently there is a thriving market in denture adhesives to overcome loose dentures, and home-applied soft relining materials to overcome painful dentures. There are also home repair materials. All of these materials used in expert hands may provide satisfactory results, but unfortunately the inexperienced patient may do more harm than good to both the appliance and the mouth in using such home remedies (Fig. 2.6).

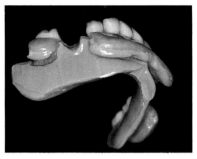

Figure 2.6 Home-applied soft relining materials may not adapt fully to the underlying denture-bearing tissues and are a potential cause of damage to these tissues.

Denture adhesives (13.6)

Proprietary denture adhesives rely on high molecular weight polymers, which form highly viscous dilute aqueous solutions which stick to denture bases and have little effect on the oral mucosa. The viscosity of the adhesive prevents its displacement from under the denture by air and therefore improves retention. Additionally, the high viscosity allows the adhesive to fill spaces existing because of poor fit of the denture, usually following continuing resorption of residual bone. The active constituents found in denture adhesives include karaya gum, tragacanth, sodium carboxymethyl cellulose and polyethylene oxide, all of which are also permitted food additives and are used as stabilizers for convenience foods. When taken in excess they can cause gastrointestinal disorders, but with the exception of karaya gum which can cause hypersensitivity, they are generally harmless when ingested. Karaya gum also has the disadvantage of producing an acidic (pH 4.7–5.0) solution which has been shown to be capable of causing decalcification of dental enamel. Adhesives using karaya gum are therefore contraindicated in partially edentulous patients. Some denture adhesives also include antimicrobial agents, for example, hexachlorophane, and most include wetting agents, plasticizer and flavourings.

Denture adhesives are usually supplied in a powder form or as a paste in petroleum jelly or paraffin oil. These are applied to the denture surface and activated by contact with water or saliva; this causes the polymer particles to swell, thereby increasing the viscosity of the adhesive. As a temporary expedient, to ensure retention of a poorly fitting prosthesis prior to its replacement, they are valuable; but their continuous use is not usually necessary except in cases where neuromuscular control of the dentures is absent because of medical conditions.

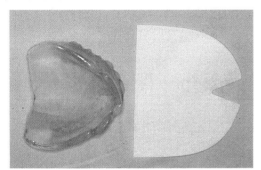

Figure 2.7 A thin paper pad containing denture adhesive has been moistened, adapted to the fitting surface of a denture and surplus paper removed with scissors.

From the patient's point of view, the major disadvantage of dental adhesives is their unpleasant feel and the difficulty of cleaning the appliance after their use. This has been partly overcome by the incorporation of the adhesive in a thin paper pad the shape of the denture fitting surface (Fig. 2.7). This is more difficult to apply to the denture but is retained on the fitting surface for longer (other materials are more easily diluted by saliva), and is easier to remove at the end of the day. Inevitably, it is also more expensive.

Temporary relining materials

The use of the word temporary implies that such a relining material will only last for a short period of time, and that it will be able to be removed in due course without damage to the relined denture. In fact, clinical circumstances where temporary relining

of dentures is used vary markedly, and the term temporary may embrace periods of time in excess of a year. For longer periods, therefore, temporary modifications, additions or relining may be carried out using self-curing higher methacrylates. Both tooth-coloured and pink versions are available (13.4) and they are sufficiently non-toxic and have a low enough curing exotherm to be used intraorally. They must not be allowed to cure in the mouth if there is any possibility of soft or hard tissue undercuts (see Chapter 7).

For short periods ill-fitting dentures are usually temporarily relined with soft, viscoelastic materials otherwise known as tissue conditioners (Fig. 2.8; 13.3).

Tissue conditioners (13.3)

Tissue conditioners consist of a polymer powder based on poly(ethyl methacrylate) and a liquid, which is a mixture of an aromatic ester with ethyl alcohol. The liquid contains no methacrylate monomer, hence these materials do not cure in the conventional sense and there is no risk of residual monomer irritating the oral mucosa. When mixed, the material first becomes a mobile fluid, appropriate for application to the denture and subsequent insertion in the mouth. It progresses from this fluid state to a coherent gel which exhibits the characteristics of a viscous fluid and an elastic solid.

In clinical use the consistency of the mix (i.e. powder : liquid ratio) and the moment of application are important in using the material. When used inside the fit surface of an upper denture, the material should be placed in the mouth within 2–3 minutes of mixing, when the viscosity is sufficiently low to enable the material to flow and form a thin layer. If a thicker layer is required under a lower complete denture, more powder may be used and/ or the insertion of the material delayed to reduce the flow under manual or occlusal pressure. The material will continue to act as a viscous fluid throughout its life, but after about 30 minutes in the mouth it becomes sufficiently elastic that it will not flow under normal loading.

The value of the material as a tissue conditioner is easily appreciated. The provision of a new fitting surface on an otherwise ill-fitting traumatic denture will itself benefit the tissues (Fig. 2.9). In addition,

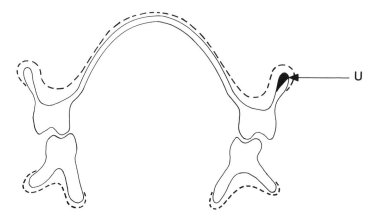

Figure 2.8 Where appropriate, undercuts (U) are removed and the temporary lining replaces the resorbed residual ridge. The material should be as thin as possible over the palate to avoid increasing the vertical dimension.

the softness of the material cushions the tissues against masticating loads and distributes the loads evenly over the whole denture-bearing area. Since the tissues will change shape as inflammation resolves, the relining procedure should be repeated frequently (preferably every 2–3 days but at least once a week) until the tissues reach a healthy condition. Even where the oral tissues appear healthy under an ill-fitting denture the use of these materials as a temporary reline for the denture increases its retention and stability and is greatly appreciated by the patient. It is also useful after surgical modification of the alveolar ridge or removal of excess soft tissue over the denture-bearing area, the healing area being covered by a layer of soft material which reduces the stress on it. The life of the material used in this way varies from 1 to 3 months and is determined by leaching of the alcohol, and to a lesser extent the ester, from the material, causing a gradual hardening and distortion. The greater loss at the surface tends to cause roughness; also the use of alkaline perborate denture cleansers is detrimental.

The versatility of these materials is increased by the addition of nystatin powder (800 000 units of nystatin per denture liner) which is extremely useful in the treatment of denture stomatitis. The slow release of the nystatin from the mixed tissue conditioner applied to the fit surface of the denture provides an antifungal effect exactly where it is required for up to 7 weeks, with much convenience to the patient.

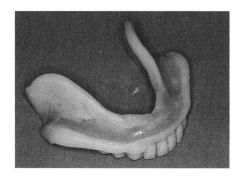

Figure 2.9 Viscoelastic gel tissue conditioner applied to a lower denture.

Emergency dentures

In a true emergency it is possible to make temporary partial dentures at the chairside. Considerable clinical time is required and the results are understandably less than satisfactory for long-term use.

A layer of pink modelling wax, softened in hot water, is adapted to the area of the mouth where the major connector of the denture is to fit, for example, the palate or lingual sulcus. To this is attached either a stock denture tooth or a tooth-coloured polycarbonate temporary crown form of appropriate size to replace the missing teeth. In the posterior regions blocks of wax may suffice to fill spaces and provide occlusal surfaces. An alginate impression is then taken over this wax-tooth trial denture. The wax is discarded and the denture teeth or temporary crown forms placed in their appropriate places in the impression. The temporary crown form has the distinct advantage of having a hollow interior which will facilitate its attachment to the denture base. The stock denture tooth may have an undercut cavity cut into it to ensure reliable retention to the denture base. Wax blocks replacing posterior teeth may be replicated using tooth-coloured acrylic temporary crown resin (4.6), and then the denture base is constructed using a pink acrylic resin (13.4) by placing a suitable quantity in the impression and reinserting into the mouth. Higher methacrylates are used in preference to poly(methyl methacrylate) because of their less irritant properties and their lower exotherm. If, however, the latter is the only resin available, protection of the oral mucosa with petroleum jelly and minimizing the time the uncured resin is left in the mouth is acceptable. The impression and the curing denture base must be removed from the mouth at the rubbery stage to ensure withdrawal from the inevitable undercuts, allowed to polymerize fully and then trimmed and adjusted to fit the mouth.

Denture repairs

Cobalt–chromium alloys cannot be satisfactorily repaired by soldering or welding. It may in some cases be possible to replace a fractured clasp or rest with wrought gold or stainless steel, soldered to the framework or attached with acrylic resin, but this is often a compromise on the original design of the denture. For this reason great care should be taken to construct the components of the cobalt-chromium partial denture framework with adequate bulk for strength, although accidental impact damage cannot be allowed for in the design (see Chapter 7).

On the other hand acrylic (poly(methyl methacrylate)) is easily repaired. The base usually breaks cleanly and reassembly is easy and accurate. The separate parts are then connected using a fresh mix of denture base material. Self-curing materials are usually used for speed and convenience, as well as to avoid distortion of the remainder of the denture which may occur at the temperatures necessary to polymerize a heat-curing material. Again, the properties of the self-curing material are inferior to the heat-polymerizing material, so that the durability of the repaired denture is limited by that of the repair material (see also Chapter 7). A very recent concept is a light-curing denture base material, similar to light-curing composite, which is claimed to have superior properties to chemically cured materials (13.8), and which may also be used for repairs.

Common reasons for denture fracture and methods of strengthening or reinforcing denture bases are discussed in Chapter 7.

Further reading

Adisman, I. K. (1989) The use of denture adhesives as an aid to denture treatment. *Journal of Prosthetic Dentistry*, **62**, 711–715

HMSO (1990) *Guidance for Clinical Health Care Workers: Protection against Infection with HIV and Hepatitis Viruses*. HMSO, London

Mellberg J. R. (1991) Fluoride dentifrices: current status and prospects. *International Dental Journal*, **41**, 9–16

Symposium (1991) Appropriate uses of fluoride – considerations for the '90s. *Journal of Public Health Dentistry*, **51**, 20–63

Welbury R. R. and Murray J. J. (1990) Prevention of trauma to teeth. *Dental Update*, **17**, 117–121

World Health Organization (1973) *Technical Report Series 512, Viral Hepatitis*. WHO, New York

Chapter 3

Treating caries and other damage to teeth

Introduction

The prevention of dental caries and methods of encouraging the remineralization of early enamel lesions have been discussed in Chapter 2. In this chapter the treatment of the irreversible, established carious lesion will be described together with the restoration of teeth damaged by trauma and toothwear (erosion, attrition and abrasion), and the management of discoloured teeth.

Isolating teeth

For many operative procedures on teeth it is helpful to isolate them from the rest of the oral environment. Some procedures require a high level of isolation, for example endodontics and restorations near the gingival margin which are harder to keep free of contamination by saliva, gingival exudate or blood. For other procedures a lower level of isolation with cotton rolls, pads and sponges is satisfactory.

Rubber dam

Rubber dam is usually supplied in ready cut sheets approximately 150 mm^2. It is also supplied in a number of thicknesses and colours. Some are flavoured to disguise the taste of rubber. Many dentists prefer the darker colours which show up the teeth in greater contrast, and there is less likelihood of leaving torn fragments behind. Rubber dam should be very elastic and not prone to tear around the punch-holes.

Rubber dam tends to cling to the tooth surface and so a lubricant helps with its application. The lubricant should be non-greasy, water-soluble and tasteless. Brushless shaving soap works quite well, as does the modifier used with temporary crown and bridge cements, but there is also a water-based lubricant specially supplied for the purpose.

Rubber dam clamps of springy stainless steel are supplied in a variety of shapes to suit different teeth and some have wings. Rubber dam can be applied in three ways:

1. It can be stretched over the wings of the clamp before the clamp is put on the tooth. `
2. A wingless clamp can be applied to the tooth first and then the rubber dam stretched over both the clamp and the tooth.
3. The rubber dam can be applied to the tooth first and then stabilized by means of a clamp, dental floss, wedges or small strips of rubber dam. With this technique both winged and wingless clamps may be used.

Rubber dam clamps occasionally spring off the teeth or break in use and this is a hazard to the patient who may inhale or swallow one of the fragments. For this reason dental floss should be attached to the clamp but with breakage this only retains part of the clamp. The risk of rubber dam clamps fracturing is greater if they have been heated and reshaped or when they have been overstretched

(Fig. 3.1). Rubber dam is also supplied already attached to a disposable frame. This can be particularly quick and convenient to apply when a single tooth needs to be isolated, e.g. for endodontic treatment. Figure 3.2 shows a tooth isolated by means of conventional rubber dam and also by means of the disposable rubber dam/frame combinations.

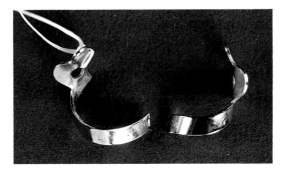

Figure 3.1 A broken rubber dam clamp with floss attached to one half. If the clamp had broken in the mouth this half could have been rescued easily, the other half is at risk of being inhaled or swallowed.

Cotton rolls, pads and sponges

Cotton rolls are commonly used for simple isolation of teeth. As well as absorbing saliva and other fluids, cotton rolls help to pack the cheek and tongue away from the operating site so that they are less likely to be caught by burs or other instruments.

A variety of pads (usually cellulose) have been produced which are applied dry to the inner surface of the cheek to assist in isolation and absorbing fluids in the mouth. These have the advantage that they are not so easily displaced by movements of the patient's muscles.

Some dentists attempt to isolate the mouth from the airway by applying a butterfly sponge to the back of the mouth. This is an oval slice of sponge material tied round the middle with cord, giving it a butterfly shape. The cord is left trailing from the mouth so that the sponge can be retrieved when necessary. These sponges are effective in the unconscious or tranquillized patient where the cough reflex is suppressed; however, the conscious

patient finds them irritating and tends voluntarily to suppress the cough reflex, which can be dangerous.

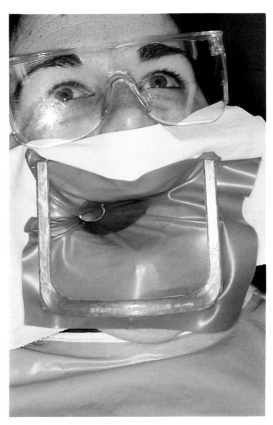

a

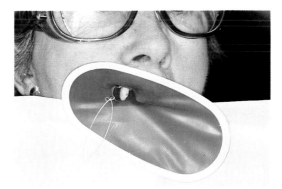

b

Figure 3.2 (a) Conventional rubber dam in place. Note the paper towel behind the rubber dam to absorb moisture. (b) Small disposable rubber dam/frame in place. Again note the paper towel.

Cavity preparation

When caries has extended to the point where it cannot be remineralized or when existing restorations have to be replaced it may be necessary to cut a combination of the following materials:

1. Enamel.
2. Dentine.
3. Carious dentine.
4. Amalgam (3.1).
5. Composite (and other tooth-coloured restorative materials, 3.2).
6. Glass ionomer cement (glass polyalkenoate; 3.4.2).
7. Porcelain (14.1–14.3).
8. Cast metal (9.1).

The methods by which teeth can be prepared include:

1. Cutting with burs or stones (1.6, 1.7).
2. Cutting with hand instruments (1.1).
3. Etching with acid.

Burs and stones (1.6, 1.7)

The cutting surfaces of dental burs are made from steel, tungsten carbide or diamond. All three may be used at conventional slow speeds in 1:1 ratio handpieces at 5000 to 20 000 r.p.m., but only tungsten carbide or diamond are used at the intermediate speeds of 12 000–160 000 r.p.m. in 1:4 ratio, friction-grip, speed-increasing handpieces or at the high speeds of 160 000 to 300 000 r.p.m. in the airotor. Slower speeds (65–5000 r.p.m.) can be achieved with 4:1 or 10:1 ratio, speed reduction handpieces, and these speeds are used for caries removal with steel burs, for drilling pin and post-holes, and for polishing and other procedures. Abrasive stones are available mounted on latch grip and friction grip shanks, and abrasive wheels or discs are available to be mounted on mandrels.

Some materials are better cut at slow speed and some at high speed but there is a grey area between the two where the personal preference of the dentist decides which speed to use.

Sound enamel is best cut with diamond or tungsten carbide burs at high speed with water spray for cooling and the removal of debris. It may be finished and smoothed with abrasive stones or tungsten carbide stones at a slower speed (Fig. 3.3).

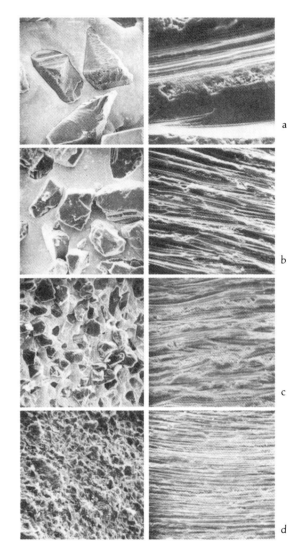

Figure 3.3 Scanning electron micrographs of four grades of diamond bur and the enamel surfaces they have prepared. The field width in each picture is approximately 350 μm. Left: The surface of the instrument. Right: The enamel surface which it has prepared. (a) A standard diamond bur with particles up to 111 μm diameter; (b) superfine diamond bur with particles up to 62 μm diameter; (c) ultrafine diamond bur with particles up to 35 μm diameter; (d) composite shaping diamond bur with particles up to 40 μm diameter. Photographs courtesy of Mr. J.R. Grundy.

Sound dentine may be prepared either with diamond or tungsten carbide burs at high speed but can also be prepared with burs of any material at slow speed. The advantage of slow speed is that the dentist has a greater sense of feel and can control the shape of the cavity rather better. The disadvantage is that the vibrating slow speed bur on the tooth can be uncomfortable for the patient.

Carious dentine is best prepared at slow speed with steel burs. Because caries tends to balloon out into dentine and produce naturally rounded cavities it is best to use round burs, as large as the cavity will accommodate, to remove carious dentine. The sense of feel is particularly important when removing caries so that there is no encroachment upon sound dentine.

Amalgam is best cut into large pieces by tungsten carbide or diamond burs at high speed and then removed from the cavity in lumps. The amalgam should be cut from the centre outwards rather than running the bur around the periphery of the old restoration. The latter technique will produce an unnecessarily enlarged cavity. Water spray and aspiration are essential to reduce the generation of hazardous mercury vapour.

Composite (and other tooth coloured restorative materials) is best removed with water-cooled diamond or tungsten carbide burs at high speed. Composite cannot effectively be cut with steel burs and so these should not be used. Silicate and acrylic resin restorations will be readily dislodged from the cavity wall once they are cut through. Acid-etch retained composite restorations and glass-ionomer restorations, however, may well need to be removed entirely by burs.

Porcelain is best removed by producing a groove in the restoration with a water-cooled diamond bur at high speed and then breaking the porcelain and removing it in pieces using a rigid instrument such as a chisel, flat plastic or a heavy scaler. Flexible instruments will flex themselves rather than fracture the porcelain.

Cast metal is best cut in the mouth with specially produced multibladed tungsten carbide burs with very small cross cuts and a low blade angle (often called a Beaver bur; Fig. 3.4). These cut cast metal quickly and effectively with a minimum of juddering or jamming and with a very low incidence of bur fracture. Diamond burs are much slower at cutting cast metal and quickly become blunt while conventional tungsten carbide burs frequently catch and break.

When removing a combination of materials, for example, a metal ceramic crown, it is worth using different instruments for the two materials so that a diamond bur is used to cut through the porcelain facing, changing to a metal cutting tungsten carbide bur to cut through the metal framework.

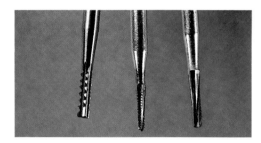

Figure 3.4 Three types of tungsten carbide, friction-grip high-speed bur. Left: a cross-cut fissure bur for general use; centre: a fine cross-cut bur used to cut cast metal in the mouth (a Beaver bur); right: a plain cut bur used for finishing and smoothing preparations.

Eye protection

Some cutting procedures in the mouth carry the risk of particles of metal, broken burs or other materials flying out of the mouth. A number of cases of damage to the eyes of the patient, the operator or the dental surgery assistant have been reported. It is good practice for all three to wear eye protection during any tooth cutting procedure, but this is particularly necessary when cutting amalgam, porcelain or cast metal.

Hand instruments (1.1)

Hand instruments may be used to prepare enamel, dentine and carious dentine and are also used to dislodge old restorations once their retention has been removed by burs.

Enamel chisels

Enamel chisels are made in a variety of shapes and the cutting edge is either steel or tungsten carbide. It is quite easy to see the difference; a tungsten carbide chisel has a small piece of tungsten carbide brazed to the tip and this is clearly visible. Chisels are used to shape and smooth enamel margins. In fact the surface left by a chisel is not particularly smooth and has a substantial enamel smear layer when viewed under the scanning electron microscope. Partly for this reason their use has declined in recent years. They are, however, still used for removing fragments of enamel near to a contact point where the use of burs would be likely to damage the adjacent tooth. Steel chisels can be sharpened on an Arkansas stone. Tungsten carbide-tipped chisels are difficult to sharpen effectively at the chairside and are best returned to the manufacturer for sharpening. However, they retain their sharp edge for very much longer than steel chisels.

Excavators

Excavators are primarily designed to remove carious dentine and if kept sharp are excellent for this purpose, particularly in patients (e.g. children) who are anxious about the use of a drill. Caries is more usually removed with slow-speed steel burs, largely because many excavators have long since lost their edge. They are still useful for a variety of purposes such as removing temporary restorations, testing the hardness of the dentine walls of a prepared cavity, applying lining materials, carving amalgam and in removing old restorations. They are made from steel. Tungsten carbide-tipped versions are not available.

Finishing cavity margins

Burs, stones, mounted wheels and discs and hand instruments are all used to finish cavity margins. Cavities are best prepared with a smooth outline to facilitate condensing the restorative material against the margin of the cavity and also the contouring and polishing of the restorative material. Defects between the restorative material and the tooth surface are more common if the cavity margin is uneven.

Cavities finished with rotating or hand instruments will be left with a smear layer on the cut surface. This remains unless it is removed chemically before the restoration is placed.

Etching enamel with acid

Acid-etching is used to prepare cut enamel cavity surfaces when the cavity is to be restored with composite. It removes the smear layer as well as etching the enamel. Acid etching is also commonly used to achieve retention in a variety of other techniques, including bonding porcelain and composite inlays and veneers, orthodontic brackets, splinting teeth temporarily and in bonding minimum preparation bridges (see later).

Conditioning dentine

The margin of the cavity sometimes consists of dentine, for example with erosion/abrasion cavities and root caries. The dentine surface may be conditioned with poly(acrylic acid) to remove the smear layer, open up the dentinal tubules and improve retention.

Handpieces

The materials used in older handpieces included a combination of non-corrodible and corrodible materials. This meant that it was not possible to sterilize handpieces effectively by means normally available in dental surgeries. Dry heat sterilization tended to congeal the lubricants and produce a high incidence of clogged and ineffective handpiece mechanisms. Conventional steam autoclaving produced corrosion while post-vacuum autoclaves (which are only available in large hospital sterilization departments) avoided the corrosion problem but not the clogging.

All handpieces produced in recent years have been made with non-corrodible materials and therefore can be autoclaved. Most handpieces are now lubricated by means of aerosol sprays inserted by means of a special adaptor into the attachment end of the handpiece. The aerosol contains a mixture of disinfecting and lubricating agents.

Retention

Depending on the material used and the size of the cavity one or more retentive mechanisms are used:

1. Physical undercuts.
2. Pins.
3. Acid-etching of enamel.

4. Dentine bonding agents.
5. Adhesion.

Physical undercuts

Gross physical retention features are incorporated into the design of most amalgam restorations. The design of an amalgam cavity must be such that the amalgam cannot be lost occlusally, buccally, lingually, mesially or distally. The approximal posterior amalgam cavity, for example, must therefore contain features which prevent occlusal and proximal loss. The alternatives are a conventional keyhole-shaped cavity with undercuts to prevent occlusal loss or a wedge-shaped cavity, without an occlusal lock, with axial grooves which prevent both occlusal and proximal loss.

Pins (4.1)

Threaded pins are made from titanium alloy or stainless steel and may be gold-plated. The least expensive are the stainless steel pins but there is some anxiety about the long-term effects of corrosion. Gold-plated and titanium alloy pins reduce the risk of corrosion. The titanium alloy pins are, however, more expensive. Earlier systems, in which pins were cemented into holes slightly larger than the diameter of the pin using either a cyanoacrylate or zinc phosphate cement, and friction retained pins are now seldom used.

Threaded pins are inserted by means of a slow-speed contra-angle handpiece, the pin being temporarily attached to a bur shank by a self shearing weakened section. Several of the threaded pin systems use plastic colour coded bur shanks to indicate the size of pin.

Acid-etch retention (4.4.1)

A number of acids in different concentrations and presentations have been used in the past but the acid which is now most commonly used is 37% buffered phosphoric acid gel, although several other concentrations of between 30 and 50% are also available. Acid in liquid form is also used, but is more difficult to control than acid gel.

Most manufacturers have standardized on a blue colour for phosphoric acid gel. However, unfortunately, one or two manufacturers use other colours,

such as pink. This is regrettable because yet another manufacturer produces hydrofluoric acid gel in a similar pink colour and this could lead to a dangerous confusion. It is to be hoped that the manufacturers will reach an international agreement on colour coding in the foreseeable future.

The acid gel may be applied with a paintbrush or can be applied more precisely through a syringe system. Several such systems are on the market and Figure 3.5 shows an example.

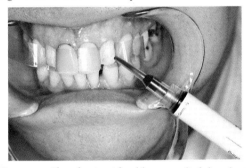

Figure 3.5 Phosphoric acid gel being applied directly to the tooth from a syringe. The tip of the syringe is disposable. A veneer is to be applied to this tooth and the coloured mylar matrix strip separating it from the adjacent teeth prevents resin which may flow behind the strip from curing.

It is important not to allow the acid to contaminate the dentine or lining surface and it is preferable not to etch beyond the prepared enamel surface. The earlier gels restricted the diffusion of acid so that they had to be constantly stirred on the tooth surface. The more recent materials are made gel-like by using small polymer particles and these allow the diffusion of acid through the material so that they do not have to be stirred on the tooth surface.

It is important to remove the acid completely from the tooth surface by washing with water spray for approximately 30 seconds (when carried out, this seems like a long time) and then thoroughly drying with oil-free air until the surface appears white and frosty (which also takes a long time; Fig. 3.6).

It is possible to achieve this frosty appearance with shorter washing and drying periods, but the risk is that debris from the etching will be left behind in the etch pits, reducing their retentive capacity.

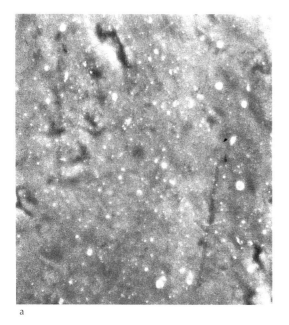

a

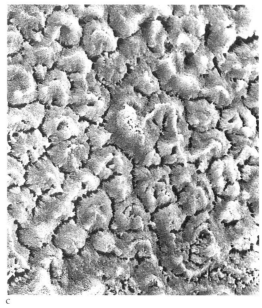

c

Figure 3.6 Scanning electron micrographs (SEMs) of: (a) unetched enamel; (b) poorly etched enamel (5 seconds); (c) well-etched enamel (15 seconds with 35% phosphoric acid gel). Field width for all three SEMs = 45 μm.

Dentine bonding agents

A substantial literature now exists on the theories, mechanisms and materials which are claimed to bond composite to dentine. Although laboratory experiments and clinical experience support the view that such bonding is now possible, the mechanism is as yet not fully understood. It seems likely that the principal mechanism is micromechanical retention rather than true chemical adhesion. It is hoped that the true nature of the bond will become clearer with further research.

With some materials the smear layer is allowed to remain and forms part of the bond; in others the smear layer is removed with poly(acrylic acid). This opens up the dentinal tubules and there is some anxiety about this increasing the risk of pulp irritation.

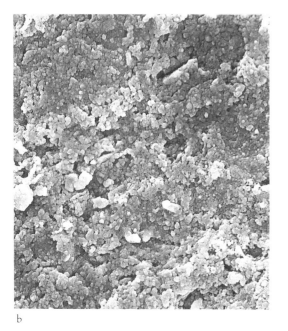

b

Adhesion

The most truly adhesive material to dentine is glass ionomer cement. The adhesion is enhanced by conditioning the surface with poly(acrylic acid).

The strength of the final restoration is limited by the cohesive strength of the glass-ionomer cement, as well as by the strength of the bond to dentine. For this reason, glass-ionomer cements are used primarily to replace missing dentine, and the enamel is then replaced by another, stronger and more wear-resistant material (see later).

Lining the cavity (2.1)

The function of a lining (sealer or base) is one or more of the following:

1. To protect the pulp/dentine from thermal stimuli transmitted through conductive restorative materials. (i.e. amalgam, gold or other cast metal).
2. To seal the dentinal tubules against the entry of bacteria and toxins, and to prevent movement of tissue fluids in the tubules, which produces discomfort.
3. To protect the pulp/dentine from chemical irritation by restorative materials or cements (e.g. zinc phosphate cement).
4. To reduce the likelihood of microleakage and consequent irritation of the pulp/dentine or secondary caries.
5. To treat the pulp/dentine therapeutically, reducing the symptoms of pulpitis and maintaining the vitality of the pulp in the short term and encouraging secondary dentine formation in the long term.
6. Shaping the floor of a cavity.
7. Replacing the bulk of missing dentine and thereby reducing the bulk of the restorative material replacing the enamel.

Cement cavity lining materials

There are five groups of these materials:

1 Calcium hydroxide-containing materials (2.1.11).
2. Materials based on zinc oxide–eugenol (2.1.1–2.1.4).
3. Zinc polycarboxylate cements (2.1.9).
4. Zinc phosphate cement (2.1.6).

5. Glass-ionomer materials (2.1.10).

Calcium hydroxide materials are used to control pulpitis either by the direct or indirect pulp capping techniques (see Chapter 2). They are also used for thin linings in shallow anterior and posterior cavities.

A large range of materials is available based on zinc oxide–eugenol. These have various mixtures of ingredients to strengthen them and to accelerate the setting reaction. They are usually supplied as a powder and a liquid which may be mixed to either a thin or thick consistency. As a lining material, the material should be mixed as thickly as possible. It is applied by rolling a suitable-sized piece of the mixed material into a ball, picking it up on the end of a probe and inserting it into the cavity. It is shaped by means of flat plastic instruments or amalgam condensers. It is important that the shaping instruments are dipped repeatedly into the powder or saliva (the patient's!) to prevent the mixed material sticking to them. Zinc oxide–eugenol linings can be made thicker than calcium hydroxide linings and so provide better thermal insulation. However, although bland, they have little therapeutic action on the pulp. They should not be used in conjunction with composite materials with which they can react. They are commonly used for moderately deep cavities in posterior teeth which are to be restored with amalgam.

Polycarboxylate cements may be regarded as an alternative to zinc oxide–eugenol. They have the property of adhering to enamel but have no therapeutic properties on pulp and indeed may be rather more irritant than zinc oxide–eugenol.

Zinc phosphate cement was at one time the universal lining material and many successful restorations were made with it. However, its low pH at the time of insertion produces irritation of the pulp and may well have produced a number of pulp deaths in teeth which would otherwise have remained vital. It is therefore no longer used as a lining material on its own but may be used over a sublining of a calcium hydroxide or zinc oxide–eugenol material.

Zinc phosphate is mixed to a thick consistency and applied in much the same way as zinc oxide–eugenol, although alcohol may also be used as a separator for the placing instruments.

Glass-ionomer cement is being used increasingly as a lining or base material. It has the advantages that it bonds to dentine, has adequate strength in bulk (as compared with the other materials mentioned so far), releases fluoride which helps to protect the dentine against further caries and, in some forms at least, has a very low setting shrinkage. This latter property is an advantage when it is planned to restore a large cavity with composite. Polymerization shrinkage will be a problem if the bulk of the cavity is filled with composite, whereas if the dentine is replaced with glass-ionomer cement and only a surface layer of composite applied, then the polymerization contraction of the composite will be less significant.

Glass-ionomer cement is used as a lining/base material in one of three forms:

1. As a relatively thin lining applied in a similar way to calcium hydroxide cement. The material is used at a fairly low viscosity.
2. A similar material to the one described above but in a light-curing version. This is convenient to use but the setting contraction is higher.
3. Materials supplied as restorative materials may be used as thick bases replacing the bulk of the dentine. They are used with a relatively high viscosity and the cavity is usually overfilled and then the glass-ionomer base is cut back to the enamel dentine junction before the final restoration is placed (Fig. 3.7).

To summarize, the two lining/base materials which are likely to continue to be used are the calcium hydroxide and glass-ionomer materials. The other three are rapidly falling out of use.

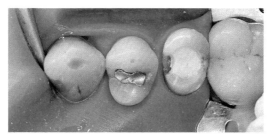

Figure 3.7 Large cavity with the dentine mostly replaced by glass-ionomer cement. This constitutes more than a simple lining.

Cavity sealers, varnishes and bonding agents

Cavity varnishes have been used for many years both to provide some chemical protection and also to reduce the initial microleakage in amalgam restorations. Cavity sealers containing fluoride have also been used in an attempt to reduce the incidence of secondary caries. There is no overwhelming long-term evidence of the value of these materials, but on the other hand they probably do no harm. Most of them are supplied in a volatile liquid carrier. The varnish is applied to the cavity walls right up to the margins and then blown dry. Evaporation of the carrier leaves pores through the varnish and so two or three coats are usually applied. Even when this is done, the varnish layer is not entirely impervious.

Dentine bonding agents have already been mentioned as an aid to retention. They are not, strictly speaking, liners or varnishes, although they are applied in a rather similar manner. The usual sequence is to prepare the cavity, apply a thin lining of calcium hydroxide material over the deepest part if necessary, acid-etch the enamel margins, apply bonding agent to the dentine walls (it does not matter if the bonding agent also flows over the enamel surface), gently blow-dry the bonding agent, apply the composite and light-cure it. Because of the contraction of the composite materials during setting, it is necessary to apply small increments of composite to different parts of the cavity and cure each increment separately.

Dentine bonding agents used in this way should serve the functions of a cavity sealer described earlier. This remains the hope, but there is as yet insufficient long-term clinical evidence to be sure that they do.

Restoring the tooth

The materials available for restoring teeth include:

1. Amalgam (3.1).
2. Composite (3.2).
3. Glass-ionomer cement (3.4.2).
4. Other cement materials (3.4.1; 3.4.3).
5. Cast gold or other metal (see Chapter 5).
6. Porcelain (see Chapter 5).

Several of these materials simply provide a plug to fill the hole in the tooth (a 'stopping'). This does little truly to restore the original properties of the tooth. For example, an MOD cavity separates the buccal and lingual cusps of the tooth which are then much more likely to break off. Also the traditional restorative materials (other than silicate cement) have done nothing to reduce the likelihood of further caries but indeed have often allowed microleakage, which has increased the risk. It is hoped that the development of restorative materials will continue to lead to restorations which not only replace the lost tissue but also get closer to duplicating the properties of the lost dentine and enamel, as well as being cariostatic.

The properties of dentine and enamel are very different from each other. A natural tooth made entirely of one or other of these materials would fail; the dentine tooth would fail through wear and the enamel tooth would be likely to fracture because of its brittleness. It is therefore somewhat naive to imagine that a single restorative material can fully duplicate the properties of these two natural materials as well as bonding to them to produce a genuine restoration. The search must therefore be for a combination of materials to restore teeth by means of systems rather than individual materials. These systems will probably have three components: a dentine substitute, an enamel substitute and an analogue of the enamel dentine junction to join the two materials together. At present, although only a crude approximation, the nearest there is to this is glass-ionomer cement to replace dentine and either porcelain or composite replacing enamel and bonded to it by acid-etching. However, these materials still have a number of significant disadvantages, including wear and polymerization contraction. The other materials are still therefore commonly used.

Amalgam (3.1)

Amalgam is one of the oldest restorative materials but has undergone a number of developments in recent times.

Traditional lathe-cut amalgam (with irregularly shaped particles of alloy) is mixed by one of the techniques described later, inserted in the cavity with a suitable carrier and then condensed either with a hand or mechanical condenser. The purpose of condensation is to adapt the very stiff amalgam paste to all parts of the cavity whilst at the same time packing together the unreacted particles of the alloy and in the process excluding all the air which, if left, would produce a porous and thus weak restoration. In addition, with older alloys and mixing techniques, condensation brought excess mercury to the surface which was then removed by carving. This is no longer necessary.

Types of amalgam alloy

Amalgam alloy is now produced with lathe-cut particles, spherical particles or a mixture of the two. The spherical alloys produce an amalgam which is very much more fluid to condense and therefore has a reduced risk of porosity. However, because it flows so easily, matrixing and wedging are particularly important, otherwise the material flows between the matrix band and the cavity margin producing overhangs. Spherical alloys have an earlier initial set and so may be used for large restorations where early strength is desirable.

The other major difference between alloys is between those that produce a $gamma_2$ (silver–tin) phase on setting and those which do not. Amalgam which is $gamma_2$-free has a greater resistance to corrosion and creep and therefore maintains better margins and surface polish. $Gamma_2$-free amalgam is produced from high-copper alloys and these are available in any of the particle shapes described above.

Properties of amalgam which limit its clinical use

Amalgam does not adhere to enamel or dentine. Artificial bonding systems are now available but long-term clinical trials have not yet established their durability. This means that the preparation of the cavity should still include mechanically retentive features and this may involve cutting away more sound tooth tissue than is desirable. Similarly, because amalgam does not bond to tooth surface, the remaining tooth structure must have its own integral strength and so overhanging enamel and weakened cusps should be removed. Amalgam does not have sufficient strength to be used in thin sections and this again limits the shape and size of the cavity which can be restored with amalgam.

Mercury is used to produce dental amalgam and this is associated with two hazards which to some extent limit the use of the material. Firstly, mercury vapour is toxic and great care must be exercised in handling liquid mercury to avoid spillages and prolonged exposure to its vapour. For this reason factory-packed capsules are preferred. When liquid mercury is used it should be stored in unbreakable plastic containers in small quantities and transferred to the mixing apparatus with great care. If a spillage does occur it should be cleaned up immediately by rolling it into a dustpan or on to paper sheets, or by sucking it up with specially produced plastic pipettes made for the purpose. Manipulations with mercury should be carried out well away from apparatus which produces heat (e.g. sterilizers), so that any spillage which does occur is not vaporized more quickly than would occur at room temperature. Also vacuum cleaners should not be used in areas where mercury spillage has occurred (or even where mercury is used at all), in case minor undetected spillages have occurred. For this reason dental surgeries should not be carpeted.

The second hazard is that a small number of patients are allergic to mercury and this may produce skin reactions both when new restorations are inserted and when old ones are cut out.

Variations in mixing and handling technique

Amalgam should not be mixed by hand because of the dangers associated with mercury vapour.

The ideal encapsulated versions require the use of an automatic vibrator. Such capsules have the advantage of accurate, factory proportioning as well as reducing the likelihood of mercury vapour polluting the atmosphere. However, care should be taken to store the empty capsules in an unbreakable sealed container after use. When full, such a container should be permanently sealed prior to disposal.

Alternatively, bulk alloy and mercury may be dispensed and mixed in a single operation in a specially designed piece of apparatus. This has a disadvantage that it is necessary to refill the amalgamator periodically with liquid mercury. The proportioning of alloy to mercury is variable and can be adjusted to suit particular techniques and different alloys. The use of bulk alloy reduces the cost.

Thirdly, alloy and mercury may be dispensed by hand into reusable capsules which are then vibrated in a mechanical amalgamator. This technique carries the greatest risk of spillage, which can occur when the constituents are being placed in the capsule. Also when the capsules get worn there is a greater risk of mercury vapour escaping from them during vibration. The method should therefore now be phased out whenever possible.

The near universal use of mechanical amalgamation has reduced the alloy to mercury ratio so that there should no longer be any excess mercury in the final mix. The proportion of mercury needed is also reduced with the spherical alloys.

Studies of hand and mechanical condensation of lathe-cut amalgam alloys have shown that if both are carried out with equal care there is no difference in the final result. However, mechanical condensation is easier and quicker and is therefore popular with busy dentists. Spherical alloys are not suitable for condensing with mechanical condensers due to their more fluid nature. They are easily and quickly condensed by hand.

For ideal carving conditions, lathe-cut alloys should be left for a few minutes before carving, whereas spherical alloys can be carved sooner. Shaping the occlusal surface but not the margins at this stage of set with burnishers is an acceptable technique.

Composites (3.2)

Composite resins are a mixture of a resin material and a particulate filler. The type of resin used and the material from which the filler is made are less important to the handling characteristics than are the particle size of the filler and the method of curing.

There are three important ranges of particle size – large, microfine and hybrid. The large particle size composites are radiopaque and reasonably abrasion-resistant but are difficult to polish and tend to accumulate plaque. The microfine composites polish well, but tend to absorb water and sometimes discolour. They have lower abrasion resistance and are not radiopaque. The hybrid materials combine the advantages of both conventional and microfine composites and there has been an emphasis in recent years on the development of hybrid materials with graded particle sizes and also particles with rounded shapes which improve particle packing within a limited amount of resin material.

Composites are either cured by a chemical reaction between two component pastes when mixed together or by the effect of light upon a single paste. Chemically cured materials have a number of major disadvantages and so their use as restorative materials has now almost completely ceased. Their disadvantages are that, with a single mix of material, the polymerization contraction is large. (This is partly overcome with light-curing materials by incremental packing.) Also, when the two components of the materials are mixed together, air is inevitably incorporated, so that the final restoration is more porous than light-cured material. The setting time is greater than the curing time for light-cured composites and there is also no control over the speed of the setting reaction. In contrast, the light-curing materials are easier to shape in the mouth as there is more time to do this.

The curing reaction on the surface of light-cured materials is air inhibited. This means that the surface should be protected by a transparent matrix during curing or, more commonly, the cavity should be slightly overfilled, the composite cured and then the surface cut back to contour and polished. A final exposure to the light improves the hardness of the surface.

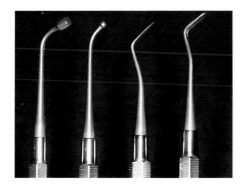

Figure 3.8 Plastic instruments coated with titanium nitride to reduce the adhesion of composite materials.

Composite materials are best placed with hand instruments which have not been previously scratched by composite filler particles and to which the composite does not readily stick. Stainless steel instruments are not ideal; nylon instruments are satisfactory but can only be made relatively bulky and so are not suitable for delicate placing of composite material, particularly approximally. Teflon-coated materials are available but the surface tends to become scratched and so the best range of instruments currently available is coated with titanium nitride (Fig. 3.8).

To prevent the possibility of eye damage when using the intense blue curing lights, care should be taken not to stare at the light. Spectacles or shields which filter out the harmful wavelength should be used.

Composites for posterior restorations

Although the early composites were developed for anterior teeth, all the major manufacturers now produce either composites specifically for use in posterior teeth or materials which can be used in either anterior or posterior teeth. The original composites were not satisfactory for restoring posterior teeth because their wear resistance was low and because marginal leakage and recurrent caries were a persistent problem. However, improvements in both materials and technique have now made posterior composite restorations an acceptable alternative to amalgam. Much of the literature comparing the materials starts with the assumption that amalgam is the standard material against which composite should be compared. This means that the criteria used often favour amalgam, for example occlusal wear. Criteria such as the conservative nature of the preparation, retaining more overhanging enamel, and the ability of composite to bond to and strengthen weakened cusps are reported less frequently. It is commonly stated that posterior composite restorations are technique-sensitive. This is true but it is equally true of amalgam restorations. The difference is that, if a mistake occurs in placing a composite restoration, the likelihood is that either the etched retentive enamel surface or the composite material will become contaminated. In the former case, retention will be lost and in the latter, if the contamination is by blood, the composite will become stained. In both cases the failure will be immediately obvious. With amalgam, the commonest form of contamination is by moisture. Initially this has no clinically observable effects. However, it increases the amount of expansion so that after a period of time a greater degree of marginal ditching occurs. The difference between materials is therefore that poor technique produces instant failure in composite and delayed failure with amalgam.

Techniques for placing posterior composite restorations have been developed and include transparent matrix and wedge systems, the light-conducting wedges being used to initiate the cure at the gingival margin rather than from the occlusal surface. The effect is to minimize marginal leakage at the gingival margin rather than cause the material to contract away from it. Manufacturers have also attempted to introduce entirely new chairside techniques for making posterior composite restorations, rather than rely on adaptations of amalgam technique. These new techniques are not yet entirely satisfactory, but development along these lines is to be welcomed in order that optimum benefit may be achieved from posterior composite materials.

Another development has been the introduction of composite materials in single dose capsules (referred to by some manufacturers as carpules or compules). The advantage of this delivery system is that it is not only more convenient, but the composite material can be introduced more precisely into the cavity with less risk of voids or contamination occurring. Because the capsules are disposable it is easier to maintain cross-infection control and there is no risk of contaminating the unset material, which is a problem with syringe delivery systems. The disadvantage of the capsule system is that the composite material must be made sufficiently fluid to be expelled from the capsule. It is claimed by some manufacturers who have not adopted the system that this fluidity is achieved by increasing the proportion of resin and that this reduces the material's abrasion resistance. The counterclaim is that this is not so and that the flow can be achieved by shaping (rounding) and grading the filler particles.

Composite inlays (3.2.2)

In attempts to overcome the inherent disadvantages of posterior composite materials, a number of manufacturers have now introduced composite inlay systems for posterior teeth. These can also be used to produce veneers (see Chapter 5).

A widely used composite inlay system produces inlays which are cured under both heat and pressure. This produces a more fully crossed-linked resin and it is anticipated that these composite inlays will be more abrasion-resistant and maintain their colour better than direct-filling composite materials.

The technique is to take an impression, make the inlay in the laboratory and cement it at a subsequent appointment. As a two-visit system, it will inevitably always be more expensive than a chairside system.

The polymerization contraction occurs in the laboratory and the laboratory technique includes a system of trimming back and adapting the distorted inlay to fit the working die. The inlay is then bonded with dual-cure composite material, the cure being initiated by light but continuing in the deeper parts of the cavity by chemical action (Fig. 3.9).

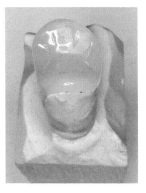

a

b

Figure 3.9 (a) A laboratory-made composite inlay on the die. (b) The inlay in place in the upper left second premolar tooth. This inlay has full cuspal protection, but this does not always need to be used.

Glass-ionomer cement (3.4.2)

Glass-ionomer cement is available in two forms – an anhydrous version which is supplied as a powder which is mixed with water on a pad, or in a capsule. They may contain poly(acrylic acid) or poly(maleic acid) in freeze-dried form as their major acidic ingredient. Both now have good resistance to initial solubility, although there is some evidence that the poly(acrylic acid) version is slightly less soluble. However, both materials have poor abrasion resistance, particularly on the occlusal surfaces of teeth and so they are either used in restoring class V cervical lesions or as a base material to be veneered with composite, porcelain or cast-metal restorations.

Early expectations of glass-ionomer materials containing silver powder cement (3.4.3) in terms of abrasion resistance have not been fulfilled. However, this cement is useful in building up cores and, because of its radiopacity, in treating root caries. It is also used as a base material.

Other cement and resin-filling materials

Silicate (3.4.1) and poly(methyl methacrylate) (3.3) were used in the past as restorative materials, but are no longer used. Silicate had the advantage of leaching fluoride which reduced the incidence of secondary caries but this advantage is now available in the glass-ionomer cements. The disadvantages of silicates were that they had a very low initial pH such that pulp death was common and they were also soluble in the oral environment.

Poly(methyl methacrylate) has a high coefficient of thermal expansion and a large setting shrinkage and so marginal leakage was common, producing stain, percolation and secondary caries. The restoration was inevitably porous and so became stained and smelly. Abrasion resistance was also low.

Finishing restorations (1.8)

The purpose of finishing restorations is to improve the marginal fit and to polish the surface so that it is less plaque-retentive and has a better appearance. In addition it is sometimes necessary to recontour the surface to suit the occlusion.

Amalgam restorations are finished by using a progression of instruments, each one less abrasive than the last. Multibladed finishing burs or abrasive stones are used first, followed by either a series of rubber points and cups or pastes of decreasing abrasivity. The usual pastes in decreasing order of abrasivity are a slurry of pumice powder in glycerine, a commercial prophylactic paste, and zinc oxide powder mixed with alcohol. These paste materials are used on a brush or a non-abrasive rubber cup in the handpiece.

Composites are finished initially by cutting excess composite material away from the margin with sharp scalpel blades or chisels. The margins are then trimmed with fine white stones or very fine diamonds mounted on friction grip or contra-angle shanks. Special multibladed finishing tungsten carbide burs may also be used. The surface of the composite is polished, again either with a progression of mounted rubber cups or points, or with flexible polymeric discs coated with different grades of abrasive. Abrasive-coated strips are also available for finishing approximal areas (Fig. 3.10).

Some dentists prefer to coat stones, discs and other abrasives with a lubricant such as petroleum jelly to reduce heat production and to stop the restoration drying out. However, if the abrasives are used dry with gentle pressure, heat production is minimal and it is possible to see more clearly where the restoration finishes and enamel starts. Improved vision also helps to avoid damaging the gingival tissues.

Glass-ionomer cements may be finished by similar techniques and then left, but it is better to protect the finished surface, at least in the early period after placing the restoration. One technique is to overfill the cavity, protect the surface with varnish and then finish and polish the surface at the next visit. Alternatively – and usually a more practical approach – the restoration is polished at the same time that it is placed and then protected with a layer of light-cured resin.

The management of discoloured teeth

Teeth become intrinsically stained during development as a result of enamel hypoplasia, fluorosis or tetracycline staining, and also become discoloured after eruption as a result of pulp death, restorations

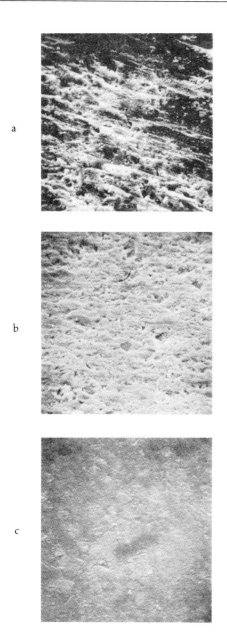

a

b

c

Figure 3.10 Scanning electron micrographs of the surface of a posterior composite restoration being shaped and polished. The field width in each picture is approximately 350 μm. (a) The surface left by a composite shaping diamond at high speed; (b) after finishing with a medium flexible abrasive disc; (c) after finishing with a fine disc. Photographs by courtesy of Mr J.R. Grundy.

and ageing. Treatment may therefore be necessary to improve the appearance of individual teeth or all the visible teeth.

If the teeth are intact or nearly so, the destructive option of crowns should be left as a last resort. Less damaging options are:

1. Microabrasion.
2. Chairside bleaching.
3. Veneers.

Microabrasion is reported as being effective in removing relatively superficial white or brown patches. The technique is to polish, under rubber dam, with a slurry of pumice in 18% hydrochloric acid and then neutralize with a saturated solution of sodium bicarbonate followed by copious irrigation.

Chairside bleaching is most effective for internally discoloured teeth resulting from the breakdown products of haemoglobin when the pulp has died. Under rubber dam, the endodontic access cavity is opened up to the base of the pulp chamber and grossly discoloured dentine is removed, leaving a roughly even layer of dentine beneath the enamel. The dentinal tubules are opened up with phosphoric acid or poly(acrylic acid) and the dentine dehydrated with ethanol or chloroform. Cotton wool with 100% hydrogen peroxide or a paste of hydrogen peroxide and sodium perborate is placed into the cavity and heated with a hot instrument and the procedure repeated a number of times. There are several variations on this technique.

Until recently home bleaching kits could be bought by patients over the counter or offered by dentists. They consisted of either carbamide peroxide or hydrogen peroxide solutions and the former may or may not contain carbopol. The dentist could carry out a quick-start first application and the patient was then provided with a custom-made applicator, rather like a mouthguard. The solution was placed in this by the patient and worn at home for specified periods over a number of weeks, returning to the dentist regularly for evaluation of progress. However, these kits have been banned in the UK to comply with a European Union directive, and similar bans are coming into force in other countries.

Veneers are dealt with in Chapter 5.

Further reading

Burke, F.J.T. (1986) Posterior composites: the current status. *Dental Update*, **13**, 227-239.

Burke, F.J.T. (1991) Dentine bonding agents – optimising the use of composite materials. *Dental Update*, **18**, 96–104

Elderton, R.J (1986) Current thinking on cavity design. *Dental Update*, **13**, 113–122

Kidd, E.A.M. and Smith, B.G.N. (1990) Pickard's Manual of Operative Dentistry, 6th edn. Oxford University Press, Oxford

Mount, G.J (1990) An Atlas of Glass-ionomer Cements. Martin Dunitz, London

Warren, K (1985) Bleaching discoloured endodontically treated teeth. *Restorative Dentistry*, **11, 132–138**

Wilson, A.D and McLean J.W. (1988) Glass ionomer cements. Quintessence, Chicago, Illinois

Chapter 4
Endodontics

Introduction

The most widely practised treatment in endodontics is root canal treatment, which is guided by three principles: the cleaning, shaping and filling of the root canal system. This review of materials will first examine instruments and solutions for cleaning and shaping root canals, before considering the choice of filling materials and their techniques of insertion. The chapter will conclude with a section on materials used in surgical endodontics.

Access burs (1.6)

The first stage of root canal treatment is entry to the pulp chamber. This may initially involve access through an artificial crown, a core of restorative material and finally dentine. Creation of a cavity through a cast crown is best achieved with a fine cross-cut tungsten carbide bur (e.g. Beaver − see Chapter 2) in the airotor; this bur will also readily cut amalgam which often forms the core. In the case of a ceramic crown or a composite resin core, a diamond bur is more suitable as it is blunted less by the extremely hard ceramic, or the filler particles in the composite resin. The bur must be able to cut on its end but otherwise its shape is not very critical. A long tapered bur is least suitable as its tip is small, and when it is deep inside the tooth, the bur may cut an unintended part of the tooth, for example while concentrating on reaching the pulp with the bur tip, the sides of the bur may overenlarge the coronal part of the cavity. The deeper parts of the access cavity are better created with a bur in the low-speed handpiece because the burs are available with longer shanks than those for the high-speed handpiece, and dentine removal is less rapid, so errors arise less quickly. When a pulp chamber is deeply placed, even longer burs may be required. After the pulp chamber has been found it can be partly enlarged with a round bur in the low-speed handpiece, which cuts dentine as it is pulled back; a safe-ended bur may be used in the high-speed handpiece to shape the access cavity without risk of damaging the pulpal floor. When the access cavity preparation has been completed, the canal orifices may be explored with a long endodontic probe which has been designed for the purpose.

Shaping instruments

The aim of root canal preparation in a mature tooth is to produce an enlarged version of the root canal which progressively tapers to the apical foramen and follows the original canal shape. This is best achieved by a filing action rather than a reaming technique which, although once popular, is no longer used. A filing action is a pull, or push and pull, movement of the file without rotation. A reaming action is a rotary movement of the file, and is usually limited to rotation through 90°.

The most widely used instrument for shaping a root canal is a *file*, of which there are different patterns. Their general shape is essentially similar -

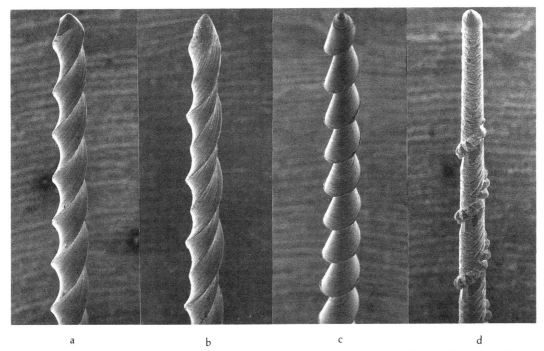

a   b   c   d

Figure 4.1 Scanning electron micrographs (× 40) of: (a) K-file, triangular section (Flexofile, Maillefer); (b) K-flex file (Kerr); (c) Hedstrom file (Kerr); (d) Shaper file for sonic handpiece (Micro-Mega)

a tapered cutting part, a plain shaft and a handle which is held between finger and thumb. Files are manufactured in standardized lengths and taper. They may be divided into two groups, ground and cut, which describe the method of manufacture. In the ground group, the facets are ground on to the metal wire before it is twisted. In the cut group, the cutting blade is machined into the wire which is not twisted. In the last two decades files have been made from stainless steel to avoid rusting and from very flexible nickel-titanium.

The cross-sectional shape of the file varies according to its type. A *K-file*, so named as it was first manufactured by the Kerr Company, is traditionally made by twisting wire of a square cross-section, although some manufacturers have used a triangular section to produce sharper cutting angles to the blade and a more flexible file (Fig. 4.1a). *K-flex* files, also manufactured by the Kerr Company, have a rhomboid cross-section (Fig. 4.1b); these have sharper angles to the blade and considerable flexibility. Their shape allows more room for dentine filings compared with a standard

K-file. The shape of the file tip varies between instruments and manufacturers. There has been a trend in recent years to produce files with non-cutting tips or rounded ends to reduce incorrect canal preparation by cutting into the apical part of the outer wall of a curved canal. Ground files are intended to be used in a push–pull motion with more emphasis on the pull stroke to avoid pushing dentine chips to the end of the canal. Rotation of ground files is not an intended method of use but may be done to a limited extent. Excessive rotation could lead to instrument fracture.

Cut files, e.g. a *Hedstrom file* (Fig. 4.1c), are intended to be used only in a pull motion, in which they cut dentine rapidly. They have no cutting ability in a push motion, and they are very likely to break if rotated. When files are used in the intended way, they should be effective for the preparation of a number of canals. However, if a file becomes excessively bent or shows deformation of the flute pattern, it should be discarded. If a small file has been rotated, it should not be used in more than two canals to reduce the risk of fracture.

Stainless steel root canal instruments must be sterilized between patients and this is effectively done in an autoclave. The process does not appear to have a significant adverse effect on the steel or the polymeric handles. Although the use of glass bead (or salt) heaters has declined because of concern about their effectiveness as sterilizers, files are not damaged by being inserted into the container of glass beads which are intended to be heated to a temperature of 225°C.

Thin files are flexible whereas thick files are stiff, therefore thin files are better able to follow curved canals. The effect of thick files straightening curved canals has been well documented. Prolonged use of a thin file in a curved canal will also show the same tendency. In a curved canal it is the outer wall in the most apical part which is cut and not the inner wall; however, a couple of millimetres back from the apical part at a place referred to as the *elbow*, canal preparation is minimal; further back, it is the inner wall which is prepared, and in a severely curved canal there is no preparation of the outer wall at this level. In the coronal part of the canal, there is more uniform preparation of all canal walls. As files are tapered, they are thicker nearer the handle and are therefore more efficient at cutting in this part. Studies have shown that when a canal is enlarged by hand files, more dentine is removed from the walls in the coronal part than in the apical part. Precurving an instrument will help it to follow a curve but there is still a tendency to straighten the canal. This is also true for mechanized files.

The most widely used files are finger-held (so-called hand files), but they are also available in long-handled versions, or for use in a contra-angle low-speed handpiece, in an ultrasonic handpiece or in a low-frequency vibratory (sonic) handpiece.

The ultrasonic handpiece vibrates files at approximately 25 kHz, which results in a wave form with several stationary (nodal) points along the file. There is marked movement of the file between the nodal points, and it is greatest at the file tip, which is referred to as an antinode (Fig. 4.2). The cutting ability of ultrasonic files is reduced as load is applied, but the extent is dependent on the energy source. When the files are used at the recommended power settings, cavitation does not occur in the solution around the file, in contrast to some manufacturers' claims. If irrigant is flowing, the ultrasonic file does not generate significant heat.

When the file vibrates freely, it creates acoustic streaming which can be regarded as flow of irrigant along the file; its effect is reduced if the file tip touches the canal wall. The file, therefore, cannot effectively clean and shape at the same time.

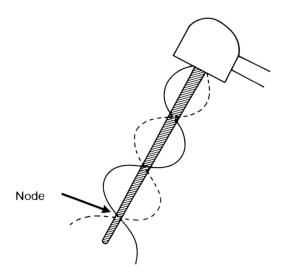

Figure 4.2 The wave pattern of an ultrasonic file. There is minimal oscillation at the nodal points. Maximum oscillation occurs at the file tip which is an antinode. After Walmsley A.D. (1987). Ultrasound and root canal treatment: the need for scientific evaluation. *International Endodontic Journal* **20**, 105–111.

The sonic handpiece vibrates at a much lower frequency (e.g. 1.5 kHz) and has only one nodal point. Specific files have been manufactured for the sonic handpiece, e.g. *Shaper* (Micro-Mega) (Fig. 4.1d).

For rapid enlargement of the coronal part of root canals, specific safe-ended burs (Gates–Glidden), which are produced in a range of sizes, may be used; some are now manufactured in stainless steel (Fig. 4.3).

Irrigation

Cleaning of the root canal system is aided by irrigation. Both the volume and type of irrigant are

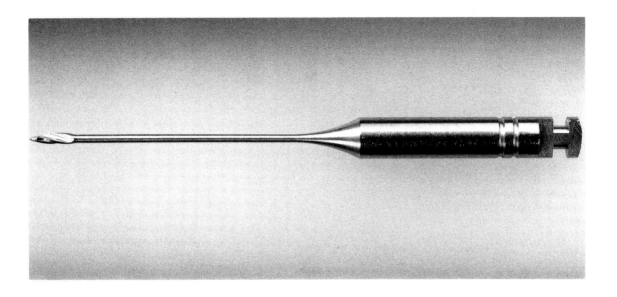

Figure 4.3 A Gates–Glidden bur used to enlarge the openings of root canals. The tip is blunt to reduce the risk of perforating the root laterally.

important; the use of a large volume is the most effective. If the irrigant is introduced by a syringe, deeper insertion of the needle produces cleaner results and therefore needles should be fine-gauged. The cleaning of the most apical part of the root canal is always the poorest. Saline has been used in the past because of its blandness; however, the use of sodium hypochlorite solution is now favoured because of its antibacterial and tissue-dissolving properties. The strength of hypochlorite solutions has varied from 0.5 to 5.0%, with little noticeable effect. The weaker solutions are less toxic, while the stronger disinfect better. Delivery of sufficient volume of hypochlorite together with mechanical agitation appear to be more important than high concentration. Mechanized handpieces, e.g. the ultrasonic system, are the most effective at delivering irrigant.

Hydrogen peroxide solution alternating with hypochlorite is no longer used as it is no more effective than hypochlorite alone. The smear layer of compacted dentine chips formed on the surface of dentine by files is not eliminated by hypochlorite; however, it may be effectively removed by a solution of a chelating agent, for example 15%

ethylene-diamine-tetra-acetic acid (EDTA).

Hypochlorite solution is corrosive and so only stainless steel root canal instruments should be used with this irrigant. Ultrasonic equipment requires special corrosion-resistant plumbing, but it is still prone to corrosion and salt deposition. It is therefore essential to wash out the system after use. In clinical use particular care should be taken to avoid hypochlorite splashing on to the skin or clothing of the patient. If hypochlorite is inadvertently forced through the apex into the periapical tissues, a severe reaction can occur; fortunately, this complication is very rare.

Various other antiseptic solutions have been used for irrigation, but none has shown superiority over sodium hypochlorite, which is effective and inexpensive.

Root canal filling materials (4.10)

Gutta-percha (4.10.1.1)

The oldest and most widely used of the root filling materials is gutta-percha in the form of tapered points; these are used in conjunction with a cement sealer in a technique of lateral condensation, that is, packing as many points as possible into the canal. It has long been accepted that preparation of the canal cannot create a perfectly round cross-section, instead its shape should reflect that of the original canal and it should taper towards the apical foramen. The first gutta-percha point, a standardized point, is selected and placed to fit the canal snugly in the apical part; it is coated with cement sealer and placed in the canal, before accessory points are inserted alongside after space has been created by pressure from an instrument – a *spreader*. The standardized point has a nominal International Organization for Standardization (ISO) size but owing to the nature of the material and the manufacturing process, its size may vary ± 0.5 mm, which is clinically significant. Accessory points have a much greater taper.

Gutta-percha points are used in root canals because they can be adapted to the shape of root canals by applying pressure from a spreader, which is a long pointed stainless steel wire on either a long handle – a hand spreader – or a short handle – a finger spreader.

Gutta-percha points consist of:

20% gutta-percha as a matrix
66% zinc oxide as a filler
11% sulphates (e.g. barium) as radiopacifiers and
 3% resins as modifiers and binders.

Individual brands vary slightly; however, manufacturers are reluctant to divulge the exact formulation of their products. There is considered to be some chemical interaction between the zinc oxide and the gutta-percha, and this may possibly explain why some points which are stated to contain only zinc oxide are stiffer than other brands.

Gutta-percha has also been widely used in Scandinavia in a solvent technique, where the points are softened by solvent and pressed together by a spreader. The technique requires care to minimize shrinkage as a result of evaporation of excess solvent. The solvent has traditionally been based on chloroform, but alternative and potentially less toxic solvents are now being sought. A recent development is a solvent based on limonene and ethyl acetate.

Chloroform may also be used to soften an existing gutta-percha root filling when its removal is required to carry out retreatment, and other solvents have also been used, for example, xylene or an essential oil such as oil of Cajaput.

Gutta-percha may be adapted to root canals by softening with heat. Either the gutta-percha may be introduced into the canal at room temperature or already heated. The simplest way of heating gutta-percha points which are in a canal is to introduce a warm spreader which has been heated in a glass bead heater; the spreader should not be heated over an open flame because its spring temper will be destroyed. The gutta-percha may also be heated by a special electrically heated spreader. Alternatively, root canal pluggers, which are blunt-ended, can be used to soften the gutta-percha before it is condensed by cold spreaders.

Another method is to use a special rotary instrument, e.g. a Gutta-Condenser (Maillefer), which is rotated at 12 000 r.p.m. in a dental handpiece. The frictional heat softens the gutta-percha points already placed in the canal, and forces the material into the entire canal space. The blade of the instrument has a reverse twist to force the molten gutta-percha forwards. Correct speed is necessary to achieve the desired amount of softening of gutta-percha, and correct rotation is essential to prevent the instrument impaling itself into the root. These instruments should only be used in a straight canal or the straight coronal part of a curved canal; in this case, the apical part may be filled by lateral condensation prior to rotary compaction in the coronal part, the so-called hybrid technique.

Two manufacturers have produced heaters which will melt gutta-percha that is then delivered into the canal by a special syringe and compressed with pluggers. This technique appears very simple; however, it does need an acquired skill to avoid overfilling in teeth with large foramina and to avoid defects as a result of premature cooling. One system uses standard endodontic gutta-percha, while the other uses a gutta-percha with a lower melting point. This is achieved by the addition of wax modifiers. Concern has been expressed about the damaging effect of heat on the cellular cementum on the root surface.

The most recent technique of filling root canals with gutta-percha uses a special filler, which consists of a handle with an attached metal shaft which has been coated with gutta-percha. This is heated and forced into the canal where the gutta-percha is condensed with pluggers. The metal carrier remains in the canal permanently and is likely to complicate subsequent post space preparation or to make retreatment, should it be required, more difficult.

Other filling points (4.10.1.2, 4.10.1.3)

Solid filling points, e.g. silver and titanium, have in the past been advocated for filling fine root canals, where their greater stiffness over gutta-percha ensures penetration to the prepared distance in a fine curved canal with minimal taper. Their use dates back to single cone techniques, which are no longer recommended because of inadequate filling of canals in three dimensions, despite the use of sealer.

The long-term success rate of using silver points has been disappointing. A large number corroded with spread of their irritating corrosion products into the tissues, necessitating their removal. Their presence also makes post space preparation difficult. Titanium points were introduced to overcome the problem of corrosion of silver points; however, they still do not fill canals three-dimensionally. Silver points, because of silver's high atomic number, are highly radiopaque; in contrast, titanium points, because of titanium's lower atomic number, are less radiopaque than silver points and the radiopacity is similar to that of gutta-percha. Radiopacity is dependent on the cube of atomic number.

Acrylic points have also been manufactured but there is an absence of information about their composition or clinical use. They have similar radiopacity to gutta-percha as a result of incorporation of heavy metal salts. As with metal points, they are too stiff and hard to be condensed into the shape of a root canal to allow for the addition of necessary accessory (gutta-percha) points.

Root canal sealers (4.10.2)

Many studies have shown that root canals are better sealed when a sealer is used in conjunction with gutta-percha points or in heated gutta-percha

techniques. Ideally, the sealer should be biocompatible, antiseptic, non-soluble, adhesive, slow setting, radiopaque, dimensionally stable, removable if required and able to achieve a good seal.

A whole range of materials from cements to resins has been recommended as sealers. None is ideal, but those based on zinc oxide–eugenol have been in use the longest. With many zinc oxide–eugenol sealers, the eugenol is usually mixed with a powder containing approximately 40% zinc oxide, 30% radiopaque filler and 30% resin binder. Grossman's sealer is widely used: it contains barium and bismuth salts for radiopacity, and natural resin as a binder.

A few root canal sealers contain several per cent of paraformaldehyde, which is a very controversial additive. The purpose of adding formaldehyde was to kill bacteria and fix remaining pulp tissue. These formaldehyde sealers have been widely used in general practice with relatively few reported clinical problems; however, in those cases where the material has been extruded through the apical foramen, or a lateral canal, into the periradicular tissues, particularly the inferior dental canal, the problems have been severe, such as sequestrum formation and permanent anaesthesia of the tissues supplied by the mental nerve. Because such extrusions cannot be predicted, it is safest to avoid potentially dangerous materials, particularly as their use is no longer recommended or indicated because of improved techniques of canal cleaning and shaping.

Sealers based on calcium hydroxide have been developed in recent years, primarily on the grounds that they could promote tissue repair at the apex. This may be possible, but in many root canals the foramen is probably obliterated by dentine chips, therefore negating the benefit of the sealer. These sealers are less antibacterial than zinc oxide–eugenol sealers so they may be less effective sealers in infected canals that have not been completely disinfected.

Medicaments

Between appointments, antibacterial medicaments may be placed in the pulp space of infected teeth to eliminate residual infection. In recent years far less emphasis has been placed on medication than formerly, and greater attention has been devoted to thorough cleaning with hypochlorite irrigants and correct canal shaping. Formerly, potent medicaments such as camphorated mono-chlor-phenol (effectively a 35% solution) were placed on cotton wool in the pulp space. Their use has declined because of their potential toxicity and the short duration of their effectiveness. Much weaker aqueous solutions have also been used as an alternative, but are not now widely employed.

Antibiotic mixtures have also been used as medicaments but their use is now very limited. Their aim was to kill a broad spectrum of bacteria, and they frequently contained antibiotics which were not used systemically to avoid the risk of sensitizing the patient. Medicaments based on antibiotic–steroid combinations have also been recommended by some authorities; the presence of steroid is intended to reduce inflammation and hence pain. These medicaments have not demonstrated greater effectiveness over traditional antiseptics, and there is some concern over the use of topical steroid (see Chapter 2).

The only medicament which is still regarded as acceptable is calcium hydroxide. It may be used as a pure powder but is frequently supplemented with up to 20% barium sulphate to increase radiopacity. The powder is normally mixed with sterile water or saline to create a stiff paste, which is condensed into the root canal with pluggers. Alternatively a commercial paste of calcium hydroxide may be used, and this is introduced into the root canal by a syringe. Studies have shown that calcium hydroxide effectively sterilizes root canals following correct cleaning and shaping.

Temporary sealing of the access cavity

When root canal treatment is spread over two or more visits, it is necessary to seal the access cavity between appointments. The purpose is to prevent oral bacteria recontaminating the root canal system. The most effective temporary seal is a reinforced zinc oxide–eugenol cement (2.1.4), which possesses adequate strength to avoid being bitten out and also prevents the passage of bacteria between it and the canal wall because of eugenol release. Cements, such as zinc phosphate or glass-ionomer, as the sole material for temporary sealing are unsuitable because they are not antibacterial. A thick layer of cement (4 mm) is less likely to be disturbed than a thinner layer. Where a large part of the tooth is missing, the temporary restoration may require the support of a stainless steel or copper band to stop it being dislodged.

If the tooth is carious or has deficient restorations, it is essential that the carious dentine is removed and the deficient restorations are replaced with permanent or temporary ones prior to root canal treatment. This is to prevent salivary contamination of the root canal during treatment or between appointments, and to prevent irrigants escaping into the mouth.

Restoration of a tooth prior to root canal treatment is only required if the tooth cannot be isolated effectively by rubber dam, since the access cavity to the pulp will destroy a large part of the restoration, and retention for the final restoration may well be gained from the pulp space.

Retrograde filling materials

In surgical endodontics, where apicectomy or perforation repair is undertaken, there is usually a large entry into the root canal system. The ideal treatment is to fill the entire root canal system but that is often not possible because of the presence of a post in the root canal and hence the reason for surgery. The solution therefore is to clean and fill the canal system as well as possible. Leaving an infected dead space in the canal system should be avoided wherever possible and so preparation of the root end should include cleaning and shaping of the residual canal as well as making a cavity to place a restorative material. The material should seal the tooth, be biocompatible, non-corrodible, non-soluble, radiopaque, antibacterial and easy to use.

Amalgam (3.1) has been widely used as a retrograde root filling material because of its ease of use, radiopacity, non-solubility and perceived sealing ability. However, clinical studies have shown only a 70% success rate of apicectomies with amalgam retrograde root fillings. A major reason for the low success rate is the failure of amalgam to provide a seal, since it is non-adhesive and when mechanically mixed contracts on setting; further, its corrosion products do not block the interface between amalgam and dentine. In some instances corrosion of the amalgam has resulted in the migration of metallic salts into the tissues and staining of the mucous membrane.

Glass-ionomer cements (3.4.2, 3.4.3) have been investigated because of their potential adhesion. However, one study (Pitt Ford and Roberts, 1990) has shown that they fail to provide an effective seal when the root canal is infected. There is concern about the use of such cements in a site that is difficult to keep dry, and most versions of the cement are not radiopaque.

Zinc oxide–eugenol cements (2.1) have been used as retrograde root fillings, but they have often been dismissed on account of their perceived solubility. A recent clinical study from the USA (Dorn and Gartner, 1990) has shown a very high success rate with a fortified version of the cement, and other histological evidence has shown good biocompatibility, and a lack of dissolution of the cement.

Composite resin (3.2) retained on the apicected root end by a dentine bonding agent (4.4.2) has also been the subject of extensive investigation in Denmark. In experienced hands the results have been very good but the success may be lower in general practice because the technique fails if there is moisture contamination when the material is being placed.

Gutta-percha (4.7.2) has also been used as a retrograde root filling material. Where access permits the root end may be prepared with files, before gutta-percha points with a sealer are condensed using an appropriate spreader; alternatively, heated gutta-percha with a sealer may be inserted.

Further reading

General

Grossman, L.I., Oliet, S. and Del Rio, C.E. (1988) *Endodontic Practice*, 11th edn. Lea & Febiger, Philadelphia, pp. 242–270.

Harty, F.J. (1990) *Endodontics in Clinical Practice*. 3rd edn. Wright, London, pp. 77–127

Pitt Ford, T.R. (1991) Endodontic materials and techniques. *Current Opinion in Dentistry*, **1**, 729–733

Root canal preparation

Ahmad, M., Pitt Ford, T.R. and Crum, L.A. (1987) Ultrasonic debridement of root canals; an insight into the mechanisms involved. *Journal of Endodontics*, **13**, 93–101

ElDeeb, M.E. and Boraas, J.C. (1985) The effect of different files on the preparation shape of severely curved canals. *International Endodontic Journal*, **18**, 1–7

Moorer, W.R. and Wesselink, P.R. (1982) Factors promoting the tissue dissolving capability of sodium hypochlorite. *International Endodontic Journal*, **15**, 187–196

Sjögren, U., Figdor, D., Spångberg, L. and Sundqvist, G. (1991) The antimicrobial effect of calcium hydroxide as a short-term intracanal dressing. *International Endodontic Journal*, **24**, 119–125

Walmsley, A.D. (1987) Ultrasound and root canal treatment: the need for scientific evaluation. *International Endodontic Journal*, **20**, 105–111

Walmsley, A.D., Lumley, P.J. and Laird, W.R. (1989) The oscillatory pattern of sonically powered endodontic files. *International Endodontic Journal*, **22**, 125–132

Root canal filling materials

Beatty, R.G., Vertucci, F.J. and Hojjatie, B. (1988) Thermomechanical compaction of gutta-percha: effect of speed and duration. *International Endodontic Journal*, **21**, 367–375

Friedman, C.M., Sandvik, J.L., Heuer, M.A. and Rapp, G.W. (1975) Composition and mechanical properties of gutta-percha endodontic points. *Journal of Dental Research*, **54**, 921–925

Kersten, H.W., Fransman, R. and Thoden van Velzen, S.K. (1986) Thermomechanical compaction of gutta-percha. I. A comparison of several compaction procedures. *International Endodontic Journal*, **19**, 125–133

Retrograde root fillings

Dorn, S.O. and Gartner, A.H. (1990) Retrograde filling materials: a retrospective success–failure study of amalgam, EBA, and IRM. *Journal of Endodontics*, **16**, 391–393

Gutmann, J.L. and Harrison, J.W. (1991) *Surgical Endodontics*. Blackwell Scientific Publications, Boston, pp. 230–264

Pitt Ford, T.R. and Roberts, G.J. (1990) Tissue response to glass ionomer retrograde root fillings. *International Endodontic Journal*, **23**, 233–238

Reit, C. and Hirsch, J. (1986) Surgical endodontic retreatment. *International Endodontic Journal*, **19**, 107–112

Rud, J., Munksgaard, E.C., Andreasen, J.O. and Rud, V. (1991) Retrograde root filling with composite and a dentin-bonding agent. 2. *Endodontics and Dental Traumatology*, **7**, 126–131

Chapter 5
Indirect restorations

Introduction

Indirect restorations are those made outside the mouth and so they normally require two appointments with a laboratory stage between. The extra time and the laboratory fee are the main reasons for the high cost of indirect restorations, rather than the cost of the materials.

Tooth preparation

In addition to the instruments described in Chapter 3 for cavity preparation, there are a number of special burs which are used for inlay, crown and bridge preparations. These fall into two groups:

1. Extra long, thin burs used for preparing the axial walls of teeth which are to be crowned.
2. Burs with specific shapes to produce tapered preparations or to produce particular crown margin configurations.

Extra long burs (1.6)

Particularly when approximal surfaces are being prepared it is an advantage to have a bur which will reach the whole length of the tooth from the occlusal surface to the preparation margin and also protrude from the handpiece sufficiently so that the head of the handpiece does not obscure vision. The bur should be thin enough to enable reduction of the approximal surface without removing too much

tooth tissue and without damaging the adjacent tooth. It should also produce the required shape and angle of margin or finish. With these very long burs, which are usually friction-fit and are used in the airotor, it is important that the handpiece runs very true. Any eccentricity in the rotation of the bur will be magnified at its tip (Fig. 5.1). Assuming that the handpiece is in good condition, there is a critical ratio between length and diameter which should not be exceeded. If a bur is too thin relative to its length it will 'whip', and although it may be thin at its tip it will cut a wide band of tooth tissue due to the eccentric movement. Moreover, the tooth preparation will be uncontrolled, there is an increased risk of damage to the adjacent teeth and also a risk of the bur bending or breaking and causing damage to the oral soft tissues.

This ratio of length to diameter varies with the material from which the bur is made and with its taper. As an example, a diamond-coated steel bur of $5°$ taper and a point diameter of 0.1 mm should not exceed 10–12 mm in length. Extra-long tungsten carbide burs are more likely to break than bend and so their diameter is greater than diamond burs of the same taper and length.

Diamond particles are graded according to the mesh size through which they will pass, and the burs are described as extra coarse, coarse, medium, fine and super-fine.

Special shapes of bur

Most friction-grip burs are produced with tapers of between $0°$ (parallel-sided) and $10°$ convergence.

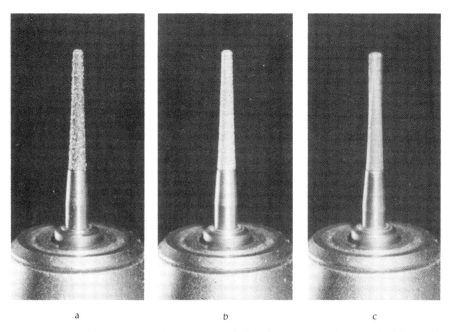

a   b   c

Figure 5.1 A long diamond bur: (a) static; (b) rotating; (c) slightly bent rotating, showing the 'whip' at the tip

Provided a tapered bur is used with a constant axial relationship to the tooth, it will produce a preparation with the same taper. However, it is impossible for the human hand to produce this degree of precision and the irregular shape of a natural tooth does not help. The average taper of a crown preparation is therefore usually at least double that of the taper of the bur.

Similarly, margin angles are subject to a number of influences as well as the bur's shape. These include the physical properties of dental enamel and the contour of the tooth surface at the point where the margin is being prepared. Figure 5.2 shows shaped bur tips and the margins they produce.

Impressions for indirect restorations (5.2)

The requirements of a satisfactory impression material for constructing indirect restorations are that at the following three stages it should fulfil these conditions.

Stage 1: Mixing and insertion

- It should be easy to proportion and mix.
- It should be biocompatible (non-toxic or non-irritant to patient, dentist, assistant and technician).
- It should flow readily around the tissues when inserted in the mouth but not when the impression tray is inverted.
- It should stop flowing when pressure is removed.
- It should have a long working time.

Stage 2: Setting and removal from the mouth

- It should have a short, snap set.
- It should have a low setting shrinkage.
- It should have a low thermal shrinkage.
- It should be flexible enough to be easily withdrawn without putting undue stress on mobile teeth.
- It should be completely elastic in its recovery after deformation.
- It should resist tearing (have a high tear resistance).

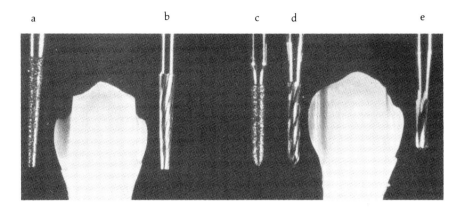

Figure 5.2 Natural teeth partly prepared with the burs shown. (a) Long tapered diamond; (b) multibladed tungsten carbide finishing bur; (c) parallel-sided diamond bur with pointed tip to produce a chamfer finishing line, together with (d) the matching tungsten carbide finishing bur; (e) parallel-sided tungsten carbide bur with round tip which also produces a chamfer finishing line.

Stage 3: Storage and die production

- It should be dimensionally stable, neither losing nor gaining volatile constituents on storage.
- It should be stiff enough to resist distortion when filled with die material.
- It should be chemically compatible with all die materials.
- It should not be affected by disinfection procedures

They should also be inexpensive.

Needless to say, no current material meets all these requirements; however, the materials available with properties approaching these requirements fall into two groups: the rubber-like elastomers (5.2.4–5.2.7) and the hydrocolloids (5.2.1–5.2.3).

With this choice, and the choice of materials within these groups, the clinician must decide which properties are desirable for a given case. It is wise to be familiar with and stock a range of two or three different materials so that the most suitable one can be chosen for a given set of circumstances. It is not, however, necessary to have the full range available.

Rubber-like elastomers

Cross-infection control procedures for rubber-like impression materials

Immediately after removal from the mouth the impression should be thoroughly washed in running water and dried. No blood or saliva should be visible. If cotton wool rolls become incorporated in the impression they should be cut out of it with scissors (rather than pulled out, which can separate the impression material from the tray). The impression should then be rewashed.

Several different regimes have been recommended for disinfecting rubber-like impressions. Some of the more intensive methods cause damage to the surface of some types of impression material, producing dies with less sharp detail. A regime which is effective and which can be used with all the materials (with a slight reservation about polyether) is to immerse the impression in a 2% solution of glutaraldehyde for 1 hour. It is then removed, washed again, dried and packed for the laboratory.

Alternatively, in centres where large numbers of impressions are processed, automatic equipment is available (Fig. 5.3).

Dispensing systems for rubber-like impression materials

The putty materials are supplied in two pots. Scoops are taken from each and mixed by hand. There is a reaction between some materials and the plasticizers of rubber gloves and so, to be safe, rubber gloves should be removed and hands washed before dispensing and mixing putty impression materials.

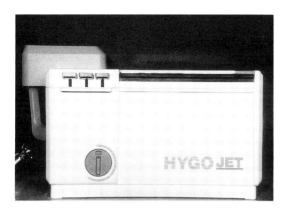

Figure 5.3 An impression disinfection unit. The impressions are marked, sprayed inside the sealed unit and can also be air-dried. With the appropriate disinfection agent the organisms which are most relevant to cross-infection control are killed within 10 minutes.

Traditionally other viscosities of materials have been supplied in two tubes which are dispensed and mixed on a pad. However, gun mixing systems have now become more popular and several viscosities of material are now available. Although this method of dispensing may be more expensive than tub and tube methods, many clinicians feel that the advantages are worth the additional cost.

The advantages include quick, reliable and bubble-free mixing. The ability to load an impression syringe directly from the gun or to inject directly into the mouth from the gun also increases speed. The waste of material is reduced, as is the time taken to clear up after taking an impression. Figure 5.4 shows a typical gun system and Figure 5.5 gives an idea of the cost comparison of the various dispensing systems.

Addition-curing silicones (5.2.5)

These are the most recent additions to the range of elastomeric materials. Most of the manufacturers produce them in a range of several viscosities and the materials dispensed from tubes may be intermixed so that it is possible to produce a very full range of viscosities. They are very accurate and can be stored for long periods without changing dimensions. In particular they remain dimensionally

stable for sufficient time to send them through the post. In fact, their great stability means that dies poured for up to a least a week after they have been removed from the mouth can be used. It is always necessary to employ die relief varnish, or a similar technique, so that the casting will both readily fit the preparation and allow enough room to accommodate a layer of luting cement.

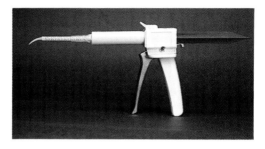

Figure 5.4 The increasingly popular automix system for addition-cured silicone impression materials and other materials. The cartridge contains the two materials to be mixed in separate barrels and the disposable automix nozzle is attached to the end of the cartridge. This photograph also shows a curved extension nozzle which can be used to inject impression material directly in the mouth, thereby avoiding the additional stage of inserting the impression material into an impression syringe.

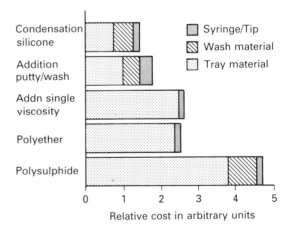

Figure 5.5 Comparative cost of full arch impressions in a stock tray. The cost of tray material can be significantly reduced by using a custom-made (special) tray. However, the laboratory charge for the custom tray is several times the cost of the material saved, even allowing for the cost of the stock tray. It may, however, be worth the extra cost to produce a better impression.

One property which some operators find difficult to come to terms with is the high surface tension. This results in difficulty in getting the materials to wet the surface of the preparation. It is also sometimes difficult to get the material to flow into a gingival crevice without vigorous and perhaps damaging gingival retraction procedures. Some materials are less hydrophobic than others, but none is truly hydrophilic.

Whilst any combination of viscosities may be used to suit the operator's preference, for example putty and wash, heavy and light or just regular on its own, a single-stage technique is essential when using two different viscosity materials (Fig. 5.6). The putty and the wash, for example, must both be fluid at the same time. The putty is just employed to force the wash into those areas where its hydrophobic nature would hinder its access.

These materials can be used with a rigid stock tray but the more fluid materials give more reliable results when rigid special trays are used. Closely adapted special trays should *not* be used with the stiffer materials because of the difficulty of removing the impression from soft tissue undercuts and tearing on removal from undercuts between and around teeth.

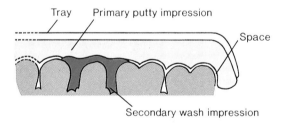

Figure 5.6 A two-stage putty and wash impression which is prone to producing a stepped impression. The putty impression is taken before the tooth is prepared and then relined with the secondary wash impression. Commonly this does not flow over all the unprepared surfaces, leaving a space. When the impression is cast, the teeth over which the secondary wash impression has not flowed will be recorded only by the putty impression, with the result that the die for the prepared tooth will be low in the occlusion. The clinical consequence will be a very high restoration.

After disinfection, impressions should be left for about 1 hour before the working model is cast to prevent the production of a porous surface from gas generated by the action of water in the die stone with unused catalyst.

No problems of biocompatability have been reported but the materials are expensive.

Polyether impression material (5.2.6)

Although available in light and heavy viscosity, the medium-viscosity material is usually used on its own. It has pseudoplastic properties and the same material used in the syringe and in a stock tray will produce very satisfactory results. It is therefore convenient and simple to use. A special tray is not required.

The disadvantages of the material when first presented were that it absorbed water so that it had to be dried as soon as it was removed from the mouth and stored dry, isolated from any alginate impressions or damp plaster casts. However, polyether in the 1990s is much less susceptible to water absorption, which facilitates disinfection, and dry storage is no longer essential for the normal transfer period from surgery to laboratory. It produces an allergic response in a significant number of people, commonly dental surgery assistants who become sensitized to the catalyst with regular use; it has relatively poor tear resistance and is a rather stiff material so that it is not suitable for use in a special tray or in some clinical conditions. For example, if it is used in patients who have mobile teeth, gingival recession and large embrasure spaces, removing the impression can be extremely difficult and might even extract the teeth. Impressions of postholes, gingival crevices and extreme undercuts can also be difficult.

The medium viscosity material is used by mixing one batch of material, loading part into a syringe and the rest into a stock tray. The tray is seated as soon as the material is syringed around the preparations. Two mixes should not be used as the purpose of the tray material is to press the syringe material around the preparations adapting it to them. If a separate mix is used for the syringe, and this mix is started before the tray mix, its set will have started by the time the tray is seated and this effect is lost. In some situations it is possible to take adequate impressions without the use of a syringe.

Polysulphide materials (5.2.4)

These were the first really accurate elastomeric materials to be introduced into general use in the early 1960s. They are available in three viscosities — light, regular and heavy — but the most commonly used technique for inlay, crown and bridgework makes use of light and heavy body material and a special tray. The two materials are mixed separately, either by two people starting the mixes simultaneously, or the light body material is mixed first followed by the heavy body material. The polysulphides have a long working and setting time, which is an advantage when impressions are being taken of multiple preparations but a disadvantage when only one or two teeth have been prepared.

Both an advantage and a disadvantage is the low surface tension of polysulphide. This means that it wets the tooth preparation well and clings to it so that the technique of blowing the impression material over the tooth surface to improve adaptation and to blow it into the gingival crevice are effective. However, should the material escape the environment for which it was intended, it also clings to patients' hair, beards and clothing and can leave permanent stains on some fabrics. Some patients dislike the smell and colour, which is brown (due to the lead peroxide catalyst) and there is some anxiety about the toxicity of lead, although there has been no reported evidence of any harmful effect.

These disadvantages are such that this material has now largely been superseded by other materials, particularly the addition-cured silicones and polyether.

Condensation-curing silicones (5.2.5)

These were the first type of viable silicones to be introduced and are still available in a range of viscosities. Whilst they are relatively inexpensive, the shelf-life of the catalyst which they employ is variable and when they set the cross-linking reaction produces volatile ethanol which causes the set impression to shrink. This shrinkage is related to the amount of silicone present and thus the heavily filled putty shrinks far less than the wash material. For indirect restorations they are frequently employed in a two-stage technique in which an impression is taken in the putty, either before or after the tooth is prepared. This is replaced in the mouth with a layer of correcting wash. A number of variables can affect the accuracy of the resulting restoration including:

1. distortion of the putty by the pressure involved in reseating it over a thin layer of correcting wash; and
2. shrinkage of the set impression, which is more marked with a thicker layer of wash material.

Whilst a certain amount of shrinkage may compensate for the distortion caused by reseating the impression, the results are unpredictable and the technique is not recommended. The only advantage of the condensation silicones is their relatively low cost compared to the other rubber-like elastomers.

Hydrocolloids

Reversible hydrocolloid (5.2.1)

Reversible hydrocolloid consists of an agar-agar gel with a filler to give it body and a degree of rigidity when in the gel state. It changes from a gel to a sol when heated in boiling water and is then stored at a temperature of approximately 60°C. It returns to a gel at a little above mouth temperature. The tray material is supplied in tubes (like toothpaste tubes) or in rods sealed in polythene. A lower-viscosity material is supplied either in glass cartridges which fit local anaesthetic syringes or in rods which fit special syringes. A blunt wide-bore needle is used to syringe this low viscosity material around the prepared teeth.

A heated water bath is necessary and this usually has three compartments. The first can be set to boil, which converts the gel to a sol and the material in its original container is then transferred to the second compartment which is maintained at 60°C as a storage bath. The material can be stored at this temperature for days or even weeks. When it is to be used, the tray material is transferred to a special water-cooled tray which is placed in the third compartment which is maintained at 50°C. This tempering allows the material to reach a tempera- ture which can be tolerated by the patient and also the material begins to thicken to a viscosity which will flow around the teeth but will not drip out of the tray. At the same time the syringe material is used straight from the 60°C bath. It cools sufficiently as it passes down the syringe nozzle not to cause damage to the pulps of the teeth.

Historically, reversible hydrocolloid was the first of the really accurate crown and bridge materials and preceded the rubber materials by many years. It still has a number of properties which are not found in the elastomeric materials. These advantageous properties are as follows:

1. It is hydrophilic and can therefore be used when it is not possible to control completely gingival bleeding or the flow of gingival exudate. In fact it is used with a wet technique, which involves spraying the teeth either with water or with a wetting agent to reduce surface tension immediately prior to inserting the impression.
2. The setting time of the impression in the mouth (when using the water-cooled trays) is rapid and because there is no mixing, once the dentist and surgery staff are familiar with the technique, the whole process of impression taking is speedy. Several impressions of the same prepared mouth are often taken at the same visit.
3. The material is relatively inexpensive.

To offset these advantages the material has a number of drawbacks:

1. If allowed to dry, the impression distorts considerably. Even when kept in a humidifier, impressions should be cast within an hour or so of being taken, preferably immediately.
2. It is not practical to disinfect reversible hydrocolloid impressions by the same techni- ques as rubber-like impressions. Therefore, preferably the impressions should be cast by the operator, or at least the technician should wear rubber gloves and use conventional cross-infection control techniques.
3. The surface of stone dies is affected by the material and so the impression has to be

soaked in potassium sulphate or alum solution to condition it before the cast is made.
4. Die materials other than artificial stone cannot be used.
5. Because the surface of the impression is translucent, it is more difficult to see the details of the preparation in the impression than with the opaque elastomeric materials (Fig. 5.7).
6. The initial capital cost of the conditioning bath and special trays is high. The process of using a water-cooled tray is cumbersome and it requires considerable practice to become efficient in its use.

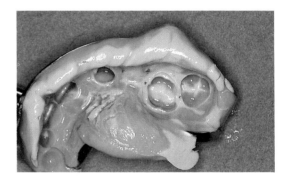

Figure 5.7 A reversible hydrocolloid impression.

Irreversible hydrocolloid (alginate) (5.2.2)

None of the present materials is sufficiently accurate or has an adequate surface texture for them to be used for inlays, crowns or bridges. This material is considered in more detail in Chapters 1 and 7.

Factors in choosing a crown and bridge impression material

Because all the materials listed above (except irreversible hydrocolloid) are capable of producing an acceptable clinical result, the factors which will influence an operator's choice are likely to be cost, convenience, experience, the laboratory's preference and the clinical circumstances. With a limited number of prepared teeth, all with supragingival margins, and with no gingival bleeding, the technique using a stock tray with fast-setting elastomeric material would be the quickest, most convenient and least expensive. However, when there are a large number of prepared teeth and there is a need for gingival retraction, then a slow-setting material will be preferred.

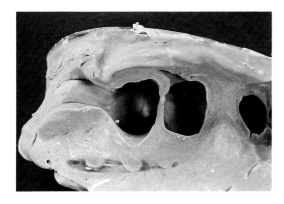

Figure 5.8 A poor, single-stage polyether impression in a strock tray. The distal part of the tray does not contain the impression material adequately, resulting in drags where the impression material flows out of the tray distally. There is a particularly bad drag on the distal surface of the last tooth and another on the buccal surface of the next tooth.

Laboratory-made rigid special trays add significantly to the cost of the impression, but are worthwhile when the distribution of missing teeth or the shape of the arch means that a stock tray is a poor fit. Special trays are particularly useful when the last tooth in the arch is to be prepared. When a stock tray is used in this situation the impression commonly fails by dragging around the distal side of the prepared tooth (Fig. 5.8).

The decision whether to use a stock or special tray will affect the choice of impression material. The materials which are more rigid when set, such as silicone putty and polyether materials, should not be used in a special tray, particularly if the teeth are mobile or have large, open embrasure spaces. In these cases, a relatively rigid set impression can result in a tooth being extracted when the impression is removed. Also the stiffer materials displace mobile teeth when the impression is being inserted and the teeth do not recover their normal

position before the impression sets. Some dentists who equip themselves to take reversible hydrocolloid impressions use the technique almost universally except when they wish to produce dies in materials other than stone (6.2–6.4), for example, with very long thin lower incisor preparations.

Special trays

The most widely used material for special trays is self-activated acrylic resin, but a very satisfactory alternative is a relatively new light-activated tray material. Trays produced in this material, which is a dimethacrylate resin (13.8.5), demonstrate excellent rigidity in thin section; good dimensional stability, even when immersed in water (or disinfectant solutions), and are easy and quick to produce. The tray blanks are, however, relatively expensive and a special light-curing unit is needed, but laboratory costs may be avoided (Fig. 5.9).

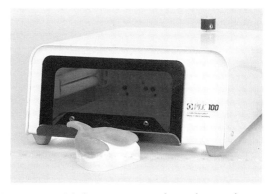

Figure 5.9 A light-curing unit used to make special trays and other restorations. The unit is switched on, showing the bright blue light.

Indirect impressions for post-retained crowns

There are two basic techniques for the posthole. Either the hole is cut to the shape of a preformed plastic or metal post which is then incorporated into the impression of the root face, or impression material is introduced into the posthole. The latter technique is used when the posthole has to be an irregular shape, either oval in cross-section or tapered along its length. Impression materials for postholes should:

- have a high resistance to tearing
- have a very efficient adhesive to attach them to a reinforcing wire (introduced to the posthole after the impression material is inserted to stiffen the impression of the posthole so that it does not distort when the cast is being poured)
- be easy to introduce into the posthole.

Reversible hydrocolloid does not comply with these requirements, particularly the absence of a satisfactory adhesive. Reversible hydrocolloid can therefore only be used when the root canal can be prepared for a preformed post.

Of the elastomeric materials, polysulphide materials come nearest to meeting these criteria but impressions of postholes are difficult with any material and the most important variable is the skill of the operator.

Direct impressions for post-retained crowns

Direct impressions may be made in fast-setting, self-curing acrylic which completely burns out, leaving no residue in the investment.

Alternatively, acrylic may be added to a cobalt–chromium–nickel wire (Wiptam, 11.3.3) and metal cast on to the wire, replacing the acrylic forming the core and any additions down the posthole to complete the shape. This technique was popular, but the different alloys (especially as at least one of them contains base metals) produce corrosion at the interface and this gives rise to discoloration and stresses within the root. In some cases root fractures have been attributed to the effects of this corrosion. It is also believed that the strength of the wrought metal post may be reduced by heating it to add the cast core. For these reasons the technique has largely been abandoned.

Inlay wax (7.1.2) may be used on a piece of wire, which is also used as the sprue. The wire is then withdrawn when the pattern is invested so that the entire post and core is of cast metal.

Preformed posts and cores (4.2)

A large variety of ready-made posts and cores is available. These are generally made of stainless steel or titanium and one has a soft brass head which is shaped to form the core once it is in the mouth.

The need for a metal core for anterior teeth is now questioned. The post and core is only as strong as its thinnest section, which is the post, not the core. If a strong, preformed, wrought base metal post is cemented and then a core added in composite in the mouth, this is quicker, cheaper and as effective as a metal core, provided that the post comes right through to the tip of the core (Fig. 5.10). This does not involve heating the post with the inherent danger of changing its properties in a detrimental way. The use of a composite core avoids the need for a laboratory stage or a temporary post crown.

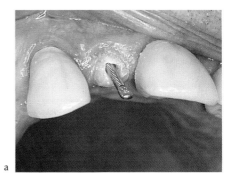

a

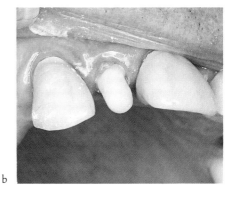

b

Figure 5.10 (a) A preformed stainless steel post being tried in. (b) The post has been cemented and light-cured composite built up to produce a core. This will now be prepared to shape.

Temporary and provisional restorations (4.6, 4.7)

Temporary inlays, crowns and bridges are either preformed (by the manufacturer or in the laboratory) or made at the chairside.

A useful distinction may be made between temporary and provisional crowns and bridges. A temporary restoration is only expected to last for a couple of weeks while the permanent restoration is being made in the laboratory. It protects the prepared tooth and maintains occlusal relationships and appearance.

A provisional restoration also serves these functions but is expected to last for longer – often periods of months and sometimes over a year. During this period extraction sockets can heal (if the provisional bridge is inserted as an immediate restoration), or other forms of treatment such as periodontal or endodontic treatment can be carried out. When the occlusion is being reorganized with large, multiunit restorations, provisional restorations are used to assess and modify the alterations to the occlusion and ensure that they are stable and comfortable before making the permanent restorations.

With modern materials the usual technique for temporary restorations is to make them at the chairside to avoid laboratory costs. It is sometimes possible to make long-term provisional restorations at the chairside, but there is the risk of them wearing or breaking, or of the colour changing unacceptably Provisional restorations are therefore more commonly made in the laboratory.

Preformed temporary crowns

Posterior temporary crowns are available in aluminium, stainless steel or polycarbonate. The aluminium temporary crowns are adjusted by trimming with scissors and stones, contouring with pliers and by the opposing teeth, and cementing with a temporary cement. At best they can only produce a mediocre marginal fit, contact with adjacent teeth and opposing teeth. They rely for their retention on a thick layer of cement and some patients complain of a metallic taste. They are, however, quick to adapt and apply. Stainless steel

temporary posterior crowns take much more time to adapt because they are harder, but they are more satisfactory than aluminium temporary crowns in that they resist corrosion more readily and hence do not create a metallic taste; they are also less likely to wear through. The polycarbonate temporary crowns are usually relined with a polymer material by means of a technique similar to that which will be described for anterior crowns.

None of these techniques is as satisfactory as custom-made temporary restorations. Temporary crowns should:

- Protect sensitive dentine.
- Allow good oral hygiene to preserve gingival health.
- Provide a stable occlusion so that axial movement of the prepared or opposing tooth does nor occur.
- Maintain contact points so that the prepared or adjacent teeth do not move.
- In some cases provide an acceptable appearance.

Metal temporary crowns serve only the first of these purposes reliably. Polycarbonate crowns serve the first and last, although with careful adjustment of the margins, occlusion and contact points, they can be made to serve all five functions. However, this adjustment often takes longer at the chairside than making the chairside temporary crowns, which will be described later.

Preformed anterior crowns are supplied in polycarbonate material and as cellulose acetate crown forms. The polycarbonate temporary crowns are tooth-coloured (one shade only) but come in a range of sizes to suit most clinical circumstances. They are relined using one of the higher acrylics in the mouth and then trimmed with stones to the occlusion and to produce a good marginal adaptation. Because they are a close fit and retentive, only a weak temporary cement is necessary.

Epimine resin of the type found in some temporary crown and bridge materials should not be used to reline polycarbonate crowns as it does not adhere to polycarbonate.

Cellulose acetate crown forms are trimmed with scissors, filled with one of the resin materials and applied to the prepared tooth. When the material has set, the temporary crown is removed, the crown form stripped off and the occlusion and margins adjusted. This technique is not as satisfactory as the polycarbonate crowns in that removing the celluloid crown form leaves the adjacent teeth out of contact. However, it is possible to make temporary crowns with a larger variety of shapes and shades with this technique.

Again, the time taken to reline and trim a preformed temporary crown is usually longer than that taken to make the complete temporary restoration at the chairside.

Laboratory-made prefabricated temporary bridges

Temporary bridges may be made in the laboratory before the abutment teeth are prepared using a prepared study cast. They may be made in self-activated or heat-activated acrylic and may include proprietary facings or denture teeth cut down to face the buccal surface. These temporary bridges are more durable and more reliable in appearance than temporary bridges made at the chairside but are time-consuming and expensive and have to be adjusted and relined at the chairside to fit the abutment teeth which are prepared after the shell of the temporary restoration is made.

Prefabricated temporary bridges of this type are usually less satisfactory than bridges made from an impression of the prepared teeth. Therefore, if laboratory costs are to be incurred in making a long-term provisional bridge, it is better to make a chairside temporary at the time the teeth are prepared, take an impression and then fit the provisional, laboratory-made bridge subsequently.

Temporary restorations made at the chairside (4.6)

Temporary restorations may be made at the chairside in one of the polymer materials either using a matrix (which is also formed at the chairside or in the laboratory), or without the use of a matrix. The polymers used for chairside temporary restorations are acrylic, higher acrylics or ethylene imine resin. Techniques for using these materials were briefly described in Chapter 2.

Matrix techniques for temporary restorations

Impressions

Impressions may be made of teeth before they are prepared, set on one side and then used as a matrix for temporary restorations. Alginate is the most commonly used material, but any of the elastomeric materials may also be used. Reversible hydrocolloid would not of course be suitable as the exothermic setting reaction of the self-polymerizing resin would soften the impression. For temporary bridges, when the patient already has a denture, the impression is taken with the denture in place and the excess crown and bridge material which flows into part of the area occupied by the denture is cut away once the temporary bridge has set (Fig. 5.11).

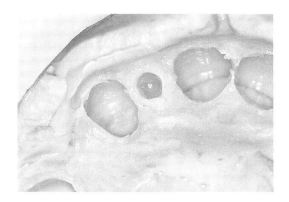

Figure 5.11 A temporary crown made in an alginate impression which was taken just before the tooth was prepared. After the tooth preparation the alginate impression has been filled with a temporary crown and bridge resin and reinserted in the mouth. This is the appearance immediately on withdrawal. The restoration will now be pulled out of the alginate impression, trimmed and cemented.

If the patient does not already have a denture it may sometimes be satisfactory to make individual temporary restorations for the prepared teeth rather than a temporary bridge. This is particularly so when the bridge is to be a fixed-movable bridge and the abutment teeth have not been prepared parallel to each other. Also with fixed-movable bridges, one preparation may be much less retentive than the other, for example, a full crown for the major retainer and an inlay for the minor retainer. In these cases arrangements should be made for the laboratory work to be completed quickly to reduce the risk of tooth movement before the permanent bridge is fitted. With posterior bridges, when there is no suitable denture, an alginate impression can be taken and the alginate cut away from the pontic area to produce a block of resin which can be trimmed to shape and adjusted to produce a stable occlusion.

Sometimes the impression is taken of a modified study cast (perhaps by the addition of a temporary pontic) prior to the clinical appointment. In this case one of the more stable elastomeric materials is preferred.

Laboratory-formed matrices

These can be made from thin poly(vinyl chloride) or polythene matrices adapted to modified study models by vacuum forming of these thermoplastic polymers. The study cast must be modified with plaster, cement or acrylic, as wax modifications would melt under the heat in the vacuum-forming machine. Alternatively, the model is modified with wax and duplicated, using an alginate impression, to produce a model on which the vacuum-moulded matrix can be made. When duplicating models with alginate in this way, the alginate should be mixed with a higher proportion of water than usual and the model soaked in water beforehand.

These matrices may be reused a number of times if necessary.

An alternative matrix material which does not require a vacuum-forming machine is polypropylene. This is simply heated in a flame and then adapted to the study cast by pressure from a mouldable pad of non-setting silicone putty.

These laboratory-made matrices may be used with any of the temporary crown and bridge resins.

Intraoral moulding

Higher acrylic resins in their moulding stage may be adapted to posterior crown or inlay preparations simply by moulding with the fingers and by the patient occluding into the material. Gross excesses will be produced, but these can be roughly trimmed with a carving instrument in the mouth and then finally trimmed with burs and stones outside the mouth once the material has set. Sometimes it is necessary to reline the first attempt at a hand-made crown, or to add to its contact points or occlusal surface. However, the technique is quick and easy and does not require any initial work before the tooth is prepared. It is suitable for teeth with amalgam or composite cores which were not carved to a realistic tooth shape and so cannot be used for the impression matrix technique. The technique is particularly suitable for inlays, and the temporary methacrylate inlay maintains the occlusion and contact better than any cement material. It is also easier to remove and if necessary replace at a subsequent visit.

Temporary crown and bridge cements (4.8)

The choice of temporary crown and bridge cement will depend upon the fit and retentiveness of the temporary restoration, the number of temporary restorations splinted together (it is common practice to join several adjacent temporary crowns together for added retention, even when the permanent crowns will be separate), and the length of time which the temporary restoration has to last.

The temporary luting cements produced specifically for the purpose consist of a fast-setting paste mixed from two tubes, which sets to a brittle consistency with a relatively low compressive strength. The cement may be further weakened by the addition of a structural modifier. Some of these materials contain eugenol and some do not. They are convenient and quick to use and are easy to clean from the tooth and temporary restoration when it is removed. The addition of varying amounts of modifier provide a range of strengths which adds to the versatility of the material. If the cement is used with the temporary restoration dry but the tooth wet, removal of the restoration later will be easier and, because the cement will adhere more to the restoration, less time will be needed to clean the prepared tooth.

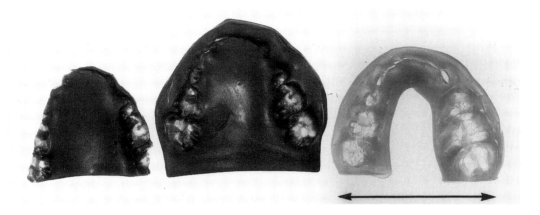

Figure 5.12. The horseshoe-shaped piece of modelling wax (right) may easily distort across the ends, as shown by the arrows. The D-shaped piece of Alminax (centre) is more stable and the trimmed record (left) may be visually checked between the teeth in the mouth or on the model.

Conventional zinc oxide–eugenol mixtures are now seldom used for well-fitting restorations because they have the disadvantages of reacting with acrylic and of not setting to a brittle consistency, which makes the removal of excess material at the temporary crown margin difficult.

When the restoration is a poor fit, for example an unlined aluminium or stainless steel temporary crown, zinc oxide, polycarboxylate or zinc phosphate may be used. They should only be used in thick layers with temporary crowns which have not been adapted to produce an accurate fit.

Occlusal registration materials (4.5)

Articulating working casts for inlays, crowns or bridges requires great precision. Many of the stages in the procedure give rise to inaccuracies which are often blamed unfairly on the occlusal registration material. The casts themselves must be accurate (in particular the opposing cast, which is often made from an alginate impression) and the occlusal surfaces of both casts must be entirely free of air bubbles. It is common for small air bubbles to be trapped in the occlusal fissures and these can prop the casts apart. This may not be apparent until the finished restoration is tried in the mouth, when it will be 'high'. This problem is common and is often

wrongly blamed on overeruption of the prepared or opposing tooth.

Sometimes simple hand-held articulation of the working and opposing models is adequate, particularly when only one anterior crown is being made; however, in the following circumstances accurate intraocclusal records will be necessary in order to articulate the models and produce the required occlusal relationships in the restorations:

1. When there are missing teeth and/or the teeth being prepared result in a lack of stability of the working casts in intercuspal position.
2. When the occlusal relationships have been altered, or will be altered, for example, when a previous, unsatisfactory intercuspal position has been adjusted by grinding the natural teeth and the new restorations are to be made in a new intercuspal relationship or in the retruded contact position.
3. When it is decided that it is necessary to simulate functional movements of the mandible using semiadjustable or fully adjustable articulators, and to construct restorations so that they are compatible with these movements.

In these cases occlusal records of wax, zinc oxide–eugenol pastes, elastomeric materials or acrylic may be used either alone or in combination.

Wax (7.1)

Pink modelling wax is cheap and convenient to use but it is difficult to soften evenly, it distorts on cooling and is not dimensionally stable. A horse-shoe-shaped piece of wax is particularly poor in this respect as distortion between the ends of the horseshoe can easily occur (Fig. 5.12). A D-shaped piece of wax is more successful and this may be reinforced either by the manufacturer by the incorporation of metal powder such as aluminium (Aluminax) or clinically by the use of a layer of gauze between two layers of wax. The cooled record should be trimmed to remove the buccal excess so that the tooth relationship may be visually checked and then reinserted into the mouth to refine the accuracy of the record.

Waxes which are relatively soft at room temperature are less satisfactory as the record will distort when the working casts are seated firmly into them. Alternatively, knowing that this is likely, the technician will not apply sufficient force and the casts will be slightly separated in the articulator, resulting in a high restoration.

Wax distorts on storage so records should be disinfected, stored in a cool environment, carefully packaged for transport to the laboratory and used with minimum delay.

Elastomeric materials (13.7)

Any of the elastomeric materials may be used to record occlusions. However, some of the materials, notably a silicone material and a polyether, have been specifically designed for this purpose and are supplied in a gun system or with a wide-nozzle, plastic, reusable syringe respectively. The material is loaded and syringed around the lower arch on to the occlusal surface of the teeth and the patient closes into whichever position is to be recorded. The materials have sufficient body not to flow off the occlusal surfaces and they set rapidly. They are most useful for patients with sufficient teeth not to need the use of occlusal rims (see Chapter 7). They are soft when the record is taken, and chemically set to a dimensionally-stable record, but when set they have a smooth surface that easily slips against a smooth wax rim. They are expensive and the need to wait for a chemical set extends the clinical procedure. Their most significant disadvantage,

however, is their lack of rigidity when set. Although heavily filled to improve rigidity, if there is more than a millimetre thickness of rubber, the relationship of the casts may be altered by manual pressure, causing displacement of the rubber material. They are thus successful where contact relationships between teeth are required but less so if precontact records are to be used.

Zinc oxide–eugenol pastes and similar materials not containing eugenol (4.5.1.1)

Conversely, the occlusal registration materials that are rigid when set need some separation between the teeth to allow sufficient bulk of material for the record to be strong enough for transfer from the mouth to the cast. For precontact records, therefore, zinc oxide–eugenol paste, self-activated acrylic resin and plaster may all be used. An exception to this rule may be allowed for the zinc oxide–eugenol pastes which can be supported on gauze on a wire or plastic framework or on an occlusal rim and used for contact relationships. These materials set to a hard brittle consistency which allow firm seating of the casts. Although the gauze framework is difficult to use, very accurate contact occlusal records may be produced in this way but they are still fragile and require careful handling in the laboratory. Where occlusal rims are to be used, zinc oxide–eugenol pastes are probably the ideal material for the production of both contact and precontact occlusal records. However, they are messy and only one record at a time may be taken in this way as paste remains fixed to the rim until the casts are articulated.

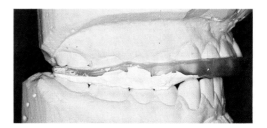

Figure 5.13 A wax occlusal record relined on both surfaces with temporary crown and bridge cement. Fast-setting zinc oxide–eugenol occlusal registration paste may also be used.

These materials may also be used to reline the surface of a wax record. The zinc oxide–eugenol materials specially designed for the purpose are ideal but the temporary crown and bridge cements are also very satisfactory (Fig. 5.13).

Impression plaster or acrylic resin registration materials

Impression plaster (5.1.3) produces accurate pre-contact records but is fragile and easily damaged during the clinical or laboratory procedures. Self-activated acrylic resin is very robust when cured. The polymerization shrinkage that occurs on hardening may be significant in thick sections; therefore records may have to be taken in two stages, the main bulk of the record being cured first and this record then being refined with a thin layer of acrylic resin or zinc oxide–eugenol paste.

Fast setting, self-activated acrylic is particularly useful to produce centric stops or incisal guidance planes when multiple tooth preparations are being carried out. For example, if all the teeth in one arch are to be prepared the occlusal vertical dimension will be lost. This problem can be overcome in a number of ways but one way is to prepare three or four selected teeth and then make small intraocclusal records in self-curing acrylic between the prepared teeth and the opposing teeth. The remainder of the teeth can then be prepared, and by reinserting these acrylic records the same vertical (and horizontal) relationship can be maintained.

Dental casting alloys (9.1–9.3)

In recent years with the increase in the price of gold and other precious metals, there has been intense activity internationally to produce acceptable alternatives to high and medium precious metal alloys for dental use. For some applications this has produced acceptable alternatives or very nearly so. In others there is still some way to go.

Gold dental casting alloys (9.1)

The traditional dental casting golds are of two types – those used alone for inlays and crowns, and those used with bonded porcelain for metal–ceramic restorations.

The ISO standard for dental casting alloys is ISO 1562 and for alloys which contain 25–75% noble metal content, ISO 8891. The ISO standard for dental ceramic-fused-to-metal restorative materials is ISO 9693. The British Standard for dental casting alloys, BS 4425, refers to types I–IV (10.1.1). Type I is a soft alloy used for Class 1 and other small restorations, where strength is less important than burnishability. Types II and III gold alloys are used for inlays and crowns. Type II is more burnishable but less hard than type III. Type IV gold may be used for partial dentures.

Alloys containing high (9.1.1), and medium (9.1.2) proportions of gold are available. Some patients still seem to derive pleasure from the idea of having precious metal alloy restorations, and few of the alternative alloys are as convenient to adjust and polish at the chairside as the gold alloys. However, the use of high-gold alloys has decreased significantly as the alternatives improve and become more acceptable.

The precious metal alloys used for metal–ceramic restorations have a high platinum as well as a high gold content (9.1.1.5). They vary in colour from yellow to silver. Their advantages are that they are relatively easy to cast and work. Although they cast at a high temperature (1200–1250°C), it is possible to control the expansion of the investments with which they are used to compensate for the contraction of the hot metal very accurately. This type of alloy casts to a fine margin, with a low incidence of miscasts. They are dense alloys, but once cemented in the mouth, the weight of the restoration is of no clinical significance.

The main disadvantage of the gold alloys is their cost and incidentally, associated with this, the need for increasingly complex and costly security arrangements in dental laboratories and organizations using gold.

Alternatives to gold alloys

In the search for less expensive cast restorations many alternative alloys have been produced. It is convenient to group these under two headings:

1. Silver–palladium and silver-free (white gold) alloys (9.1.3; 9.3.2)
2. Nickel–chromium (base metal) alloys (9.2.2)

Silver–palladium and silver-free alloys (9.1.3; 9.3.2)

These may be cast using conventional investments and casting techniques at convenient temperatures. They are less dense than the precious metal alloys and so when cast by the centrifugal process a larger bulk of alloy is required. The material degrades with repeated melting and so, as with many of these materials, 50% new alloy should be included with each casting, and this together with the large bulk of alloy needed means that if the manufacturer's recommended techniques are followed, a considerable wastage occurs which should be returned to scrap. This factor increases the overall cost of the material which, although lower than high-gold-containing alloys, is not negligible. The material is sluggish to cast and until technicians become familiar with it, miscasts are common.

Silver–palladium and silver-free alloys can be used either alone or in the metal–ceramic process.

Nickel–chromium alloys (9.2.2)

Nickel–chromium alloys cast at 1150–1250°C and so require oxy-gas, induction or electrical resistance melting of the alloy. The investments used are usually phosphate-bonded. The thermal compensation with these alloys is not so precise as with the gold alloys and this means that when measured in the laboratory, castings in nickel–chromium are slightly less precise than those in gold alloys. However, many clinicians regard the difference as insignificant, and this difference is getting less with improvements in the base metal alloys and their casting investment.

Also improving are the other properties of the base metal alloys. They can now be cast to fine margins and in thin sections, and they are becoming easier to finish. It seems likely that, although not yet fully developed, these materials will replace precious metal alloys in inlay, crown and bridge work within the foreseeable future to the same extent that cobalt–chromium has replaced gold in partial denture construction.

There are two hazards with nickel–chromium alloys which need to be considered. Firstly, the earlier alloys which contained beryllium produced a toxic dust when polished and these materials are banned in some countries even when efficient dust extraction is used. Secondly, there has been anxiety about a possible allergic response to nickel, and nickel-containing alloys have also been banned in some countries. However, this latter anxiety should not be overstressed as only a few cases of allergy have been reported, despite the millions of nickel–chromium alloy restorations which have now been made.

Nickel–chromium alloys are stronger in thin sections than the gold or white gold alloys and can therefore be used for long-span bridges or in other situations where strength is important, particularly in the production of minimum preparation (resin-bonded/ Maryland) bridges and splints. The higher strength in thin sections is ideal for the retention wings and, if the bridge is to be bonded with a conventional bonding resin, nickel–chromium alloy can be etched in an electrolytic bath containing nitric and sulphuric acid or at the chairside with hydrofluoric acid gel to produce a micromechanically retentive surface for resin-based cements.

If the bridge is to be bonded with one of the chemically adhesive resin cements (for example, Panavia Ex (2.1.13.1)), the surface is sand-blasted for as short a time as possible before the bridge is fitted. Sand-blasting cleans the surface and produces an irregular but not undercut surface. It also appears to increase the surface activity and therefore the adhesion of the cement.

One disadvantage of nickel–chromium alloys in minimum-preparation bridges is that their colour can produce a grey discoloration of the abutment teeth if the teeth are thin.

Factors in selecting a dental casting alloy

Cost

The cost of precious metals as a proportion of the total cost of the restoration is not insignificant and direct and third-party payment schemes for dentists often take account of the cost of precious metals in the fee structure.

Appearance

Most patients who are concerned with the appearance of their teeth do not like the appearance of any metal. At one time the display of a certain amount of gold was fashionable and perhaps represented a certain status in society. However, this is now much less true and so the difference in appearance of the various alloys is of little relevance.

Laboratory handling characteristics

Laboratories require special casting and finishing equipment in order to produce base metal and white gold bonding alloy castings, in particular efficient dust extraction because of the risk to health of the dust from grinding alloys containing nickel and other base metals. Once they have acquired this equipment and have become experienced in its use, laboratories with a high turnover of crown and bridge work can produce a consistently high standard of base metal and white gold castings. However, the small laboratory will usually find gold alloys easier and safer to work with.

Clinical handling characteristics

Base metal and white gold alloys are more difficult to adjust and polish at the chairside than gold alloys. However, the differences are reducing and these problems can be surmounted provided the dentist is equipped with suitable finishing instruments (see later).

Preparation design for cast restorations

Traditionally the margins of preparations for cast restorations have been prepared with bevelled cavosurface line angles. This was partly to allow for burnishing of the metal margin and to reduce the likelihood of acute or right-angle enamel margins chipping. Although the latter reason still exists, the newer, harder alloys cannot be burnished in the mouth, and in any case burnishing margins is no longer recommended as it damages the integrity of the cement at the margins. The recommended cavosurface angle for cast restorations is now about 135°C.

On the occlusal surface, gold alloys wear at a faster rate than nickel–chromium and so a greater thickness of material is needed (and so the occlusal reduction of the preparation needs to be greater) if the occlusal surface is subject to wear from opposing natural or restored teeth.

Dental porcelain (14)

Dental porcelain is used as a restorative material on its own in the construction of porcelain jacket crowns, as porcelain veneers and inlays, and in conjunction with a suitable alloy in the metal–ceramic system.

Conventional dental porcelain is reinforced with alumina particles which are present to reduce crack propagation through the material. Unfortunately they add to the opacity of the porcelain and so the proportion of alumina is reduced in the surface layers of porcelain.

As well as conventional feldspathic porcelain, which has been used for well over a century, there have been a number of recent developments in ceramic materials aimed at increasing their strength. These include castable ceramics, systems for producing alumina cores by building ceramic materials up on dies poured in refractory die material and 'mouldable' ceramic cores.

Conventional porcelain crowns (14.1)

Tooth preparations for porcelain jacket crowns are designed to be compatible with the properties of porcelain. A thick layer of enamel and dentine is removed, leaving a shoulder, at the margin with a 90° cavosurface angle. The best compromise for a junction between the two relatively brittle materials, enamel and porcelain, is a butt joint. Adequate enamel and dentine must be removed from the occluding surface, and with upper incisor crowns this part of the porcelain jacket crown is made of high alumina porcelain, increasing its strength but reducing its natural appearance. Fortunately in this position this does not matter.

The porcelain jacket crown is built up in several layers on to a thin platinum foil, A high alumina core is applied followed by 'dentine' porcelain which gives the crown its basic colour, and then 'enamel' porcelain, which is more translucent and gives the crown a natural appearance (Fig. 5.14).

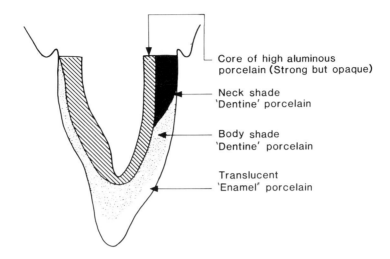

Figure 5.14 Porcelain build-up of an aluminous porcelain jacket crown.

The crown preparation is also designed to reduce internal stresses within the porcelain as it contracts on firing. Sharp external angles on the preparation give rise to sharp internal angles in the crown, producing stress concentration and an increased risk of fracture. Similarly, the surface of the preparation should be smooth and free of defects such as those resulting from previous restorations which have been lost during the preparation of the tooth. If such defects do exist they should be restored before the impression is taken.

Castable ceramic crowns (14.3.1)

These semicrystalline glass crowns are suggested for use where full coverage is required as an alternative to cast metal or metal–ceramic restorations. Whilst they are claimed to be stronger than conventional porcelain, they cannot be used in thin sections. Their appearance is somewhat monolithic, despite the stains which are applied purely as a surface coating.

The first commercially available cast ceramic material was popular for a while, despite the relatively high cost of the restorations initially. Expensive equipment is necessary together with long, and therefore expensive, processing time. Once the laboratories recovered the initial capital cost of the equipment, many of them reduced the price of the restorations, but at the same time alternative high-strength ceramic restorations were coming on to the market and clinicians began to question the claim that this material was an acceptable alternative to metal–ceramic restorations as clinical failures began to occur.

There are now new versions of castable ceramic materials, but there is, as yet, very limited clinical experience with these materials.

Systems to produce strong alumina cores by build-up techniques

There have been a number of systems which are designed to be used in ordinary dental laboratories without expensive capital investment. One of these is Vita Hi-Ceram (14.2.1). An investment die is made and the material built on to this and fired. Conventional porcelain is then built up on to the high strength core. Initial results with this material were promising (Fig. 5.15a) but the same manufacturer has now produced In-Ceram (14.2.1) and claims that the strength of the core material is even greater. Small bridges can be made with this material, which has so far given good clinical results (Fig. 5.15b).

a

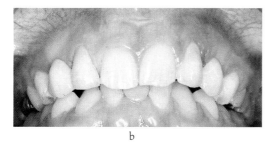

b

Figure 5.15 (a) A Hi-Ceram crown. The core material is rather opaque; (b) Two In-Ceram, three-unit bridges replacing the upper canine teeth. The retainers are partial veneers on the first premolar teeth and full crowns on the lateral incisor teeth, which were peg-shaped.

With the In-Ceram technique fine-grain aluminium oxide powder is mixed to a wet slurry consistency and applied to a special plaster model. The plaster absorbs moisture from the 'slip', leaving a densely packed material which can be carved with a scalpel. This is then fired for 10 hours. The fragile sintered framework is carefully adjusted and a thin slurry of glass powder mixed with distilled water is flooded over the surface and fired. This process is repeated four to six times, during which the sintered aluminium oxide framework is infiltrated with glass. Conventional porcelain is then built up on to this core.

Moulded cores (14.3.2)

Specialist equipment is necessary for these systems, but the capital outlay is not as great as for cast ceramic equipment.

A wax pattern is made on a conventional die, invested in special investment and heated. The hot investment ring is placed in a special press with ceramic tablets in the sprue hole. The furnace is heated to 1100°C and a pneumatic plunger presses the ceramic in its pyroplastic state into the mould.

When used as a core material, conventional

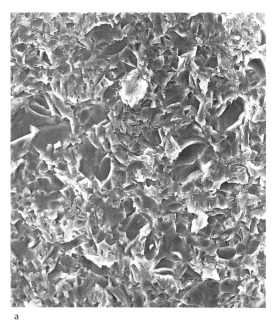

a

b

Figure 5.16 (a) A scanning electron micrograph (SEM) of the fit surface of a porcelain veneer sandblasted with 50 μm aluminium oxide particles; (b) A similar surface etched with 7% hydrofluoric acid for 5 minutes. (Field width for both SEMs = 90 μm.).

porcelain is then applied, but it is possible to use this technique to produce the complete crown, adding a thin layer of surface porcelain to produce the required appearance by a similar technique to that used with cast ceramics.

Porcelain veneers and inlays (14.1.2)

Although it is possible to make porcelain veneers with a platinum foil technique similar to the conventional porcelain crown, the more common technique is to use a refractory die and this technique is universally used for porcelain inlays.

Porcelain veneers have no conventional mechanical retentive features, such as opposing, near-parallel walls, as is the case with most porcelain inlays, but are bonded to the etched enamel surface with composite luting resin. The preparation of the fit surface of a porcelain veneer is therefore crucial to its retention. There are a number of techniques for making the porcelain surface retentive and these include sand-blasting (which is done anyway to remove the refractory die material) and this is sufficient with some porcelain materials such as Hi-Ceram core material. A more retentive surface can be obtained by etching the porcelain with hydrofluoric acid. When this is to be done the first layer of porcelain applied to the refractory die is a layer of glaze porcelain followed by dentine and enamel porcelains. The glaze layer is then etched, once the die has been removed (Fig. 5.16). In either case a silane coupling agent may be applied to the porcelain to enhance the bond to the resin luting cement.

Porcelain veneers can produce a good and durable improvement in appearance (Fig. 5.17a,b), but they also have a rather high failure rate and should only be used when the appearance is sufficiently poor to justify the risks involved in making veneers (Fig. 5.17c).

The same bonding techniques may be used with porcelain inlays, but in this case the main objective of using a silane coupling agent is to reduce microleakage and enhance the bond to the remaining tooth structure, thereby increasing its strength, rather than to assist with retention, which is usually adequate in any case.

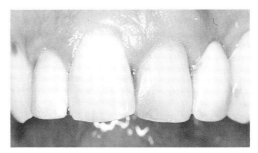

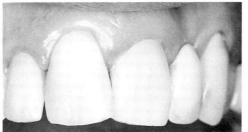

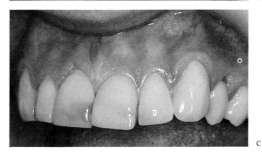

Figure 5.17 (a) A discoloured upper left central incisor. (b) A porcelain veneer in place. Because of the shape of the tooth, no preparation was necessary in this case. (c) Six porcelain veneers (canine to canine) which are beginning to leak and stain.

Porcelain restorations made by computer-aided design/computer-aided manufacture (CAD/AM) (14.1.4)

There are a number of systems being developed in different countries (some of which are already commercially available) which produce a porcelain restoration in one visit at the chairside. Although the equipment is at present expensive and limited in its range of application, it is a breakthrough for chairside computer technology and is likely to be the forerunner of more versatile and affordable systems if computer development continues at its present pace. The eventual real reduction in cost will come from the ability to produce one-visit, rather than two-visit indirect restorations.

The material from which the restorations are milled is a dense, porosity-free ceramic material which in early laboratory studies appears to behave rather more like enamel than other porcelains, particularly in the way it wears opposing teeth.

Porcelain used in the metal–ceramic system (14.1.3)

Porcelain used for metal–ceramic restorations is similar to the porcelain used for conventional porcelain jacket crowns. However, it contains components to adjust its coefficient of thermal expansion almost to match that of the cast metal substrate to which it is to be bonded. It is also necessary to apply an opaque layer of porcelain to the metal to prevent its colour affecting the final restoration. This also acts as the bonding layer. Partly because of this additional opaque layer and because the thickness of metal encroaches into the crown, the appearance of metal–ceramic restorations may be less satisfactory than porcelain jacket crowns unless substantially more enamel and dentine is removed. It is often not possible to remove a sufficient layer of tooth tissue from a healthy tooth without endangering the pulp. This means that very many metal–ceramic crowns, for example, for lower incisor teeth, have a rather dense, opaque, unrealistic appearance. It is usually not difficult to spot the 'metal–ceramic smile' of many entertainment personalities who had their teeth capped in an attempt to improve their appearance.

This is one reason for the continuing interest in finding a sufficiently strong all-porcelain system for at least individual crowns and preferably for small anterior bridges as well. However, it is likely that the metal–ceramic system will need to be used for more extensive bridges for the foreseeable future.

Bonding mechanisms of porcelain to metal (14.1.3)

The mechanisms by which porcelain bonds to metal

are complex and are described more fully in Part Three. Briefly they are:

1. Chemical bonding to a metal oxide layer on the surface of the casting.
2. Mechanical (compression) bonding to the irregularities of the metal surface.
3. Van der Waals forces.

Of these, the one that affects the preparation of the tooth most is the compression force.

In the early days of metal–ceramic restorations, when technicians were only familiar with the techniques of making facings of acrylic or porcelain which were then cemented directly to the buccal surface, they applied bonded porcelain facings just to the buccal surface of the metal. This did not maximize the compression bonding effect and was one of the reasons for porcelain facings commonly being lost. Now the ceramic material is wrapped around the metal as far as possible so that when it contracts it grips on to the metal, improving the bond. The implication for the dentist preparing the tooth is that sufficient clearance for metal and ceramic material should be allowed on at least two and preferably several surfaces of the restoration. Contrary to early belief, porcelain carried across the occlusal surface of posterior restorations increases the strength overall by increasing compression bonding, even though porcelain is in contact with the opposing teeth. It also improves the appearance of the restoration, in particular with lower posterior crowns and bridges, where in many cases the occlusal surface shows more than the buccal surface (Fig. 5.18).

Repairs to metal–ceramic restorations in the mouth (14.5)

Agents are available which chemically bond light-cured composites to dental porcelain. These silane bonding agents are applied to the roughened porcelain surface followed by the composite, which is then shaped and cured (Fig. 5.19).

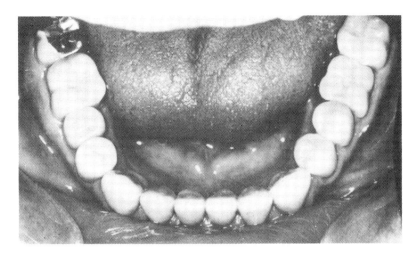

Figure 5.18 A complete lower arch reconstruction in metal–ceramic crowns. All have porcelain occlusal surfaces except the lower second molar. This tooth had a short clinical crown and a metal occlusal surface was used to limit the need for occlusal reduction.

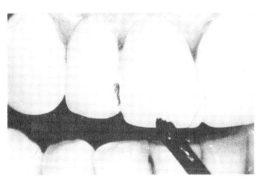

a

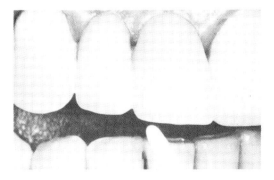

b

Other crown and bridge facing and veneer materials

A variety of polymers have been used to face cast restorations. The only materials currently available are unfilled acrylic and composite resins. Acrylic resin has a low abrasion resistance and stains and wears rapidly. It should no longer be used as a facing material for permanent crowns or bridges, but is a less expensive alternative than composite resin for provisional restorations. It requires mechanical retention to be cast into the metal framework as it cannot be bonded directly to the metal.

Light-cured composite facings (13.8.4) also require mechanical retentive features in the cast metal, a light-curing unit similar to that shown in Fig. 5.9 and a complete, expensive stock of different shades has to be purchased. They seem to offer little advantage over metal–ceramic restorations other than the capability of repairing them in the mouth.

Figure 5.19 Repair of a chipped porcelain facing on a metal–ceramic bridge. (a) The chipped surface has been slightly roughened and the conditioning agent is being applied with a paintbrush. (b) The bonding agent has been applied and repair completed with a light-curing composite, shaped with a plastic instrument. The composite material will now be polished.

Light- and pressure-cured composite materials have now been developed which appear, in relatively short-term clinical trials, likely to be acceptable as permanent restorations. They still require mechanical retention to the metal framework and this takes space, meaning that the thickness of the final restoration is at least as great as a metal–ceramic crown and therefore the preparation needs to be at least as extensive.

The colour stability and wear resistance are good and the materials have a slight flexibility which will perhaps mean fewer examples of chipped facings than with metal ceramic restorations.

These materials can also be used without a metal framework as inlays and veneers. They are much quicker to produce in the laboratory than porcelain inlays and veneers and the result, initially at least, is also good.

Dental solders (9.4)

Larger bridges and splints are sometimes cast in a number of separate units and soldered together. This is because some casting techniques are not sufficiently precise to produce multiple unit castings of the same accuracy as can be obtained by soldering smaller units together. Gold solders are used with gold alloys and also (using special techniques) with silver–palladium alloys. Special solders must be used with nickel–chromium alloys and are also available for palladium-based alloys. With metal–ceramic restorations the metal castings may be soldered (before the porcelain is added) with a high-fusing solder which will not melt at the temperatures used to fire the porcelain. When large bridges are assembled in this way it is preferable to solder sections of the bridge together in the middle of a pontic. This allows a large surface area for the solder joint and the joint will also be covered (at least partially) with porcelain, which will further reinforce the joint. Solder joints at the interdental connectors are weaker. Alternatively, metal–ceramic units may be soldered together after the porcelain is added, or metal–ceramic units may be soldered to gold alloy units using a low-fusing solder which melts at a temperature below the fusing temperature of porcelain (Fig. 5.20).

If it is necessary to divide a metal framework at the chairside at the try-in stage, it is best to do this with a fine fretsaw blade which will leave a gap to be soldered of approximately 0.5 mm. Using burs or discs produces a larger solder gap which can distort as the large bulk of solder contracts.

Luting cements (2.1)

The function of a traditional luting cement is to provide retention by interlocking between the minor irregularities on the prepared tooth surface and the restoration surface. This means that the important physical properties of a traditional luting cement are its compressive and shear strength. More recently, truly adhesive cement systems have been introduced but it is too early to say whether these will radically alter this concept of the retentive role of luting cements.

Biological properties of luting cements

Luting cements are applied directly to cut dentine surfaces, which in many cases have not been modified by the formation of secondary dentine as a result of the progressive development of a carious lesion. It might be supposed therefore that irritant cements would have a profound effect upon the pulp. However, it appears that even zinc phosphate cement (with a pH of less than 4 when placed as a fluid luting cement) only causes pulpal problems in a limited number of cases. Millions of restorations have been cemented with zinc phosphate cement and with other apparently irritant materials without a high incidence of clinically detectable harm to the pulp.

An advantageous biological property of a luting cement is to provide resistance to caries by means of leachable fluoride. Only glass-ionomer cements offer this as an inherent advantage and some polycarboxylate cements contain fluoride additives.

Physical properties of luting cements

As well as having high compressive and shear strengths, luting cements should have low solubility and possibly adhesion to the tooth tissue. The advantage of adhesion, provided the material adhered to the restoration as well, would be to improve retention. A second advantage would be to

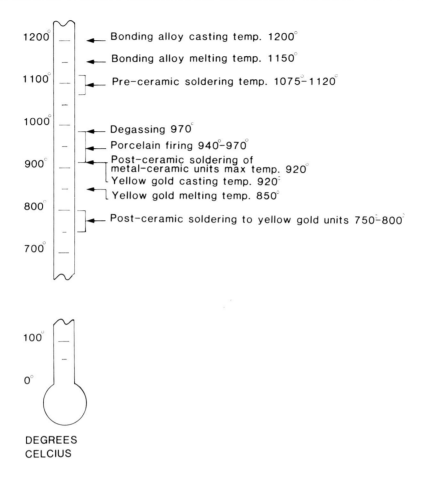

Figure 5.20 Typical temperature ranges (°C) for the metal–ceramic process. These temperatures vary according to the metal, porcelain and solder used, and with the type of furnace, in particular its rate of temperature rise.

reduce the likelihood of microleakage between the cement layer and the tooth surface. Microleakage here may produce secondary caries and/or pulp sensitivity. It is claimed that glass-ionomer cement achieves both these aims.

Available luting cements

Zinc phosphate cement (2.1.6)

This has the major advantage that it can be mixed to provide an extended working time when large numbers of restorations or large bridges or splints are being cemented. The mixing technique used in this case is to use a cooled, thick glass slab, to add very small increments of powder, mixing the material over a large surface area to dissipate the heat of reaction and to extend the mixing time to 1.5 or 2 minutes, adding small increments of powder throughout.

A further major advantage of zinc phosphate cement is that it will produce the thinnest cement film of any luting cement.

Glass-ionomer luting cements (2.1.10)

These are claimed to adhere chemically to both

dentine and enamel and may also adhere to base metal oxide layers on the fit surface of restorations. It is therefore possible (in theory) to produce a truly adhesive system via dentine to glass-ionomer cement to metal oxide layer and thus to the restoration. The strength of this layer and the likelihood of it breaking down with the stresses produced within it, resulting from differential rates of expansion and contraction of the restoration and the tooth preparation, have yet to be established. In the meantime it is unwise to modify the retentive design of tooth preparations and rely too extensively on the adhesive properties of the cement. Glass-ionomer cements also have a high cement film thickness (greater than 40 μm) and, although the early versions were relatively soluble at the margins, the current anhydrous and capsulated cements are much less soluble, even very soon after the initial set, and they can be used with similar precautions to protect them from saliva while setting, as are used with zinc phosphate cement.

The slow release of fluoride from glass-ionomer luting cement is an advantage of the material.

Resin-based luting cement (2.1.12)

Resin-based cements, mostly chemically curing bis-GMA resins, may be used to cement any permanent restoration, but were developed primarily to cement Maryland and other minimum-preparation bridges and splints. As they only contain a small amount of fine-particle-size filler and have low viscosities, small cement film thicknesses are possible. With Rochette retainers, where the cement is in contact with the mouth through the holes, it is better to use conventional, more heavily filled, chemically curing composites in view of their greater abrasion resistance.

Adhesive cements (2.1.13)

A new generation of genuinely adhesive cements is now available, and these may also be used to cement any permanent restorations, but are again used primarily with minimum-preparation bridges and splints. It is still necessary to etch the enamel surface, but instead of etching the metal surface it is sand-blasted to produce a clean, irregular surface which readily adheres to the cement. The cements contain either 4-META or a phosphonate derivative.

The setting of these cements is significantly inhibited by oxygen and so air must be excluded from the margins by means of an aqueous jelly material while the cement sets. If the cements are used with an etched metal surface, it appears air becomes trapped in the depths of the etched surface and inhibits the set of the cement. It is therefore not wise – although it might appear to be a logical way of improving retention – to use these cements in conjunction with etched metal surfaces.

Resin-based luting cements are either entirely chemically curing or dual-cure. Dual-cure materials are initiated by light and continue to cure chemically. An advantage of dual-cure is that translucent restorations, such as veneers, can be 'tacked' into position and the unset resin cleaned from the margin before the cure is complete.

Reinforced zinc oxide–eugenol cements (2.1.3; 2.1.4)

These have the advantage that they are potentially less irritant to the pulp and so are often used with deep preparations. They have lower compressive strengths than zinc phosphate cement but are within an acceptable range provided the design of the preparation is retentive and the restoration is a good fit. They are slightly more soluble than zinc phosphate at the margin and produce a thicker cement film thickness. There is less control over the working time.

Polycarboxylate cements (2.1.9)

These were introduced as the first truly adhesive cement. They have a fairly low pH when unset but it is claimed that the large molecule size of the acid prevents this being an irritant to the pulp as in the case of the unreacted acid in zinc phosphate cement. The cement film thickness is high, often two to three times that of zinc phosphate cement. Polycarboxylate cements also absorb water and if the cement film thickness is excessive it appears that the luting cement may in some cases soften, allowing the restoration to be lost. For these

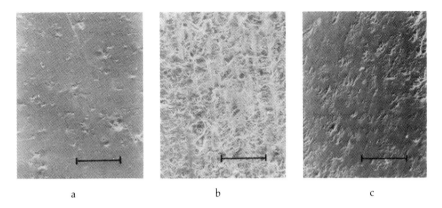

a   b   c

Figure 5.21 Scanning electron micrographs of the same porcelain surface. The marker equals 100 μm. (a) After glazing; (b) after grinding with a heatless porcelain stone; (c) ground surface has been polished with a composite finishing disc. Even better finishes can be obtained using porcelain polishing kits consisting of a series of mounted rubber wheels or points of different abrasivity.

reasons polycarboxylate cements are used less frequently as a permanent luting cement than when they were first introduced.

The choice of luting cement

All the available luting materials are capable of working successfully. The choice of which to use in a given case will depend upon the clinical circumstances (e.g. the proximity of the pulp, the age of the patient, the need for additional retention, the caries incidence of the patient, etc.) and on the relative importance the dentist attributes to the chemical and physical properties of cements.

For conventional crowns and bridges the major choice is between zinc phosphate and glass-ionomer cement. Unless the particular properties of zinc phosphate are required, for example, a long working time, then it seems increasingly that glass-ionomer cement is the material of choice for individual crowns and small bridges. There has been no significant improvement in the properties of zinc phosphate cement for decades, but there have been significant improvements in the properties of glass-ionomer cements and these developments are likely to continue.

For minimum-preparation, resin-bonded bridges and splints, the choice is between a chemically curing or dual-cure resin-based luting cement or one of the adhesive cements. The adhesive cements

have the major advantage that the restorations can be returned from the laboratory completed, tried in the mouth and then cemented. If a conventional resin-based luting cement is to be used, the metal is preferably etched after the restoration is tried in the mouth. If not, the etched surface becomes contaminated by salivary proteins and the delicate etched metal surface can be damaged physically. These factors reduce the retention and so ideally the restorations should be tried in, returned to the laboratory for etching or etched at the chairside, and then cemented. This adds an additional laboratory stage or considerable chairside time to the procedure and is therefore less cost-effective than using an adhesive cement.

Although in the laboratory adhesive cements perform well in tensile and shear tests, they perform less well than conventional resin-based cements in stress-cycling (fatigue) tests. There have not yet been any satisfactory long-term clinical trials comparing these cements.

Metal and porcelain finishing instruments and materials for use at the chairside (1.7, 1.8)

A range of discs, wheels and mounted points is available to adjust and polish metal and porcelain at the chairside.

Metal is adjusted by grinding with pink or green stones containing relatively hard coarse abrasives. These are followed by rubber wheels containing mild abrasives in a range of particle sizes and these can produce a very fine finish on gold. Alternatively, the final polish can be produced by jeweller's rouge on a felt wheel.

Dense, vacuum-fired porcelain can also be satisfactorily polished to a satin or gloss finish which does not accumulate stain or plaque and which is perfectly acceptable clinically. The technique is to shape the porcelain with a fine heatless wheel which does not chip the porcelain. The surface is then smoothed with composite finishing discs in descending order of coarseness, or by a sequence of rubber wheels specially made for the purpose (Fig. 5.21).

Further reading

Atta, M.O., Smith, B.G.N. and Brown, D. (1990) Bond strengths of three chemical adhesive cements adhered to a nickel chromium alloy for direct bonded retainers. *Journal of Prosthetic Dentistry*, **63**, 137–143

American Dental Association (Council on Dental Materials, Instruments and Equipment) (1990). Polyvinylsiloxane impression materials: a status report. *Journal of the American Dental Association*, **120**, 595-600

Brown, D. and Curtis, R.V. (1992) Alternatives to gold. *Dental Update*, **19**, 325–330

McLean J.W. (1979, 1980) *The Science and Art of Dental Ceramics*, vols I and II. Quintessence, Chicago, Illinois

Mount, G.J. (1987) *An Atlas of the Glass-ionomer Cements; A Clinician's Guide*. Martin Dunitz, London

Smith, B.G.N. (1990) *Planning and Making Crowns and Bridges*, 2nd edn. Martin Dunitz, London

Tay, W.M. (1992) *Resin Bonded Bridges*. Martin Dunitz, London

Chapter 6
Periodontology and oral surgery

Introduction

In this chapter procedures which are unique to periodontics or oral surgery are dealt with separately but in some cases, for example, sutures and grafting materials, they share common ground and are therefore considered together.

Instruments for scaling and root planing (1.1)

Periodontal hand instruments are made of steel which may or may not be tipped with tungsten carbide. Tungsten carbide, being rather brittle, is difficult to produce in thin section so the finer instruments tend to be produced in steel only. The most commonly used instruments are scalers (pointed tip and triangular cross-section) and curettes (rounded tip and more rounded cross-section; Fig. 6.1). They are made in a wide variety of designs – larger instruments are used for supragingival scaling and surgery, finer instruments for subgingival scaling and root planing. The complex design of the shanks of some instruments permits instrumentation in areas with difficult access (Fig. 6.2).

Steel curettes and scalers can be sharpened at the chairside using an oiled flat stone on the sides of the blade (Fig. 6.3). Alternatively the blade face can be ground using an abrasive stone in a handpiece or using a hand-held tungsten carbide blade such as the Nievert Whittler (Fig. 6.4).

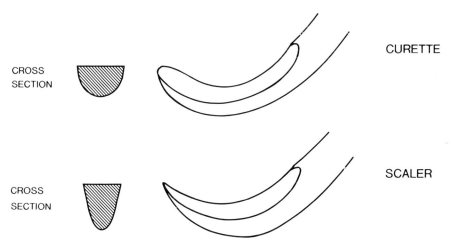

CROSS SECTION

CURETTE

CROSS SECTION

SCALER

Figure 6.1 Diagram to compare the pointed and triangular tip of a scaler and the rounded tip of a curette.

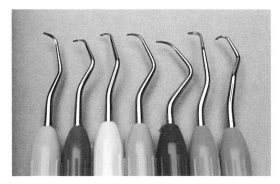

Figure 6.2 A set of Gracy curettes designed for subgingival instrumentation of specific tooth surfaces.

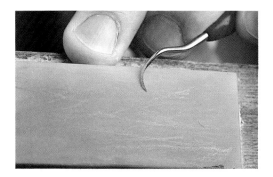

Figure 6.3 Sharpening the side of the blade of a scaler with a flat stone.

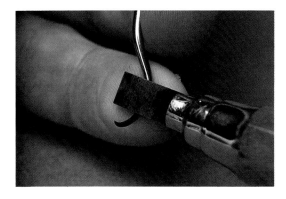

Figure 6.4 Sharpening with a Whittler on the blade face.

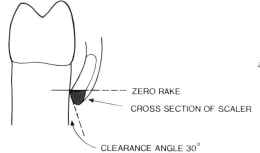

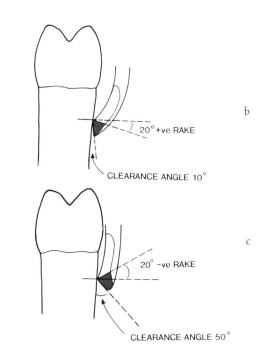

Figure 6.5 (a) Diagram illustrating zero rake angle where the blade face is at 90° to the root surface. Assuming a blade edge angle of 60°, the clearance angle is 30°. (b) Positive rake of 20° and reduction of clearance angle to 10°. (c) Negative rake of 20° and clearance angle increased to 50°.

Grinding the face of the instrument requires a higher degree of precision to maintain the contour. A sharp edge will not reflect light and sharpness can also be tested on purpose-designed plastic rods. Cutting efficiency is controlled by blade rake and edge clearance (Fig. 6.5a). If the blade face is perpendicular to the tooth surface, the rake angle is zero and the clearance angle is the angle between the side of the blade and the tooth.

The best cutting action is achieved with zero rake or slightly positive rake where the blade face is turned away from the tooth surface, thus reducing the clearance angle (Fig. 6.5b). Although zero rake is preferable, a great deal of root instrumentation is carried out with negative rake (Fig. 6.5c).

Other hand instruments such as hoes (Fig. 6.6) and files are used for subgingival scaling and root planing, although the latter instruments are not commonly used in the UK.

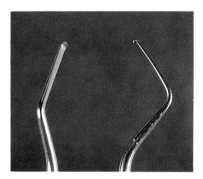

Figure 6.6 Hoe tips.

Scaling is the removal of calculus, both supragingival and subgingival. Root planing is the removal of cementum from the root surface within the pocket to ensure complete removal of calculus, plaque and bacterial contaminants. In reality it differs little from thorough subgingival scaling. The term curettage is usually applied to the intentional removal of the soft tissue lining of the pocket. It is rarely advocated as it does not appear to produce better results than root planing alone.

Ultrasonic scalers use stainless steel tips which do not need to be sharp. They vibrate at very high frequencies and will remove stain, plaque, calculus, cementum and soft tissue. They work mainly by micromechanical movement but also by cavitation (rapid changes in pressure within the coolant fluid) and acoustic streaming (Fig. 6.7). The vibration of the tip is produced by a ferromagnetic stack in a high-frequency magnetic field, a piezoelectric unit whereby an oscillating current is applied to a quartz crystal, or an air-driven mechanism activating a vibrating rod. The latter mechanism is found in sonic scalers which vibrate at a lower frequency.

Clinical trials have shown similar results when comparing these instruments with hand instrumentation. Ultrasonic scalers reduce the tactile feedback to the operator but produce a good washed field. Because an aerosol is created they are not recommended in the treatment of high-risk patients.

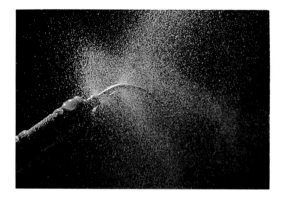

Figure 6.7 The water coolant is converted into a fine spray at the tip of an ultrasonic scaler where cavitation and acoustic streaming occur.

Materials used to replace or regenerate bone and periodontal ligament (16.3)

A wide variety of materials (in place of actual bone grafts) has been used to substitute for lost bone or to enhance repair of bone defects in periodontology and oral surgery. Very similar procedures and materials have been used to augment edentulous ridges to provide support for removable prostheses and to improve the appearance of bridge pontics where there are localized alveolar deformities or there has been excessive resorption. This section is divided into bone substitutes and guided tissue regeneration.

Bone substitutes (16.3.2)

Certain materials allow bone ingrowth (osteoconductive) whereas others claim to promote bone regeneration (osteoinductive). Hydroxyapatite has been extensively tested and can be manufactured in a variety of ways to alter its properties. The solid form is extremely dense and non-resorbable and the porous forms allow tissue ingrowth and are biodegradable. It can be manufactured in block form or as particles. Dense solid hydroxyapatite is difficult to cut and therefore needs to be prepared in the laboratory. It has been used to stabilize osteotomies as an interpositional graft. It needs good bone contact as it is not osteogenic; it can be displaced because there is no tissue ingrowth and it may cause resorption of superficial bone. It therefore has very limited applications.

Porous hydroxyapatite blocks are easier to cut and shape. It can be used to augment a deficient edentulous ridge to improve the appearance of a pontic (Fig. 6.8). In this situation it will allow tissue ingrowth and will therefore remain stable. Similar materials have been made using various combinations of hydroxyapatite, collagen, PTFE, vitreous carbon and alumina.

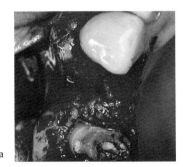

a

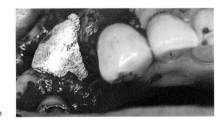

b

Figure 6.8 (a) A surgically exposed bone defect in the upper premolar region where a bridge is planned. (b) An hydroxyapatite block has been carefully trimmed to fit the bone defect.

Particulate forms of hydroxyapatite and resorbable materials such as tricalcium phosphate are more commonly used in periodontal bone defects (Fig.

6.9) and extraction sockets in an attempt to preserve ridge form and preprosthetic ridge augmentation (Fig. 6.10) where block forms may lead to complications such as wound dehiscences and infection. It is difficult to keep the particulate material localized and therefore in procedures such as ridge augmentation, attempts are made to produce a fibrous tissue capsule to prevent dissemination. Alternatively, a matrix such as collagen is used to bind the particles together.

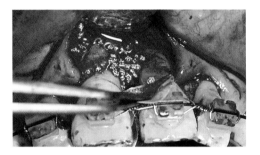

Figure 6.9 Hydroxyapatite particles placed into a surgically exposed periodontal defect. It is difficult to prevent them being displaced.

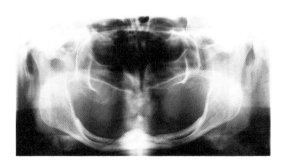

Figure 6.10 Radiograph of ridge augmentation using particulate hydroxyapatite.

Ridge augmentation often produces only negligible improvements and is not favoured by many prosthodontists. In periodontal bone defects there is also a tendency for the material to be lost, particularly if the soft tissue coverage is inadequate. Results with periodontal defects are contradictory, with many studies showing no additional benefit, whereas others have shown small clinical advantages mainly in terms of the radiographic density of the site. It is assumed that bone fill occurring in periodontal defects using these techniques does not include regeneration of lost ligament and new cementum. The attachment to the tooth surface is mediated through a long junctional epithelium produced by the rapid downgrowth of epithelium. Similar variable results have been reported with porous particulate non-resorbable composites of poly(methylmethacrylate), poly-(hydroxyethylmethacrylate) and calcium hydroxide.

Guided tissue regeneration materials (16.4)

An alternative approach to promote regeneration of bone and periodontal tissues is to utilize the regenerative capability of the existing tissues by facilitating ingrowth of the required tissue and preventing ingrowth of adjacent tissues using physical barriers. This is achieved by the placement of occlusive membranes of inert materials such as expanded PTFE (Gore-Tex) or resorbable materials such as polylactic acid, polyglactin and collagen (type 1 human and bovine). It has been suggested that the membranes need to be biocompatible, cell occlusive and able to maintain space, stabilize the wound and prevent epithelial downgrowth. These membranes have been used locally to augment ridges by producing a space into which adjacent bone can grow. In some situations it is necessary to support the membrane from collapsing by using struts of hydroxyapatite. This same principle is used to produce bone fill around osseointegrated implants where there is inadequate bone volume.

In periodontal defects the technique is used to produce a new attachment consisting of cementum, periodontal ligament and bone on a previously disease-affected root surface. Most work in this area has been with PTFE membranes (Fig. 6.11). Following elevation of full-thickness mucoperi-osteal flaps, the periodontal defects are thoroughly prepared by removing all inflammatory tissue and all root surface deposits by meticulous root planing (Fig. 6.12a). A membrane of the appropriate shape is trimmed to fit around the root face and to cover the defect and surrounding bone by a margin of about 2 mm (Fig. 6.12b). The membrane is secured tightly around the tooth with a PTFE suture (this is not used with resorbable membranes) and the membrane carefully covered with the flaps using vertical mattress sutures.

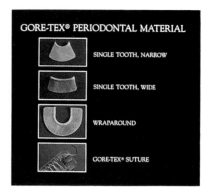

Figure 6.11 Configurations of PTFE (Gore-Tex) membranes designed for use with various shapes and sizes of periodontal defects.

The membrane is left buried for a period of 4–6 weeks to allow ingrowth by cells of the remaining periodontal ligament and bone, whilst excluding ingrowth by gingival connective tissue and preventing epithelial downgrowth, which is thought to be a major preventive factor in the establishment of a connective tissue attachment. The PTFE membranes have a microporous collar at the tooth margin which prevents epithelial down-growth by contact inhibition (Fig. 6.12c). The technique provides good protection for the organizing clot. At the time of surgical removal of the membrane the periodontal defect is filled with organizing connective tissue and has a jelly-like consistency (Fig. 6.12d). This is carefully protected by replacing the gingival flap which was covering the membrane (Fig. 6.12e).

Because the membrane has to be surgically removed it is not surprising that efforts are being made to produce a suitable resorbable material with similar mechanical properties. However, it should be remembered that resorption involves inflammatory responses which may not be conducive to optimum healing. Guided tissue regeneration has demon-strated that it is possible to regain lost periodontal connective tissue and therefore this offers great promise (Fig. 6.13). The most favourable results are obtained in situations where the three-dimensional morphology of the defect allows contribution of

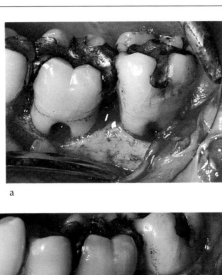

a

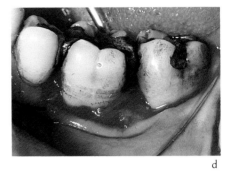

d

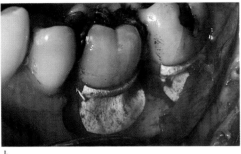

b

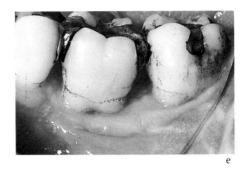

e

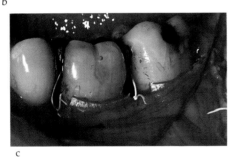

c

Figure 6.12 (a) Surgical preparation of a lower molar furcation for guided tissue regeneration. (b) The bone defects and instrumented root surfaces are covered with a PTFE membrane. (c) The microporous collar is exposed after flap closure. Ideally the membranes should be completely covered. (d) Six weeks after the initial surgery, the membrane is removed to reveal the healing tissue filling the defect. (e) The result 2 months after membrane removal.

Periodontal packs (16.1)

ligament cells from several aspects. Therefore it is recommended in grade 1 and 2 furcation lesions and infrabony defects, whereas in horizontal defects, supracrestal gain in connective tissue attachment is very limited.

In attempts to enhance the predictability and magnitude of regeneration, many reports have been published describing combinations of all the existing techniques. None of these combination therapies has been shown to be clearly superior. Further research to identify and exploit the appropriate growth and adhesion factors may improve the results of these treatment methods.

Packs are indicated in the apically repositioned flap procedure and gingivectomies. In the former, a full-thickness mucoperiosteal flap is cut with an inverse bevel incision and elevated beyond the mucogingival junction. Following removal of the pocket lining, inflammatory tissue and careful root surface preparation, the flap is apically displaced and supported around the teeth by a continuous suture. This prevents further apical displacement and the pack prevents coronal movement and produces close adaptation. Packs are used in other flap procedures to help to adapt closely a flap margin to the tooth surface, where there is

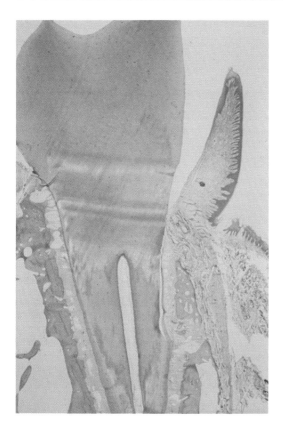

Figure 6.13 Histological section of guided tissue regeneration in an experimental animal model. The PTFE membrane is visible on the exterior surface of the alveolar bone. The alveolar bone crest has regenerated, together with periodontal ligament and new cementum on the root surface. An artefactual split has arisen during processing between the newly formed cementum and the root surface.

considerable denudation of bone or simply because of operator preference (Fig. 6.14).

Gingivectomies produce considerable exposure of connective tissue (and occasionally bone) and a pack is placed to protect the wound, help with haemostasis and to reduce postoperative discomfort. There is considerable debate as to how effective or necessary a pack is in reducing postoperative pain.

Packs are usually available as a two-paste system similar to zinc oxide–eugenol impression paste but with substitution of the eugenol because it causes

tissue irritation (16.1.1.2). It is necessary to lubricate the operator's gloves to prevent the pack sticking to them. A small quantity of pack is placed to cover the flap margin and pushed into the interdental spaces to help retention. A careful check is made to ensure that it does not extend on to the occlusal surface of the teeth and that it is not overextended into the buccal or lingual sulcus. Border trimming is therefore recommended by moulding the material with the cheeks and lips.

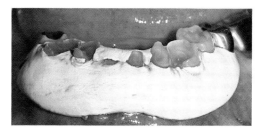

Figure 6.14 A periodontal pack in place 1 week after surgery.

The more recently introduced single-component light-cured system (16.1.4) is applied directly from a purpose-designed syringe and is therefore easier to handle. It is pink and slightly translucent and produces a better appearance. It sets quite firmly after light-curing and may be a little more difficult to remove from undercut embrasure spaces. Packs are left on for about 1 week.

The development of packs containing slow-release medicaments may provide further indications for their use. Antiseptics, antimicrobials, anti-inflammatories and other pharmacological agents could be incorporated to modify and enhance the healing response.

Slow-release polymers have also been developed for placement subgingivally as an adjunct or even substitute for scaling and root planing. For example, chlorhexidine, metronidazole and tetracycline have been incorporated in acrylic strips for placement into pockets. One of the most promising recent systems is an ethylene vinyl acetate fibre containing tetracycline. This is claimed to disinfect the pocket by releasing bactericidal concentrations over several days but with a total dose that is a fraction of that which would be required if the drug were given systemically. Further experimental evaluation of these products is required before general clinical use.

Splints for mobile teeth

Tooth mobility may be due to a reduction in height of support (attachment loss and bone loss due to periodontal disease), an alteration in the quality of support (inflammatory changes in the marginal tissue and/or periodontal ligament) or an increase in width of the ligament (as a result of occlusal trauma). Mobility may be either increased but stable, or increasing in severity. The former situation may not give rise to any symptoms or problems but may be of such magnitude as to interfere with function or comfort of the patient, in which case permanent splinting is indicated. An increasing mobility is usually due to progressive periodontal disease or it may occur in the adaptive phase of occlusal trauma. In rare instances it occurs in a treated healthy periodontal ligament which has been reduced to such a degree that forces from occlusion exceed its adaptive capacity. This is a further indication for permanent splinting.

Permanent splints

Permanent splints can be made by attaching a cast metal plate made to fit the lingual surfaces of the unprepared or minimally prepared teeth by acid-etch-retained composite using a technique similar to that of the minimal-preparation (Maryland) bridge (Fig. 6.15; see Chapter 5).

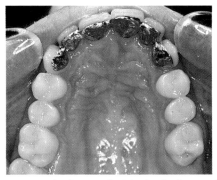

Figure 6.15 Palatal view of a Maryland splint on the upper incisors following orthodontic repositioning.

An alternative technique (Rochette − Fig. 6.16) gains retention from the cast splint by making six to 10 undercut holes through it, rather than etching the metal surface as in the Maryland technique.

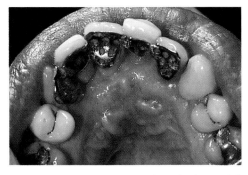

Figure 6.16 Palatal view of a Rochette bridge used for stabilization after periodontal treatment and to replace missing teeth.

The Rochette technique has advantages for splinting if it is to be used in the medium term as it is more readily and less traumatically removed, simply by drilling the composite from the holes. It is also easier to recement if debonding occurs and it can be adapted by adding a denture tooth or composite material to make a very good immediate-replacement provisional bridge/splint if a tooth has to be extracted later. Special chemically activated, microfine composites with low viscosity have been developed for attaching the Maryland type of splint, but conventional chemically curing composite should be used to attach Rochette splints to reduce the degradation of the composite which passes through the holes and is in contact with the mouth. In some cases permanent splinting can only be reliably achieved by partial or full coverage cast or metal−ceramic restorations (see Chapter 5)

Temporary splints

When a splint is necessary for a short period of time, for example after a tooth has been loosened by a blow, after reimplantation or transplantation of a tooth or when an uncomfortable tooth has to be stabilized during a course of periodontal treatment, temporary splints can be made by applying acid-etch-retained composite to adjacent teeth and simply bonding a series of teeth together. A potentially stronger splint can be made by incorporating a length of wire or wire mesh into the splint (Fig. 6.17) – a technique that has been advocated for long-term postorthodontic retention.

This technique maintains a reasonably good appearance and is so successful that it has replaced many other forms of temporary splinting, such as wire ligatures and acrylic, cemented acrylic and metal foil splints.

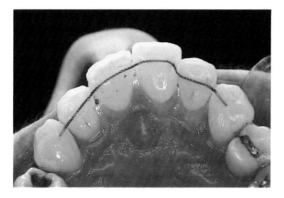

Figure 6.17 Palatal view of a wire and composite splint for post-orthodontic retention.

Composite splints function better in the lower incisor region where most of the forces are directed apically, but there is a higher failure rate with the upper incisors where there is a tendency towards splaying. Failure is also greater where there is a marked variation in mobility of the teeth which are to be joined. Subsequent removal of these splints carries the risk of damage to the enamel as high-speed cutting instruments are usually necessary.

Suture materials (16.2)

Suture materials are of two basic types, resorbable and non-resorbable. Both types are readily available bonded to needles of various shapes and sizes. Most needles are a cutting design and should be carefully rotated through the tissues taking adequate bites from the wound margins to avoid tearing. The size of suture material is given by a numerical code, known as USP (United States Pharmacopoeia), which is gradually being replaced by a metric code. The sizes most commonly used in periodontal

and oral surgery are 3/0 and 4/0 and the finer sizes (5/0 and 6/0) are more commonly used for the closure of extraoral wounds in maxillofacial surgery.

The equivalent sizes are given below

Metric	USP
1	3/0
1.5	4/0
2	5/0
3	6/0

Non-resorbable materials are either monofilament synthetic fibres (polypropylene, nylon, PTFE) or multifilament braided materials (black silk, braided nylon). The monofilament polypropylene and nylon sutures are springy and therefore 4/0 or finer are used for intraoral use. In addition, three throws are recommended to make sure the knot remains tied. PTFE sutures are very soft and flexible, tie very well and remain taut over extended periods of time. They are particularly useful in guided tissue regeneration procedures where a membrane is tied around a tooth for 4–6 weeks.

Resorbable sutures include plain gut and chromic gut which has a higher tensile strength and delayed resorption. More modern resorbable materials such as polylactic acid, polyglycolic acid, polydioxanone and polyglactin are more flexible and therefore more useful for intraoral use. Resorbable sutures are used where deep layers are closed and the suture remains buried or in situations where the operator does not want to remove them, such as in small children or where there is likely to be considerable swelling or postoperative discomfort, for example in the lip or the floor of mouth.

Mucous membrane dressing materials (16.1.5)

A material which adheres for a period of time to the oral soft tissues is available in paste or powder form. It is a mixture of natural and synthetic gels (carmellose sodium, gelatin, pectin) and is also produced containing various medicaments such as corticosteroids. It is used in the treatment of such conditions as aphthous ulcers and minor trauma.

Implants (16.3)

Dental implants are being used more routinely as a result of much improved success rates following careful research and longitudinal clinical evaluation. The major advance has been the predictable union of the implant surface with bone. The term osseointegration is a histological definition: 'a direct structural and functional connection between ordered living bone and the surface of a load-carrying implant' (Brånemark, 1985). This was originally described with implants of commercially pure titanium used in the Brånemark system. Alloys of titanium (Ti–6Al–4V) have been claimed to give similar success rates and research has also been directed at producing coatings of hydroxyapatite and tricalcium phosphate to improve compatibility and speed of osseointegration. They have not been shown to have any advantage over pure titanium. Clinically successful implants have also been produced using Al_2O_3 and crystal sapphire.

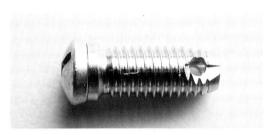

Figure 6.18 A threaded titanium implant fixture (Brånemark).

The techniques for inserting implants place great emphasis on avoiding trauma to the bone. In particular it is essential that there is minimal heat generation during the procedure. Therefore copious irrigation and slow drilling speeds are used. The implants (fixtures) are often threaded (Fig. 6.18) and are placed after tapping the site or, alternatively, self-tapping fixtures are used, especially in areas of poor-quality bone. In most systems emphasis is also placed on avoiding loading in the first 3–6 months, during which time osseointegration is taking place and therefore the implant is left buried beneath the oral mucosa during this period. It is subsequently uncovered and connected by a transmucosal abutment to a bridge, denture attachment or single tooth replacement (Fig. 6.19). In some systems the implant is left exposed following initial installation.

Particular care has to be paid to the occlusion as osseointegrated implants are rigidly connected to the bone and do not have the physiological mobility and adaptability afforded by a periodontal ligament.

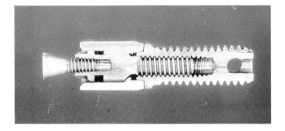

Figure 6.19 Cross-section through an assembled fixture and transmucosal abutment. The small screw on top is used to connect a fixed-bridge prosthesis.

Good plaque control by the patient is obviously important to maintain healthy peri-implant tissues. If scaling of the transmucosal component is required then it is important to use only specially designed instruments made from plastic as the titanium surface is relatively soft.

Splints for fractured jaws

Mandibular fractures

Cast silver cap splints (Fig. 6.20) are nowadays rarely used in the UK and many fractures are still treated with eyelet wiring (Fig. 6.21). This is a system where stainless steel wire loops are made around the teeth in each jaw and connected with wire ligatures (intermaxillary fixation). Soft stainless steel wire is used; this is prestretched to produce a

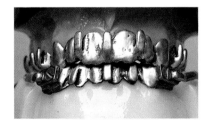

Fig 6.20 Cast silver cap splints

material which will remain tight when the ends are twisted together but it is not springy and therefore handles more easily. Stainless steel wire is also used to attach preformed or custom-made arch bars to the teeth (Fig. 6.22) and for directly wiring bone fragments together (intraosseous wiring) at the upper or lower border of the mandible.

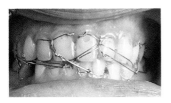

Figure 6.21 Eyelet wiring in both jaws joined by wires to provide intermaxillary fixation.

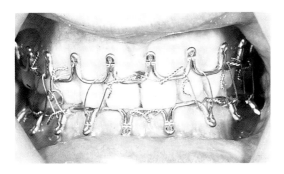

Figure 6.22 Arch bars wired to teeth in both jaws and connected by intermaxillary fixation.

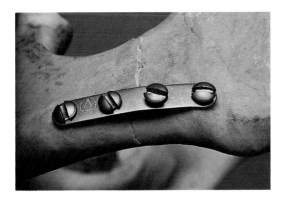

Figure 6.23 A non-compression plate screwed across a fracture in a dried mandible.

With the development of miniplating systems (non-compression plates and screws) for intraoral use, bone segments can be readily joined without the need for intermaxillary fixation (Fig. 6.23). This allows better and more rapid recovery of jaw function and carries only a slightly increased risk of infection. Miniplates and microplates are usually made of nickel–chromium–molybdenum alloy, stainless steel or titanium and experiments have also been carried out with resorbable systems.

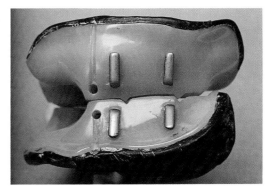

Figure 6.24 Custom-made Gunning splints lined by black gutta-percha.

Compression plating systems are rarely used in the UK. Extraoral plating and external pins and bars are also rarely used.

In edentulous mandibles, splints may be made from existing dentures or custom-made Gunning splints retained by circum-mandibular stainless steel wires (Fig. 6.24). These splints are made of acrylic lined with black gutta-percha which, although slightly elastic, shows plastic properties and will flow under pressure. The gutta-percha lining is initially shaped by softening in a water bath at 60 – 70°C, flaming the surface to be attached to the plate to encourage adhesion, and moulding the fit surface on to a model made from the old denture or an impression of the mouth. Final fitting occurs in the mouth, and gutta-percha will continue to respond to localized pressure by flow rather than causing soreness.

Midfacial fractures

These are commonly treated with extraoral fixation

using halos and pins. Stainless steel wires are used for intermaxillary fixation and internal suspension wires. Plating is uncommon because of the very thin bone and difficulty of exposing the fracture site. When deficiencies in the orbital floor need to be repaired, the choice is between grafted bone, lyophilized dura, or sheets of Silastic, PTFE or Supramid. Complications such as extrusion of synthetic materials are occasionally seen.

Many of the methods mentioned in this section on mandibular and mid facial fractures are also used in the stabilization of osteotomy fragments.

Further reading

Periodontology

Brånemark, P.I., Zarb, G.A. and Albrektsson, T. (Eds) (1985) *Tissue Integrated Prostheses.* Quintessence, Chicago, Illinois

Kieser, J.B. (1990) *Periodontics – a Practical Approach.* Wrights, London

Minabe, M. (1991) A critical review of the biological rationale for guided tissue regeneration. *Journal of Periodontology,* **62,** 171–179

Paquette, O.E. and Levin, M.P. (1977) The sharpening of scaling instruments: I. An examination of principles. *Journal of Periodontology,* **48,** 163–168

Oral surgery

Frame, J.W. and Brady, C.L. (1987) The versatility of hydroxyapatite blocks in maxillofacial surgery. *British Journal of Oral and Maxillofacial Surgery,* **25,** 452–464

Hardman, F.G. and Boering, G. (1989) Comparisons in the treatment of facial trauma. *International Journal of Oral and Maxillofacial Surgery,* **18,** 324-332

Rowe, N.L. and Williams, J.Ll. (1985) *Maxillofacial Injuries.* Churchill Livingstone, London

Chapter 7
Partial and complete dentures

Introduction

Partial dentures may either be tooth-supported, mucosa-supported or both tooth- and mucosa-supported, while complete dentures are necessarily mucosa-supported. The materials of which dentures are constructed and the handling of those materials used in the clinical stages are closely related to the oral anatomy and physiology of the individual patient. It is only possible to deal with the materials in any detail if a knowledge of the clinical criteria is assumed. The component parts of partial dentures are shown in Fig. 7.1, although many designs may exclude one or more components. Each individual design is planned with the assistance of articulated study casts (see Chapter 1) and the materials used may be strongly influenced by the design.

Preparation of the mouth

The handling of materials used in ensuring a healthy oral environment in which to place the dentures has already been discussed (see Chapter 2). Tooth rest seat preparations or modifications of tooth contour that are required are carried out using suitable burs for cutting either enamel or metal restorations (see Chapter 3). The design of these tooth preparations

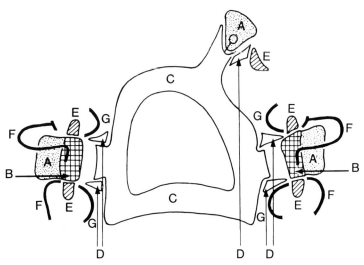

Figure 7.1 Component parts of a partial denture. A = saddles and artificial teeth; B = retentive grid on metal framework; C = major connector; D = minor connectors; E = rests; F = clasps; G = reciprocal bracing arms.

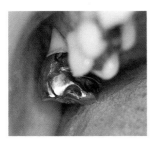

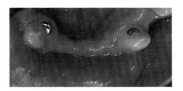

Figure 7.4 Cast metal cingulum rest seats bonded to the lingual surfaces of lower canines.

Figure 7.2 Mesial occlusal rest seat incorporated into a full gold crown.

is outside the scope of this book but care must be taken to avoid penetration of either the enamel or metal restorations, which may need to be replaced if they are of insufficient thickness. For this reason, planning the denture should precede the planning of restorations. Cast metal restorations demonstrate the ideal properties for resting surfaces as amalgam restorations will creep over long periods (Fig. 7.2). Composite resins can be etch-retained on to enamel surfaces to form cingulum-type rest seats or suitable undercuts for retentive elements (Fig. 7.3). However, these do not have ideal wear properties and due to the abrasive nature of their fillers can also wear metal components of the denture with associated discoloration of the composite. Cast metal rest seats may also be bonded to enamel surfaces using etch retention (Fig. 7.4).

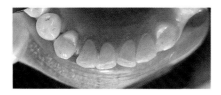

Figure 7.3 Composite resin build-up of both lower canines prepared to provide cingulum rest seats.

Restorations should be polished after preparation as should prepared enamel surfaces using rubber cones or discs containing progressively finer abrasives (1.7). It may also be appropriate to apply topical fluoride preparations (15.2; see Chapter 2) to prepared enamel surfaces.

Impressions for dentures

Primary impressions

Primary impressions for the partially dentate mouth have been discussed in Chapter 1. For edentulous patients suitable-shaped trays are also available in metal and polymers. The former are able to be sterilized and therefore can be reused while the latter are usually disposable. Some more expensive polymer trays are available which can be autoclaved and reused. All types are suitable for alginate primary impressions, but only the metal trays are rigid enough to be satisfactorily used with composition.

Primary impression materials

Composition (5.1.2) is easy to handle and requires minimal support from the stock tray. It must be adequately heated to ensure satisfactory flow, coated with petroleum jelly to protect the oral mucosa and facilitate flow and preshaped prior to insertion in the mouth. Vigorous border moulding is required or overextension is certain to occur, although trimming of the periphery with a sharp knife, reheating with a pin flame, reinsertion and further border moulding are possible. Additions are also easy using the same material provided in a stick form suitable for softening in a flame. Being non-elastic, it is unsuitable for undercut residual ridges and the apparatus required for softening is inconvenient, often messy, and must be sterilized between patients.

Silicone putty materials (5.2.5) provide a good alternative to composition, having a similar viscosity, but longer working time. They cannot easily be added to, although reduction with a sharp knife and relining with a lower-viscosity silicone rubber or alginate is possible, but rarely necessary. They do not require any special equipment for their use, are elastic, thus allowing withdrawal from undercuts, but may be more expensive than composition (Fig. 7.5). Problems with mixing and handling of silicone putty may be experienced because contact with the plasticizers used in latex rubber gloves inhibits polymerization.

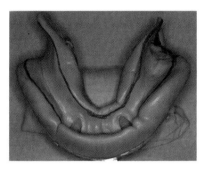

Figure 7.5 Silicone putty used as a primary impression for a complete overdenture (only the roots of the lower canines are retained).

Irreversible hydrocolloid or alginate (5.2.2) is cheap and will record undercut areas accurately. However, alginate does not readily flow into areas into which the stock tray does not extend. The stock tray may therefore require modification with pink modelling wax (7.1.1) or composition. Carding or red wax (7.1.5) can also be used but is too soft for all but the smallest extensions.

As previously noted (see Chapter 1), neither alginate nor composition is compatible with recommended disinfection procedures, while silicone putty is, and this may encourage its use.

The prescription for the construction of the special tray is best provided by marking the extension of the required tray on to the impression with indelible pencil. Undercut areas which require blocking out may also be marked in this way.

Working impressions

Fitting surface impressions

A working impression for a partial denture should record accurately both the remaining natural teeth and the mucosa surfaces upon which the denture will also be supported or will cover. Where the denture is planned to be totally tooth-supported a *mucostatic* impression of the mucosa surface is appropriate so that no load is applied to this surface when the denture is subjected to occlusal loading. Conversely, where the denture is to be partially or wholly mucosa-supported, a *mucodisplacive* impression is necessary so as to ensure displacement of thicker soft tissue layers and distribution of occlusal load over as wide a supporting area of residual bone as possible. In order to achieve this objective the impression material should either be sufficiently viscous on its own or be confined within a close-fitting tray to restrict its flow.

In addition, although the retention of the partial denture is not dependent upon the peripheral seal, so necessary in complete dentures, maximum extension of the denture base allows the utilization of the maximum support from the residual bone that is available.

Peripheral impression

The impression of the periphery should therefore be an exact prescription to be copied by the technician as the periphery of the denture. Slight displacement of the peripheral tissues is also desirable but the periphery must, of course, rest on non-moving tissues. In order to achieve a good impression of the periphery a close-fitting tray is required.

Well-extended special trays do not require peripheral extension. There may, however, be advantages in recording the peripheral impression separately from the main impression. Green stick composition (5.1.2) may be used, completing small lengths of the periphery at each insertion of the tray, or border-moulding acrylics (13.4) may be used, to complete the whole periphery at one insertion (Fig. 7.6). The latter material must be allowed to reach the dough stage before use to ensure sufficient stiffness to record a displaced peripheral impression and a delay is needed for polymerization to take place before the working impression is completed (this may be hastened by placing in warm water). In both cases, any border moulding material that enters undercut areas must be trimmed and the closeness of the fit of the new periphery of the special tray is an indication for the use of a lower-viscosity impression material.

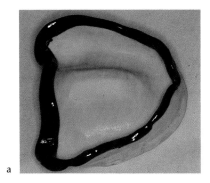

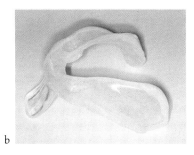

Figure 7.6 Border moulding of special trays to give a peripheral impression prior to completing the working impression using; (a) green stick composition; (b) border-moulding acrylic.

Posterior border seal (post-dam)

An adequate seal at the posterior border of the complete and some partial dentures is essential for satisfactory retention. Adequate displacement of the softer tissue areas may be obtained with the impression procedure, especially if a border-moulding material is used across the posterior border of the tray extending into the buccal sulcus, prior to the main impression. However, polymerization shrinkage of most polymeric denture base materials has its greatest effect in the midline of the palate (Fig. 7.7), and additional trimming of the cast is required to compensate for this. The area to be trimmed should be marked on the impression with an indelible pencil as a prescription for the technician.

Close-fitting or special tray

The use of special trays has a number of advantages,

particularly when either only a few or no natural teeth remain. The accuracy of fit of a special tray ensures correct recording of the periphery of the denture-bearing area without the distortion often caused by a poorly fitting stock tray. The closeness of the fit of the tray over the mucosa surfaces allows the recording of a *mucodisplacive* impression of these surfaces, where appropriate, provided the correct impression material is used. In this respect, if a viscous or stiff impression material is used, it is essential that the special tray is sufficiently rigid, as any distortion of the tray while making the impression will be released on removal from the mouth, thus distorting the impression. The closeness of the fit of the special tray also limits the quantity of impression material necessary, significantly reducing the cost where expensive elastomeric impression materials are used.

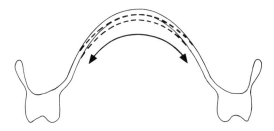

Figure 7.7 Linear shrinkage in the direction of the arrow reduces the height of the palatal vault, as shown by the broken outline. A groove cut in the cast (post-dam) compensates for this, ensuring an adequate fit in the mouth.

Newly available light-activated resin materials (13.8.5) provide rigid and stable trays which are easy and quick to produce (see Chapter 5). Self-activated acrylic resin (12.1.2) or shellac (7.2) trays are cheaper, but need to be thickened over the crest of the ridge to improve rigidity. Acrylic resin trays must be left for at least 24 hours after being made, to ensure complete polymerization and dimensional stability and, in addition, immersion in water will cause further distortion. All of these require a correctly extended primary impression for their construction.

A metal tray is sufficiently rigid, but is unlikely to be close-fitting unless a very wide selection is available. Metal trays may be modified at the chairside using composition or silicone rubber putty

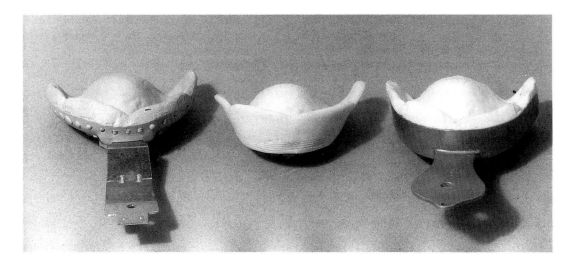

Figure 7.8 Special trays for complete denture impression. Left: a disposable plastic stock tray modified with composition. Centre: an acrylic resin tray thickened over the crest of the ridge. Right: a metal stock tray modified with silicone rubber putty.

suitably trimmed with a sharp knife to the correct peripheral extension. Disposable plastic stock trays are too flexible and if used they should be modified and reinforced with composition or acrylic (Fig. 7.8).

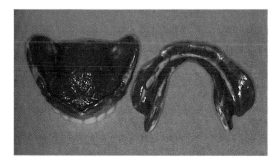

Figure 7.9 Working impressions made at the trial denture visit within the self-activated acrylic resin bases using a thin layer of silicone rubber material to avoid disturbing the carefully recorded occlusal relations.

Although it is usual to make the working impression prior to the construction of occlusal rims, an alternative procedure for complete dentures is to construct the occlusal rim on a self-activated acrylic base made on a cast taken from a primary impression. Shellac is a less satisfactory alternative. The working impression is then made at the trial denture visit, taking great care not to disturb the carefully recorded occlusal relations (Fig. 7.9).

Working impression materials for partial dentures

When choosing an impression material for a partial denture working impression, the properties to be considered are as follows:-

1. The packaged material should have an adequate shelf-life.
2. It should be compatible with the oral tissues, for although it is only in contact with these tissues for a short period of time, hypersensitivity reactions have been known to occur. A pleasant taste and odour are also desirable.
3. The working time should be long enough for mixing, loading in the tray and placing in the mouth before setting commences, while a

short setting time is desirable to limit the total time taken for, the impression procedure and the time the patient needs to have the impression in the mouth. The viscosity of the unset materials is also relevant – a more viscous material is desirable where a *muco-displacive* impression is required.

4. It must be elastic when set in order to record undercut areas, should be reasonably compliant so that removal from the mouth and the subsequent casts will not stress mobile teeth in the mouth or fracture teeth from the cast, and should be sufficiently stiff when adequately supported by the tray to avoid distortion on casting the dental stone (6.1.2). Dental stone should always be used for partial denture casts to withstand the extensive laboratory procedures necessary.

5. It must have an adequate tear strength so as not to tear when removed from important undercut areas, although it should ideally tear from between the teeth without excessive force being necessary or the impression may be distorted, the natural teeth unduly stressed or the cast fractured. In practice, unwanted undercuts between the teeth may be blocked out with soft wax (Fig. 7.10) and this, together with the removal of impression material from between the teeth on the set impression, produces a stronger cast with less chance of fracturing stone teeth on impression removal. There must also be adequate adhesion to the tray so that removal from the mouth does not cause separation of the impression material from the tray.

6. It must be dimensionally stable. Changes in dimension can occur on setting, on removal from the mouth temperature to room temperature and on storage. The latter dimensional changes may be overcome by rapid pouring of the cast, but this is not always convenient.

7. It should not be significantly affected by the moisture with which it will inevitably come into contact, although it must be noted that a satisfactory impression of the oral tissues can rarely be obtained if they are covered in a layer of saliva. Even the newer so-called hydrophilic impression materials, whilst demonstrating better wettability, are not de-

signed to absorb oral fluids. For this reason the oral cavity should always be dried prior to impression taking. The impression material must also be compatible with the dental stone with which it is to be cast.

8. Impressions will be rinsed free of blood and saliva and should be capable of being disinfected prior to transfer to the laboratory. The World Health Organization recommend (*Viral Hepatitis* 1973, Technical Report series 512. New York, WHO) a 1-hour immersion time when using 2% glutaraldehyde solution or hypochlorite solution with 10 000 p.p.m. of available chlorine. This will only be acceptable if no change in dimensions or surface detail occurs during the disinfection process.

9. Finally, the cost of the material should be considered.

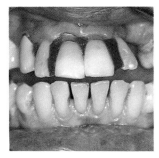

Figure 7.10 Large interdental spaces between the upper incisors have been blocked out with soft red carding wax. These teeth are not involved in the denture designed for this patient and the elimination of these undercuts will facilitate the removal of the master impression and strengthen the resultant master cast.

Naturally, none of the available materials is ideal for every impression and the material chosen will be based partly on the clinical conditions prevailing and partly on the clinician's preference. However, for partially edentate patients, the choice is limited to the hydrocolloid and elastomeric impression materials because of the need for elasticity.

Hydrocolloid impression materials

Reversible hydrocolloid impression materials (5.2.1) are not usually used for partial denture impressions because the need for a water-cooled tray conflicts with the desire to use a tray adapted to fit the partially edentulous mouth. The advantages and disadvantages of this material are covered in Chapter 5.

Irreversible hydrocolloid (alginate; 5.2.2) impression materials have been widely used for partial denture impressions since their introduction in the 1940s. Their viscosity when unset is low which, together with the use of a spaced tray (see later) means that they will only produce a *mucostatic* impression. Their elasticity is adequate, although clinical handling is important in this respect. Withdrawal from the mouth should be rapid otherwise permanent distortion of the alginate may occur and this clinical requirement conflicts with the rather poor adhesion of the material to the tray and with its low tear strength (see Chapter 1). A perforated tray has the added advantage that any separation of the alginate from the tray is easily visible so that a failed impression may be discarded. The poor tear strength is partly overcome by the use of a spaced tray as thicker layers of material obviously have greater resistance to rupture.

Silicone-reinforced alginate is also available (at an increased cost), and this appears to have an improved tear strength. However, it should be noted that if the material did not tear out of deep undercuts, it would probably separate from the tray; deep undercuts are therefore an indication for the use of a different impression material.

Even when set, the stiffness of alginate is not great, so withdrawal of the impression from shallow undercuts is easy, but this lack of stiffness also means that alginate extensions must be adequately supported when the impression is cast. Ideally, this support is provided by adequate extension of the tray, but in difficult cases extra support may be added by placing a backing of impression plaster (5.1.3) on the outer surface of the unsupported alginate.

The poor dimensional stability of alginate on storage and on disinfection are important failings of this impression material. Proper precautions should therefore be observed in the laboratory if this material is used. The high proportion of water in the material also means that the impression is unaffected by small amounts of moisture in the mouth. The impression may be cast in dental stone with little difficulty and the cost of the material is low. In this latter respect, it is worth considering the consequences of a failed impression, in the sense of a denture or denture framework that does not fit because of dimensional changes in the impression. The cost of a cobalt–chromium framework (see later) in particular is high and a small saving in cost on the impression material becomes irrelevant if even a small proportion of such castings fail to fit.

Elastomeric impression materials (5.2.4–5.2.6)

It is the disadvantage of the alginate impression materials, in terms of dimensional stability and in terms of the cost of the production of the denture, which has led to a wider use of the more dimensionally stable elastomeric impression materials, even though the material cost is higher. Four main types of elastomeric impression materials are available: condensation-curing and addition-curing silicone rubbers, polysulphide and polyether impression rubbers. As supplied, all of these materials have an adequate shelf-life, although condensation-curing silicones are less reliable than the others because of the instability of the catalyst. Their biocompatibility is generally satisfactory but hypersensitive reactions to the dibutyl tin dilaurate catalyst used in condensation silicones and to the dichlorobenzene sulphonate catalyst of the polyether material have been reported. In addition, the polysulphides in common usage have a lead dioxide catalyst which, whilst not being identified as a biological hazard, has an unpleasant taste and odour and is dirty to mix or clean from work surfaces, hands and faces.

There is a range of working and setting times available to suit individual preference and further, a range of viscosities both within and between the different materials. A medium viscosity is most appropriate for a special tray impression and may be used in conjunction with a low viscosity (fluid) material to record the detail of tooth preparations if desired. Heavy-bodied or high-viscosity materials are rarely used in partial denture impressions as their use in a close-fitting tray would lead to excessive mucodisplacement and overloading of the mucosal surfaces, as opposed to distribution of load between the teeth and soft tissues.

All of the elastomeric impression materials demonstrate excellent elasticity and adequate tear strength and this makes them suitable for the recording of significantly undercut areas. As they are less compliant than alginate, this makes their withdrawal from the mouth more difficult and possibly uncomfortable if any of the remaining teeth are mobile. In this respect the single-viscosity polyether material and medium-viscosity addition silicones are particularly stiff when polymerized. With these materials difficulty may be experienced in removing the impression from the mouth or the resultant cast unless a tray spaced around the teeth has been used to allow more room for the material to deform as it is removed. Care should also be taken with larger soft tissue undercuts and the tray may need to be modified by shortening the flanges in these regions (Fig. 7.11). This may limit their application in certain patients. The lower stiffness of the other materials means that, like alginate, parts of the impression unsupported by the tray may be distorted when pouring the dental stone cast. All elastomeric impression materials require the use of an adhesive to assist their retention in the impression tray.

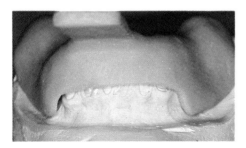

Figure 7.11 Modification of a special tray by shortening the flange to avoid the large soft tissue undercut labial to the lower incisors not required to be recorded for the construction of the denture.

Moisture must be carefully controlled during the impression procedure as all of the elastomeric materials are hydrophobic and the presence of any moisture will lead to lack of surface detail on the impression. In dry conditions, surface detail of the impression is excellent and, although problems have been reported with the poor wettability of silicone impression materials by dental stone, with care casts with excellent surface detail may be produced. In this respect the so-called hydrophilic materials are easier to cast since they are more readily wetted by the wet stone.

The dimensional stability of all impression rubbers is more than adequate to ensure a well-fitting denture and they may be stored for periods of up to a week without significant distortion, thus making transfer to the laboratory much more convenient. In general they withstand disinfection without dimensional or surface changes.

Factors in choosing a partial denture impression material

Because all of the materials discussed above are capable of producing an acceptable clinical result, the factors which will influence the operator's choice are once again likely to be cost, convenience, experience, the laboratory's preference and the clinical circumstances, including the type of denture to be provided. Where a few teeth are to be replaced with a simple, low-cost, acrylic denture, an alginate impression in a stock tray is often used, although the difficulty of disinfection is a real disadvantage. The replacement of a greater number of teeth increases the indications for the use of a special tray and a *mucodisplacive* impression technique, thus shifting the balance in favour of an elastomeric impression material. In the production of a complex, high-cost, cast cobalt–chromium denture the use of an accurate, dimensionally stable elastomeric impression material should be mandatory. In addition, the presence of significant undercut areas in the mouth is a strong indication for the use of the elastomeric impression materials.

Special impression techniques for the free-end or distal extension saddle

This type of partial denture must of necessity be partially mucosa-borne. For this reason a *mucodisplacive* impression technique is important to prevent rocking of the denture about the distal tooth abutment. The use of elastomeric impression materials in most cases fulfils this requirement. However, an alternative technique, most commonly known as the altered-cast or modified Applegate technique, is claimed to have some advantages over the more conventional approach.

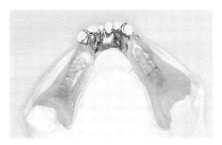

Figure 7.12 Modified Applegate technique. The partial denture framework is constructed using a conventional impression technique and to this is added, in the free-end saddle region, a close-fitting self-curing acrylic resin base, in which a *mucodisplacive* impression is made.

The partial denture framework is constructed using a conventional impression technique and to this is added, in the free-end saddle region, a close-fitting self-curing acrylic resin base (Fig. 7.12). This base is then relined in the mouth using an impression wax (7.1.2). These impression waxes are dimensionally stable at room temperature but will flow under load at mouth temperature. Even at mouth temperature they have a high viscosity so a *mucodisplacive* impression of the soft tissues covering the free-end denture-bearing area is obtained. Different viscosities of wax are available, the stiffer versions being used initially for the peripheral impression and the softer versions for recording the surface detail of the impression. The wax is first melted in a dish kept over a water bath at 60°C, painted on to the base, inserted into the mouth and left for up to 4 minutes to flow. No direct pressure is applied to the base but manual pressure is used to ensure the denture framework is seated on to the teeth. It is then removed and inspected, a matt surface indicates a satisfactory impression and a shiny surface an area where more wax is required. This procedure is repeated until the whole of the impression surface is successfully recorded. The master cast on which the framework is constructed is then sectioned to remove the saddle area of the cast. The framework plus the new

free-end saddle impression is reseated on the cast, and the free-end saddle portion cast in dental stone. The denture may then be completed.

This technique is claimed to have the advantage of a more functional mucodisplacement than that obtained using a setting impression material. The impression material will flow for as long as it is left in the mouth, thus permitting some recovery of displaced soft tissues until a balance is obtained between the soft tissue shape and the impression shape. The technique is, however, complex; great care must be taken in handling, transporting and casting the completed impression and there is no firm evidence that a free-end saddle denture made by this technique is any more stable than one made using a conventional impression. It does, however, have the clinical advantage of being able gradually to build the impression with repeated visual checks rather than attempting to record the whole impression surface at one time.

Since impression waxes are rarely used, some difficulty may be experienced in obtaining them and, in addition, the effect of disinfectant solutions on these waxes is unknown. Some of the advantages of the technique may still be gained using setting impression materials, such as impression rubbers or zinc oxide–eugenol impression paste (see below).

Working impression materials for complete dentures

Many of the properties considered for partial denture impressions are also of relevance in the choice of an impression material for complete dentures. In contrast to partially edentate patients, the denture-bearing area of completely edentulous patients rarely demonstrates severe undercuts and those that are present are often in soft tissue. Hence the choice of impression materials can include both rigid and elastic materials.

Impression plaster (5.1.3), alginate (5.2.2), zinc oxide–eugenol impression pastes (5.1.4) and impression rubbers (5.2.4–5.2.6) are all sufficiently accurate for this procedure. Plaster and zinc oxide–eugenol pastes are non-elastic and are not suitable for undercut residual ridges although plaster will fracture cleanly and may be reassembled. Plaster and alginate are not suitable for use in a close-fitting tray and require a spaced tray. They therefore record *mucostatic* impressions which are only appropriate where the residual ridge is noticeably fibrous or 'flabby' in nature. The effect of disinfectant solutions on plaster has not been reported, while their effect on alginate has already been discussed.

Zinc oxide–eugenol pastes are cheap but messy and the eugenol may cause mucosal irritation. Hence eugenol-free materials are also available (5.1.4). The operator's fingers, patient's lips and all instruments require liberal coating with petroleum jelly to facilitate cleaning. They require no adhesive but are difficult to remove from the tray if the impression requires repeating (a solvent or impression paste remover is available but is not very effective). Small additions can be made but care must be taken to ensure that the additions are not proud of the surface of the main impression, thus leading to pressure areas in the completed denture. Impression pastes are often slow setting and the setting point is difficult to determine. When the residual paste on the mixing pad fails to adhere to itself the impression is sufficiently stable to be removed from the mouth. The resultant impressions are compatible with glutaraldehyde and chlorhexidine but hypochlorite solutions are destructive.

All the elastomeric impression materials may be used, but the condensation silicones are used most frequently as they are sufficiently accurate and the least expensive. The closer the fit of the special tray, the lower the viscosity of the rubber required. Intermediate viscosities between the light-bodied or 'wash' materials and medium-bodied materials may be obtained by mixing appropriate proportions of the two materials. For a very close-fitting tray such as one made of silicone putty, a 'wash' material is appropriate, while for a special tray made on an alginate (mucostatic) primary impression a medium-bodied material is more suitable. No adhesive is necessary as impression removal forces are low (unless there is significant undercut) and the material is easily removed from the tray if repeat impressions are required. The material is clean, well-tolerated by the patient, sets rapidly and decisively, and small additions may be made, usually with a low-viscosity version of the material. As noted above, the mouth does need to be dry before using these materials, but overall the advantages in clinical handling and their compatibility with disinfection solutions easily outweigh the slightly increased cost of these materials.

Occlusal registration

Occlusal records will be necessary at several stages in the construction of a partial denture. Initially, study casts of the mouth will need to be articulated to help in designing the partial denture (see Chapter 1). Where the denture is to be provided with a cast cobalt–chromium framework, occlusal records are necessary to articulate the master casts prior to the construction of this framework in order to prevent the framework interfering with the occlusion. Finally, both the partial and complete denture master casts need to be articulated to allow the artificial teeth to be set in a harmonious occlusion.

Occlusal registration rims

Occlusal registration rims may or may not be necessary depending on the number of natural teeth remaining in occlusion. Where necessary, these should be constructed of hard modelling wax on a baseplate which is constructed of wax, shellac or self-activated acrylic resin. After a cobalt–chromium framework has been constructed, this is used as the base for the wax rim and forms the most stable base available. For complete dentures, permanent or heat-activated acrylic resin bases are almost as stable and the retention and stability of the final denture may be assessed at an early stage. However, they are expensive to construct, the master cast is destroyed so that overtrimming in the mouth is difficult to correct and they must not be allowed to dry during subsequent laboratory stages or distortion will occur. Wax or shellac on the other hand is notoriously unstable at mouth temperature and should therefore be kept cool during use, spending only short periods in the mouth, and avoiding excessive occlusal loading which may easily cause distortion.

The clinical handling of self-activated resin bases is less demanding as they are stronger and sufficiently rigid to withstand the normal clinical procedures. However, care must be taken both in their construction and in placing and removing them from the stone cast to prevent abrasive damage to the accurate cast. The use of self-activated acrylic resin (12.1.2) adapted to the master cast by the 'sprinkle' technique offers some advantages in closeness of adaptation by controlling curing distortion. Undercut areas can be dealt with either by simple blocking out, which leaves a space in the mouth and spoils the retention, or by filling these areas with a viscoelastic tissue conditioner. The latter is preferred to other elastic materials because of the good bond to the acrylic.

All of the materials used in the construction of occlusal registration rims are capable of disinfection by immersion for the recommended time, and this procedure is recommended in all transfers of appliances between the clinical site and the dental laboratory.

Occlusal registration materials

The occlusal registration material should be evenly soft during the recording procedure to allow the mandible to move to the desired registration position without the need for significant occlusal force. A harder material can displace mobile teeth, soft tissue-supported occlusal rims or even the mandible from its normal path of closure. The material should then set (or cool) to a rigid record without dimensional changes, and remain dimensionally stable on removal from the mouth, during disinfection, during transport to the laboratory and during the laboratory stages of articulating the stone casts. The use of wax, zinc oxide–eugenol pastes, plaster, self-activated acrylic resin and elastomeric registration materials has already been covered in some detail in Chapter 5.

Choice of occlusal registration materials

There is clearly no ideal material for recording the occlusion in every circumstance. The variety of materials available and the ingenuity and range of techniques developed and used are a clear indication of the problems involved. The choice of registration material is therefore essentially a matter of operator preference, with cost and convenience being strong influencing factors. Where sufficient natural teeth remain, both contact and precontact records will probably continue to be recorded in wax which, used in the manner described, with adequate precautions, will give satisfactory results. If a higher level of accuracy is required then contact records may be taken in elastomeric materials or supported zinc oxide–eugenol pastes, the latter also being suitable for precontact records while, if occlusal rims are necessary, zinc oxide–eugenol pastes are nearly ideal.

Reciprocal impression techniques (piezography)

These techniques are almost exclusively reserved for edentulous patients. Where adverse clinical conditions make the assessment of the denture space difficult a reciprocal impression or piezograph of this space is helpful. Since this space is a dynamic functional space changing from function to function a viscoelastic material, which responds to prolonged or repeated forces but not short-term forces, is desirable (Fig. 7.13). Tissue conditioner materials (13.3) which gel rather than set are therefore suitable for this purpose but must be mixed with a higher powder content than when used for tissue conditioning or temporary relining. This produces a stiff gel which can be handled with moistened fingers to produce a shape on a denture base for insertion into the mouth and subsequent moulding by the lips, cheeks and tongue. After 10–15 minutes in the mouth the impression is disinfected, coated with impression plaster at the chairside to stabilize the gel and then sent to the laboratory for conversion to a wax registration rim. Other materials have been used for this technique such

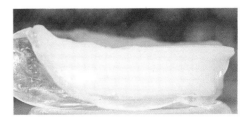

Figure 7.13 A reciprocal impression or piezograph of the denture space, recorded in a viscoelastic tissue conditioner supported on a mandibular acrylic denture base.

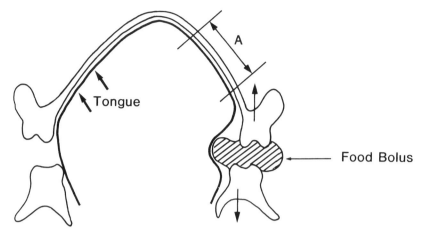

Figure 7.14 The thinner the denture base in area A, the greater the flexing under occlusal loading and the more locally concentrated the load.

as alginate or polysulphide impression rubber (supported by a thick wire rather than the denture base), but these have not received wide acceptance.

Denture base materials

Major (and minor) connectors

These may be constructed in acrylic (12.1), cobalt–chromium alloy (9.2.1), stainless steel (11.1) or occasionally gold alloy (9.1). All connectors should be rigid in order to transmit occlusal stresses to as wide a distribution of supporting tissue as possible. Since increasing bulk tends to increase rigidity, patient tolerance of this bulk is important in the choice of material. Similarly the material must be capable of being constructed to fit the mouth accurately and capable of being finished to a smooth surface.

Heat-activated poly(methyl methacrylate): acrylic

The need to provide a rigid major connector limits the design of such connectors in acrylic to the form of a plate of considerable thickness and extension. This, together with the poor thermal conductivity of this material, may reduce the patient's tolerance to these connectors. Care should be taken to map

out the areas of the mouth to be covered using palpation to assess tolerance.

Rigidity and mechanical strength

It is desirable that dentures do not significantly distort under masticatory loads. Acrylic has a relatively low modulus of elasticity and therefore the denture base should not be constructed less than 1 mm thick. The temptation to reduce this thickness to improve patient tolerance and comfort should be resisted as increased flexibility will lead to local concentration of loads (Fig. 7.14) and locally-accelerated residual ridge resorption. Fatigue failure, which is the result of constant flexing across the weakest area of the denture base, is also more likely. Impact resistance of denture base materials has also received considerable attention, although the most common reason for failure is fatigue rather than impact.

Dimensional stability

Acrylic shrinks on polymerization, expands on absorption of water and will distort if exposed to high temperatures. Polymerization shrinkage is reduced significantly by the 'dough' technique and the rigid mould used in the heat-activated technique, to the extent where it is only noticeable in the vault of the palate (see posterior border seal p. 102), although internal stresses will be created in the polymerized base. The absorption of 2% by weight of water into acrylic is only relevant if the denture is allowed to dry out repeatedly when it is not in the oral environment. This will result in crazing and distortion of the denture base. High temperature distortion may only occur if the patient is not warned against cleaning the denture in very hot water or if a local concentration of heat is produced by careless polishing procedures.

Appearance and maintenance of the denture base

Colour matching of acrylic to the oral mucosa is generally satisfactory and coloured fibres may be incorporated to give a veined appearance. Pigmentation is, however, difficult to achieve and the use of clear acrylic may produce a more satisfactory result in these circumstances. A contoured and stippled surface to the labial flange will give a better appearance than a highly polished and reflective surface but this does produce significant difficulties in cleaning the denture surface (Fig. 7.15). Over-enthusiastic cleaning with toothpaste or other abrasive cleanser may lead to noticeable abrasion of the surface and patients should be encouraged to use non-abrasive pastes (13.5) or soap, with a rotating rather than a scrubbing brush action (for denture cleansers, see Chapter 2).

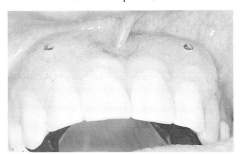

Figure 7.15 A contoured and stippled surface to the labial flange will give a better appearance than a highly polished and reflective surface. In this two-part partial denture the two metal tubes placed in the flange accommodate a key used to remove this part of the denture.

Patient tolerance

True allergy to acrylic is extremely rare. However, hypersensitivity to the residual monomer in the denture base is more common and may be characterized by soreness or burning sensations in the oral mucosa. An overnight or slow curing cycle used with the heat-activated materials produces the lowest residual monomer and rapid curing cycles should be discouraged. Denture-related stomatitis is usually associated with poor denture hygiene and/or other denture faults rather than any oral reaction to the denture base material itself.

Microwave-activated poly(methyl methacrylate)

This method of activation is used with the same materials designed for heat-activation. In general the properties of the resultant polymerized material and the processing changes are very similar for both methods of activation.

Self-activated poly(methyl methacrylate) (12.1.2)

The pourable denture base materials are the only self-activated materials which have been regularly used for permanent denture bases. These use an increased liquid to powder ratio to facilitate pouring the uncured mix into the mould which is usually a reversible hydrocolloid or soft plaster and their main advantage is a less time-consuming technique.

In pourable acrylic the monomer has only 20 minutes to wet and diffuse into the polymer beads so a less homogeneous polymer is produced. This results in a less rigid material with inferior fatigue and impact resistance. Dentures made from this type of material contain a higher percentage of residual monomer and this may act as a plasticizer, reducing the temperature at which distortion occurs, and increasing the tendency to creep under load. Dentures of this type undergo more processing shrinkage and are more porous. Although both these effects may be reduced by polymerization under hydraulic pressure in a hydroflask, the porosity means that they are more likely to stain in normal use. In addition, the chemical activators used may lead to poor colour stability.

Light-activated poly(methyl methacrylate) (13.8.2)

These materials have the convenience of self-activated acrylics but require specialized equipment. Their clinical performance is yet to be evaluated, but experimental work has shown lower values for mechanical properties than heat-activated materials and processing dimensional changes intermediate between heat-activated and self-activated materials.

High-impact acrylics

The incorporation of metal mesh or wires into acrylic acts to concentrate stress at the metal–acrylic interface and thus tends to weaken the denture base. High-modulus fibres such as carbon fibres when chemically treated to improve their bonding to the polymer matrix produce improvements in rigidity, impact resistance and fatigue properties. The carbon fibres are non-irritant but, although their use is restricted to the non-visible surfaces of the denture, their black colour reduces their acceptance. Recent developments using translucent organic fibres (ultra-high modulus polyethylene) with similar mechanical properties may overcome this problem. These fibres can be used either in the form of a woven mat (Fig. 7.16) or as cut fibres mixed with the acrylic dough.

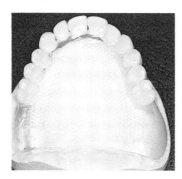

Figure 7.16 Translucent organic fibres (ultra-high-modulus polyethylene), incorporated into the poly(methyl methacrylate) denture base in the form of a woven mat, increase both impact and fatigue strength.

Commercially available high-impact denture base materials usually incorporate a microdispersed rubber phase into the polymer, although one type uses a rubber/methacrylate co-polymer. This produces improvements in both impact and fatigue resistance but there may be a consequent reduction in rigidity.

Radiopaque acrylics

The need for a radiopaque denture base material is related to the likelihood of fragments of fractured appliances being inhaled or swallowed, which is most likely to occur during accidents or fits accompanied by loss of consciousness. Sufficient barium sulphate cannot be incorporated into the polymer to give good X-ray opacity without serious loss of mechanical properties. A co-polymer containing 36–40% poly(2,3-dibromopropyl methacrylate) has been reported to possess satisfactory properties (Davy and Causton, 1982). Until this is commercially available patients at risk are best managed by using a high-impact denture base material.

Polycarbonates (12.2)

These are an alternative to poly(methyl methacrylate) as a denture base material and their impact resistance is up to nine times greater than that of acrylic. However, injection moulding techniques are required to process polycarbonate; that is expensive and few dental laboratories have the necessary facilities.

Cobalt–chromium alloys

Cobalt–chromium alloys are the ideal material for a major connector of a partial denture. They are rigid and strong in thin section, thus allowing a wide variation in major connector design. They are well-tolerated by patients, particularly because they can be used in thinner section than acrylic resins; they have good thermal conductivity and a low density for a metal, so that the resultant denture is light; and they may be finished to a high polish. They are very tolerant of the oral environment (and it of them) and, although they may be affected by some denture cleansers (see Chapter 2), they have an excellent life span in the mouth. They may be cast accurately and the material is inexpensive. However, the rather difficult laboratory procedures involved in casting and polishing the material tend to increase the cost of the denture so that they are significantly more expensive than an acrylic denture. They are rather difficult to adjust at the chairside. Abrasive stones or discs produce only slow removal of the hard material and it is impossible to add new material if underextension or overtrimming occurs.

Cobalt–chromium alloys may also be used in both upper and lower complete dentures to improve the rigidity and fatigue resistance of the denture base. In the upper denture the palate of the base is constructed in the alloy with a retentive framework for the acrylic teeth and flanges, while in the lower denture a lingual plate or internal framework is used. Fracture of the attached acrylic, especially on impact, is still a risk in either case but since the major cause of failure in an acrylic denture base is fatigue, this method of strengthening is clinically successful. Dimensional stability is excellent and there is no need for a compensating post-dam at the posterior border of the maxillary denture. However, adjustments of the hard alloy are more difficult and relining is impossible so some operators prefer to have the post-dam area added in acrylic to facilitate adjustment of this crucial area (Fig. 7.17). The alloy is denser than a polymer base and achieving retention of the maxillary denture is consequently more difficult. The laboratory procedures are more time-consuming and the denture consequently more expensive but there are no extra clinical stages in the construction of the denture. The metal base is incorporated by the laboratory during processing of the trial denture, thereby ensuring an appropriate positioning of the metal–acrylic junction related to the position of the artificial teeth.

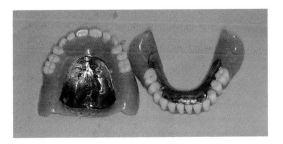

Figure 7.17 Cobalt–chromium alloys may be used in both upper and lower complete dentures to improve the rigidity and fatigue resistance of the denture base. An acrylic post-dam area has been used in this case to facilitate adjustment of this crucial area.

There is an occasional incidence of sensitization of the patient to the nickel contained in some cobalt–chromium alloys. For this reason, many alloys are now produced in a nickel-free form, which has the disadvantage of increasing the difficulties in producing a satisfactory cast. In addition, rare sensitivity to cobalt and chromium may occur. While sensitization to the alloy may not have serious consequences in the mouth, placing a metal prosthesis into the mouth of a patient already sensitized by a previous orthopaedic prosthesis may cause the primary implant to fail, with disastrous results. Before choosing this type of denture base, patients who have any implants of any kind should be patch tested for sensitivity to nickel, cobalt and chromium. Where positive results are obtained, an alternative denture base should be used.

Gold alloys (9.1)

Type IV gold alloys are now rarely used as a denture base material. Their modulus of elasticity is approximately half that of cobalt–chromium alloys so a denture in gold is much less rigid than one of a similar thickness in cobalt–chromium. The gold alloy is also denser and this, combined with the need to construct thicker, more extensive connectors to ensure rigidity, may lead to a very heavy denture, and a very expensive one. Consequently the gold alloy base is only rarely used for partial denture frameworks where sensitization to other metals has developed.

Stainless steel (11.1)

Wrought stainless steel has occasionally been used in the form of thin sheets as a maxillary connector, or in the form of a mandibular lingual bar connector. Swaging of the thin sheet is achieved by explosive or hydraulic pressure while the lingual bars are hand-formed with the use of pliers. The equipment necessary for the former method is now rarely available and the use of hand-bending of major connectors is to be discouraged because it is impossible to construct a rigid connector in this way.

Rests and reciprocals or bracing arms

These may be considered together because they are both required to be rigid in thin section to perform their supporting and bracing functions. They may, therefore, only be constructed in metal alloys and both cast cobalt–chromium and cast type IV gold alloys are suitable. As for major connectors, cast cobalt–chromium alloys are usually preferred.

Wrought stainless steel rests are occasionally used in conjunction with acrylic partial dentures (Fig. 7.18). These consist of short pieces of bent stainless steel wire (11.1.2) and, although they are less rigid and more likely to fracture than cast rests, they are clinically satisfactory and much cheaper to produce than cast alloy rests. The rather crude method of construction means that they may be used only where there is adequate space between the occluding teeth. Longer lengths of wrought stainless steel wire are not usually sufficiently rigid to be used as reciprocals or bracing arms, so acrylic plates are usually preferred for this function in this type of partial denture.

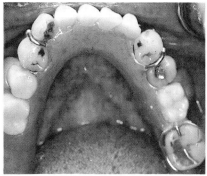

Figure 7.18 A wrought stainless steel rest used in conjunction with an acrylic partial denture providing support mesially on a lower molar. Ball-ended wrought stainless steel clasps provide some support by passing over the embrasures between the canines and first premolars.

Clasps

There are many factors influencing clasp design which are outside the scope of this book. However, the different materials available for the construction of clasps both limit the shape of certain clasps and allow versatility to overcome natural anatomical variation.

Cobalt–chromium alloys (9.2.1)

The very properties that make conventional cast

cobalt–chromium ideal as connectors are those that limit their usefulness as clasps. A clasp must be flexible, have a high proportional limit so as to deform repeatedly when entering and leaving the undercut area of the tooth and demonstrate complete recovery of the original shape.

The high modulus of elasticity of conventional cast cobalt–chromium alloys limits the undercut that a clasp in this material may engage to less than 0.25 mm. They are also easily permanently distorted so that clasps which no longer engage the relevant undercut are a common clinical finding on recall. In addition these materials demonstrate a low elongation at break (6% at best) and such clasps commonly break when adjustments are made or even in normal clinical use. Despite these failings, this type of clasp is still commonly used and this reflects the simplicity of casting the whole denture framework (major and minor connectors, rests, reciprocals and clasps) in one material, whereas the addition of clasps of a different material to the cast framework involves extra time and expense. In 1970 a new cobalt–chromium casting alloy called Crutanium, containing 4–10% titanium, was introduced. This was claimed to have an elongation at break of 10–15% and undercuts of up to 0.5 mm may be used, while the properties of the material are still perfectly satisfactory for the production of the other components of the framework. Clasps in this material are therefore much easier to adjust and are more effective both in short-term and long-term use.

Unfortunately, the casting of Crutanium involves a more demanding technique in which the alloy is cast under vacuum, and since its success depends upon the production of a good cast, only a limited number of laboratories will provide cast frameworks in this material and they are naturally more expensive.

Gold alloys

Gold alloy clasps may either be cast in type IV gold alloy (9.1) or cold-worked in gold wire (11.2). The lower modulus of cast gold alloys allows the engagement of a larger degree of undercut than conventional cast cobalt–chromium alloys but they are only conveniently used when the whole framework is being cast in the gold alloy.

Wrought gold wire clasps, on the other hand,

may be attached either by soldering or with acrylic resin, to a conventional cobalt–chromium alloy framework. Their design is limited by the round cross-section of the gold wire as supplied but the variety of shapes may be extended by soldering two pieces of wire together. The modulus of elasticity of wrought gold is even lower than that of the hardest cast gold alloys, so deeper undercuts may be engaged and adjustments are easily made. The only disadvantage of this easy adjustment is that they may be inadvertently adjusted by careless handling by the operator or the patient.

The extra cost of the gold alloy and extra laboratory stages involved in adding the gold clasp to the cast framework increase the cost of the final denture. However, the colour of gold is more acceptable to some patients than that of the base metal alloys and consequently they are commonly used for gingivally approaching clasps in the anterior part of the mouth.

Stainless steel (11.1)

Stainless steel clasps are commonly used in conjunction with acrylic dentures as they are not considered sufficiently precise or robust for use with the more expensive cast dentures. They are formed of cold-worked stainless steel wire, and as soldering of stainless steel reduces its corrosion resistance the variety of clasp shapes that may be formed is limited. However, a more expensive form of stainless steel clasp is available which is preformed by the manufacturer in a variety of designs and these require less work to adjust them to fit the individual tooth. A certain amount of skill is required in cold-working the clasp to fit the tooth as the process reduces the ductility of the material. The greater the number of adjustments made to the clasp to fit the tooth in the laboratory the more likely the clasp is to fracture both on subsequent clinical adjustment or normal use. Although their inherent flexibility will allow them to engage the same degree of undercut as wrought gold clasps, they are less likely to fail if slightly shallower undercuts are used.

Prefabricated attachments

Prefabricated attachments are sometimes used to provide retention for partial dentures although their

cost and complexity do limit their applications. It is not appropriate to consider the wide range of available designs in this text but they include spring-loaded devices which act to engage natural undercuts and devices with both male and female parts, one of which is attached to the natural tooth to create a retentive feature, the other being attached to the denture to engage it. Consequently, the requirements of the materials used in their construction are somewhat similar to those for a denture framework. Parts of the attachments will need to be rigid, while others will need to be flexible. They are therefore most commonly constructed in cast hard gold alloys, although non-precious alloys, stainless steel and nylon components are also used. The choice of alloy depends in part on how the parts of the prefabricated attachment will be fixed to the denture, and the tooth or cast restoration respectively. Attachment to the denture can be by soldering or by the use of self-activated acrylic, while attachment to the tooth can be by composite resin (using the acid-etch technique), by soldering to a cast restoration or by casting a cast restoration against the attachment. In the latter case the alloy of the attachment should be compatible with the alloy used for the cast restoration.

The properties of the hard gold alloys are quite satisfactory for this purpose with the possible exception of their abrasion resistance. Quite large stresses are often placed on rather small components which are precisely fitted together. As wear occurs they become less effective and this may be a serious disadvantage where one component is permanently fixed to a tooth and replacement is a major clinical procedure. To overcome this problem, bearing surfaces are sometimes made replaceable, or combinations of materials with different abrasion resistance are used: for example, stainless steel and nylon, with the component which is designed to wear preferentially being placed in the denture where it may be easily replaced. In a similar fashion the stainless steel springs that are usually used in spring-loaded devices are always easily replaceable.

Saddles

These are almost always constructed in acrylic as there is usually sufficient room to provide adequate bulk for rigidity and strength; acrylic is easy to process to the correct shape, easy to polish and it is an appropriate colour to replace gingival and mucosal tissues. Constructing the fitting surface of the saddle in acrylic has the advantage that this surface may easily be adjusted to refine the fit in the mouth and further, may be relined with a new layer of acrylic to compensate for resorption of the residual ridge. Where space is limited a metal alloy may be used for the fitting surface to provide strength in thin section and this is recommended in the totally tooth-supported stable base appliance. However, if resorption cannot be discounted the use of a metal fitting surface should be avoided as relining a metal fit surface is very difficult.

Artificial or denture teeth (13.1)

Artificial teeth are set into the wax rims for trial in the mouth prior to processing of the denture. They are available in numerous different tooth colours and moulds and posterior teeth are available with different occlusal forms ranging from 30° cusp angles to flat or inverted cusp forms. The choice of tooth form and colour is largely a matter of individual preference but the more expensive teeth are usually more carefully and accurately characterized in both colour and form.

Either porcelain or cross-linked acrylic teeth may be used. Porcelain teeth do not chemically bond to the acrylic denture base and require mechanical retention which in turn requires adequate space in the denture saddle – usually available in acrylic-based dentures but not often present in association with cobalt–chromium-based dentures. Acrylic teeth should form an adequate chemical bond to the acrylic base, but because of the high level of cross-linking of the acrylic used for these teeth, the chemical bond is not always reliable and mechanical retention is often advised for these teeth as well. Roughening of the surface of the acrylic tooth has been shown to increase the bond strength. Porcelain is more brittle than acrylic but shows better resistance to abrasion (Fig. 7.19). However, porcelain teeth are more difficult to adjust.

Special note may be made of the effect of peppermint oil (mint sweets) on acrylic teeth. Excessive use of such sweets causes softening of

the acrylic surface and often results in excessive wear.

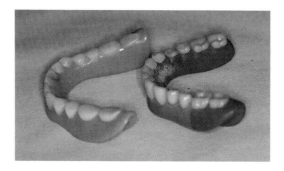

Figure 7.19 Two old and well-used mandibular dentures, clearly showing the different wear properties of (right) porcelain (on a vulcanite base) and (left) acrylic (on an acrylic base) teeth.

Teeth made with the occlusal and buccal portions utilizing a large molecular weight cross-linking agent (urethane dimethacrylate) enriched with 27% microfill silica are also available and these have an abrasion resistance intermediate between porcelain and conventional acrylic teeth. The remainder of these teeth are made of conventional cross-linked acrylic bonded to the modified resin during manufacture, thus facilitating the bonding of the teeth to the denture base. The need for such complexity may be questioned since, in general, the wear properties of acrylic teeth are sufficiently good to last the clinical life of most dentures.

In partial dentures where the artificial teeth occlude with natural teeth in the opposing dental arch, particular care must be taken to provide a material which does not wear too rapidly, as this may allow the overeruption of the opposing tooth. Since there is rarely sufficient space to accommodate porcelain teeth, cross-linked acrylic teeth are most commonly used and regularly reviewed for replacement when wear has become significant. Alternatively, if wear is likely to be rapid, a metal occlusal surface may be used, most simply by placing amalgam alloy (3.1) into the acrylic teeth at the point of occlusal contact, or by casting an individual cobalt–chromium alloy or gold occlusal surface (Fig. 7.20). This latter occlusal surface can only be used where it is not visible as it is aesthetically unsatisfactory and great care must be taken with occlusal registration as adjustment is difficult. Occasionally, the use of a metal occlusal surface will negate the need for a saddle – a hygienic pontic (similar to a bridge pontic) providing both the occlusion and the connection between other components of the denture on the abutment teeth.

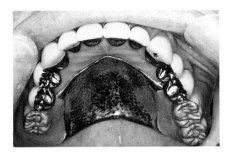

Figure 7.20 Gold occlusal surfaces on an upper precision retained partial denture used to reduce wear in function. (Courtsey of Mr D.L. Aitken and with permission of A.E. Morgan Publications).

Adjustment of dentures at the chairside

Adjustments to dentures may be required on insertion or subsequent recall to the fitting surface, the polished surface or the occlusal surface. The use of indicator materials (13.7) to diagnose the area that requires adjustment has been discussed in Chapter 1, and the difficulty of adjusting cobalt–chromium alloys compared with the ease of adjusting acrylic already referred to in this chapter. Fine adjustment of the mucosa-supported denture occlusion is particularly difficult because of the displaceable nature of the denture-supporting tissues which will mask small premature contacts by allowing the denture to tip or move horizontally. Ideally, the use of a central bearing device attached to the dentures to centralize the occlusal forces while recording a check occlusal record gives the most satisfactory results. However, this procedure involves an extra visit and laboratory rearticulation and adjustment of the occlusion.

It is usually unnecessary to polish adjustments made to the fit or occlusal surfaces, as a precise fit to

the mucosa or opposing occlusal surface is considered desirable. Further, a slightly rough fit surface is more easily wetted by saliva to form a protective and retentive layer between the denture and the oral mucosa. Only in cases of xerostomia may a polished fit surface be of benefit to the comfort of the patient, since any movement of the dentures is not being lubricated by saliva.

Polishing procedures used in the laboratory are outside the scope of this text but occasionally it will be more convenient to polish the adjusted denture at the chairside. Polishing is of course only appropriate once a smooth surface has been obtained using abrasive stones of varying dimensions and abrasivity. Acrylic may then be effectively polished using tripoli (1.8) on a small felt wheel in the dental handpiece. Gold alloys may be polished as described in Chapter 4, but cobalt–chromium alloys cannot be satisfactorily polished at the chairside.

An alternative method of restoring the polished surface of small areas of acrylic surface utilizes the unfilled resin (3.2.1) supplied with composite resin filling materials. This can be flowed on to the acrylic surface in a thin layer and cured (usually by light) to give a durable smooth surface. Small additions to the contour of acrylic teeth may be made in the same way using a composite resin of the appropriate shade.

Relining/rebasing dentures

Temporary relining materials are considered in Chapter 2.

Intra-oral relining materials

Polymerizing self-activated poly(methyl methacrylate) (12.1.2) in the mouth is to be discouraged because of the irritant effect of the monomer on the oral mucosa and the exotherm associated with its polymerization.

Higher acrylics such as a co-polymer of ethyl and butyl methacrylate (13.4) have an acceptably low exotherm and a non-irritant monomer and have been used as direct relining materials. Apart from the clinical difficulties of ensuring an evenly thin layer of relining material (thus avoiding changes in the occlusion), and the distortion that may occur when removing the partially polymerized material from undercut areas, the intraoral properties of these materials are not as good as those of heat-activated acrylic. Comment has already been made about the inferior properties of self-activated acrylic but these higher acrylics are weaker, distort at lower temperatures (around 70°C) and are more prone to staining and colour changes. They are thus best considered as intermediate between temporary and permanent materials.

Laboratory relining of complete dentures

This is carried out using heat-activated (12.1.1), self-activated (12.1.2) or light-activated (13.8.5) acrylic, the former giving the best result. The clinical procedure is similar to making a master impression for a complete denture in a close-fitting tray and the same impression procedure and materials are therefore appropriate. Again care must be taken to ensure a thin, even layer of impression material to avoid disturbing the occlusal relationships, and all undercut areas on the denture must be removed, otherwise the impression and denture cannot be removed from the master cast without breaking one or the other.

One technique for obtaining the impression which cannot be used with a special tray is the use of a viscoelastic gel (tissue conditioner; 13.3); as the impression material. This is applied to the denture as for temporary relining in a consistency which will allow sufficient flow to create a thin even layer, allowed to gel for 5–10 minutes, removed from the mouth for trimming of the periphery and then returned to the mouth for a minimum of 24 hours. The long-term viscous flow of these materials allows changes to occur in the impression in response to functional loading, while the elastic properties prevent short-term forces causing excessive distortion of the impression. The minimum period of wear is 24 hours because these materials are initially too sticky to allow a satisfactory cast to be made. Even after 24 hours, storage of the impression is not recommended because distortion may occur if the material is inadvertently loaded. Transport to the laboratory is therefore difficult and the impression should be cast as soon as possible.

Fitting and occlusal adjustment of the relined denture follow the same procedure as for new dentures.

Relining of partial dentures

The materials used in the relining of partial dentures in order to refine the fit surface of the acrylic saddle areas are very similar to those used for relining complete dentures. Of vital importance in the partial denture is the relationship between the fit of the saddle area and the fit of the tooth-borne part of the denture. Sufficient space must be made under the saddle for the impression material when the remainder of the denture is fully seated. Free-end saddle dentures most commonly need relining and in this case a mucodisplacive, reline impression is most appropriate.

Permanent soft denture lining materials (13.2)

These must not be confused with temporary soft lining materials or tissue conditioners (13.3; see Chapter 2). Unfortunately, the manufacturers do not always make this distinction clear but in general self-activated soft acrylic materials may be considered as temporary materials while the acrylic materials polymerized by heat and the silicone rubber materials are usually referred to as permanent lining materials. Since the displaceability of the lining is restricted by its bond to the rigid acrylic portion of the denture, a thickness of at least 2 mm is essential to achieve clinically acceptable softness. This can only be obtained by laboratory construction as it is impossible to control the lining thickness adequately if it is added to the denture in the mouth. Since the benefit of the lining is achieved by displacement of the lining from areas of high pressure rather than actual compression of the lining, it is necessary to extend the lining to the peripheries of the denture (Fig. 7.21), a boxed lining being restricted and therefore allowing less displacement (Fig. 7.22). The reduction of the hard acrylic portion of the denture to make room for the soft lining obviously reduces the strength of the denture. Where space is limited therefore, the denture may require strengthening, usually by the

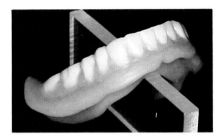

Figure 7.21 Soft lining material extended to the periphery of a lower complete denture.

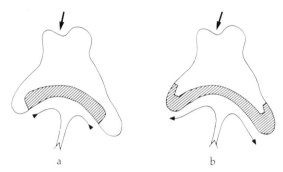

Figure 7.22 (a) Boxing the soft lining restricts its displacement and therefore its effectiveness. (b) Correct placement of the lining for maximum efficacy.

use of a cobalt–chromium alloy lingual plate (Fig. 7.23), these materials being most frequently used in the mandibular denture. Another occasional use is to replace a portion of the denture flange where the ridge is undercut, often in the tuberosity region. Here sufficient overlap of the hard and soft materials must be provided to ensure adequate bonding of the lining to the denture base acrylic.

Choice of permanent soft lining material

Self-activated silicone rubber materials (13.2.2) demonstrate high levels of water absorption, poor dimensional stability, poor strength, poor wettability and poor adhesion to the acrylic denture base, and are not therefore considered satisfactory as permanent soft lining materials.

Heat-activated soft acrylic resin materials (13.2.1) are initially satisfactory. As they are harder at room temperature than at mouth temperature, adjustment and polishing are possible. They demonstrate good

adhesion to the denture base but, unfortunately, the plasticizer, which confers softness to the acrylic, leaches out of the material in the moist environment of the mouth and the lining hardens and distorts, often after only 6 months' use.

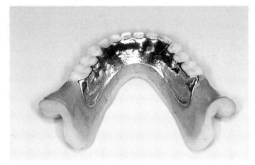

Figure 7.23 Lingual plate cobalt–chromium strengthening is often required in conjunction with the use of a soft lining.

Heat-activated silicone rubber materials, on the other hand, maintain their softness almost indefinitely and demonstrate low water absorption, giving good dimensional stability. Their adhesion to acrylic is unreliable but this can be overcome by careful processing, preferably against a part-cured acrylic resin, and utilizing mechanical undercuts if possible. They are difficult to adjust and finish, and polishing is impossible. This, together with their poor wettability, may lead to frictional damage to the oral mucosa, particularly if salivary flow is deficient. Despite these disadvantages, heat-activated silicone rubber is the soft lining of choice in most instances.

A new material based on a powdered synthetic elastomer, polyphosphazine fluoroelastomer, has recently become available but although laboratory studies demonstrate satisfactory properties, no independent clinical studies are available.

Duplication of complete dentures

There are many different methods of copying or duplicating dentures, some of which are laboratory-based and rely on the use of plaster masks of the (relined) existing dentures to produce wax trial dentures which are later conventionally processed.

One useful chairside technique (Fig. 7.24) allows the production of an acrylic replica of the existing denture which may then be modified by relining and/or occlusal addition/adjustment in the mouth prior to the production of the trial denture. An alginate mould of the existing denture is produced in a rigid box (either a suitably sized plastic box or two opposed stock trays) by making impressions of both the fit surface and the polished/occlusal

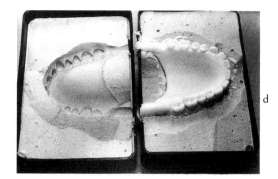

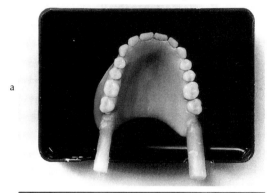

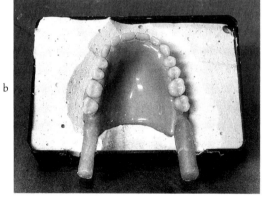

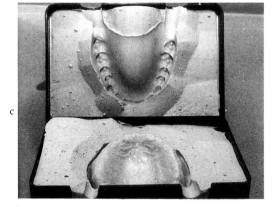

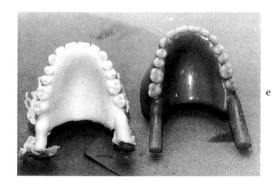

Figure 7.24 Production of an acrylic replica of an existing denture. (a) The denture to be duplicated is placed in a rigid box with wax sprues attached to the heels passing through holes in the side of the box. (b) An alginate mould of the fit surface and the periphery is made and trimmed with a sharp knife from around the teeth. (c) An alginate mould of the teeth and polished surface is made in the other half of the rigid box and the denture removed. (d) The box is secured together with elastic bands and a thin mix of self-activating acrylic is poured through the sprue holes, while at the same time the box is vibrated. When the acrylic is cured the box is opened. (e) An acrylic replica of the original denture is then formed which, after trimming, can be modified by relining and occlusal adjustment in the mouth. The teeth are then replaced with stock denture teeth and, after trial, the duplicate is flasked and new heat-activated acrylic denture produced by conventional means.

surfaces. The denture is removed and the duplicate denture produced by pouring self-activated poly(methyl methacrylate), e.g. pourable acrylic resins, special tray material, one of the intraoral relining materials, or a peripheral border-moulding acrylic (13.4) into the mould. The polymerization shrinkage and distortion that occur are compensated for by making a reline impression in the duplicate and adjusting the occlusion prior to the production of a trial denture in the laboratory. This simple technique has the major advantage of not needing to adjust the existing dentures in any way and involving the minimal time in which the patient has to be without the dentures.

Further reading

Barco, M.T. and Flinton, R.J. (1988) An overview of four removable partial denture clasps. *International Journal of Prosthodontics*, **1**, 159–164

Basker, R.M and Tryde, G. (1977) Connectors for mandibular partial dentures: use of the sublingual bar. *Journal of Oral Rehabilitation*, **4**, 389–394

Bergman, B. (1989) Disinfection of prosthodontic impression materials: a literature review. *International Journal of Prosthodontics*, **2**, 537–542

Burns, D.R. and Ward, J.E. (1990) A review of attachments for removable partial denture design: Part 1: classification and selection. *International Journal of Prosthodontics*, **3**, 98–102

Clayton, J.A. (1980) A stable base precision attachment removable partial denture: theories and principles. *Dental Clinics of North America*, **24**, 3–29

Davy, K.W.M. and Causton, B.E. (1982) Radio-opaque denture base: a new acrylic co-polymor. *Journal of Dentistry*, **10**, 254–264

Gunne, J., Hogstrom, J. and Nilson, H. (1990) Impression technique for RPDs. *Swedish Dental Journal*, **14**, 225–231

Kaaber, S. (1990) Allergy to dental materials with special reference to the use of amalgam and polymethylmethacrylate. *International Dental Journal*, **40**, 359–365

Ladizesky, N.H. and Chow, T.W. (1992) Reinforcement of complete denture bases with continuous high performance polyethylene fibres. *Journal of Prosthetic Dentistry*, **68**, 934–939

Lyon, H.E. (1985) Resin bonded etched metal rest seats. *Journal of Prosthetic Dentistry*, **53**, 366–368

Takamata, T. and Setcos, J.C. (1989) Resin denture bases: review of accuracy and methods of polymerization. *International Journal of Prosthodontics*, **2**, 555–562

Warren, K. and Capp, N. (1990) A review of principles and techniques for making interocclusal records for mounting working casts. *International Journal of Prosthodontics*, **3**, 341–348

Winkler, S., Monasky, G.E. and Kwok, J. (1992) Laboratory wear investigation of resin posterior denture teeth. *Journal of Prosthetic Dentistry*, **67**, 812–814

Wright, P.S. (1981) Composition and properties of soft lining materials for acrylic dentures. *Journal of Dentistry*, **9**, 210–223

Chapter 8
Orthodontics

Introduction

Recent advances in materials have had a marked impact on the delivery of orthodontic treatment. In particular, the ability to bond brackets directly and the development of aesthetic brackets and resilient wires have made orthodontic treatment available to a wider range of patients, including more adults.

The aim of this chapter is to give a general guide to the materials that can be used in orthodontic treatment without going into the specific requirements of any particular technique.

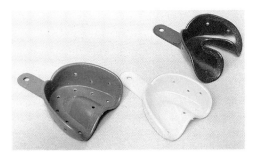

Figure 8.1 Disposable orthodontic impression tray.

Impressions (5.2)

When dealing with young patients, impression materials need to have a firm consistency to minimize the possibility of escape at the back of the tray, which is uncomfortable for a child. They also need to set rapidly to ensure that the procedure is carried out quickly. Disposable trays, which are designed for orthodontic use, should be used whenever possible, and these should carry extensions into the buccal sulcus to ensure that the study models include an adequate area of the reflection of the mucosa (Fig. 8.1). This is not merely for appearances sake, but it helps in the assessment of the underlying shape of the supporting alveolar bone. Models should be cast using gypsum mixed under vacuum to ensure that they are free of bubbles. Working models should be cast in dental stone (6.1), and study models in a hard white die stone (6.1.2).

Waxes

Occlusal registration to record intercuspal position can be made satisfactorily with standard modelling wax (7.1.1). When occlusal registration is required to record a postural position of the mandible, for example for functional appliances, then a combination of modelling wax and soft carding wax may be used. Modelling wax is firm enough to enable sufficient occlusal separation and for posture to be recorded, while softer carding wax (7.1.5) added to the lower occlusal surface of the bite block gives a more accurate index of the occlusion. This can be readily removed and replaced when a patient is required to rehearse a postural position, without any influence on the overall vertical dimension.

A soft white wax (comfort wax) should be given to patients who have had fixed appliances fitted to enable them to protect their cheeks from abrasion from the appliance. An alternative to this is to use a silicone elastomer (13.2.2)

Wires (11)

An essential requirement of any wire is that it is *biocompatible*. This is associated with the tolerance of the tissues to the alloy used to produce the wire, which must itself possess a high resistance to corrosion (sometimes called showing good *environmental stability*).

The wire must be capable of being formed into the required shape. This *formability* is related to the ductility of the alloy, which is an indication of its ability to be bent into the desired configuration without fracturing. If the alloy can be joined by either soldering (using an alloy with a lower melting point to form a metallurgical bond) or by welding (forming a metallurgical bond by localized melting without the use of a second alloy), it is said to have good *joinability*, and this is also a desirable property.

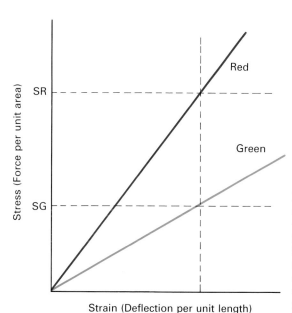

Figure 8.2 If the red and green wires have similar dimensions and are deflected the same amount, the strain in each will be the same. However, the force (SR) needed to deflect the stiffer (red) wire will be much greater than that required (SG) to deflect the less stiff (green) wire.

The elastic properties of the wire are those employed by the orthodontist to apply forces to teeth. It is easy to appreciate that, for the same

material, thicker wires are stiffer than thinner ones.The *stress* in a material is given by dividing the applied force by the cross-sectional area over which it acts, and the *strain* produced by this stress is related directly to the deformation that the stress produces. When the stress is divided by the strain it produces a unique value for each material – the *elastic modulus(E)* . This gives the *stiffness* of the material from which the wire is made, and in orthodontics it is sometimes known as the *load deflection range*. These properties are illustrated in Figs 8.2–8.4.

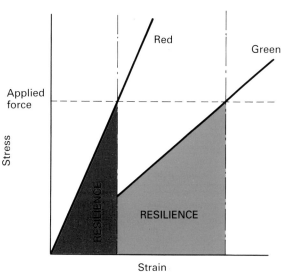

Figure 8.3 If the red and green wires are employed to apply a similar force to a tooth, the ranges of deactivation will be quite different. During deactivation, the force on the tooth (which is applied as a result of deflectin the wire in an elastic manner) falls as the tooth moves. Because the red wire is the stiffer of the two, this movement results in a more rapid drop in the force than it does for the green wire. Hence, appliances made from the red wire will require adjustment at an earlier date than those made from the green wire.

This figure also demonstrates the difference in *resilience* of the two wires. Resilience is defined as the amount of energy required to deform the wire elastically, and it is represented by the area under the stress/strain curve. Thus the green wire is seen to have a higher resilience than the red.

In practice, the useful range of activation of a wire is limited by the point at which a wire ceases to behave in an elastic manner and starts to show permanent distortion. This point is represented by the *yield strength (YS)* of the alloy from which the wire is made. If this value is divided by the elastic modulus (E), it provides an indication of the property known as the *springback (YS/ E)*. This is known by a variety of alternative names, including those of maximum elastic deflection, maximum flexibility, range of activation, range of deflection and working range.

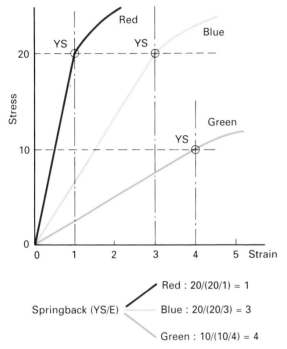

Red : 20/(20/1) = 1

Springback (YS/E)   Blue : 20/(20/3) = 3

Green : 10/(10/4) = 4

Figure 8.4 The red wire has a high yield stress (YS), but because it has a high elastic modulus its springback value is only 1. The blue wire has a similar yield strength, but because it has a lower elastic modulus, its springback value is 3. The green wire has a lower yield strength than the other two wires, but because it has an even lower elastic modulus, its springback value is 4. High springback means that the appliance has a long working time, which from a practical viewpoint means fewer visits for the patient to have adjustments made.

A further property, which is sought in wire for use in fixed orthodontic appliances, is a *low coefficient of friction*. If friction between a wire and a bracket is too high there may be little or no tooth movement due to binding, and anchorage may be compromised. However, the factors that control friction between the bracket and the archwire are numerous, with the slot size, bracket width, composition and dimensions of the archwire being just a few of the important variables.

It must be remembered that all of the mechanical properties described so far are fundamental properties of the materials from which the wires have been manufactured. The mechanical properties of wires in clinical use are highly dependent not only on the material, but on their diameter, length and shape.

Removable and functional appliances.

The wire that is most commonly and appropriately used for these is cold drawn stainless steel wire (11.1.2). The diameters that are used are from 0.5 mm for active springs to 0.7 mm for clasps and retainers, and up to 1.5 mm to give the rigidity necessary for connectors or extraoral face bows. In view of its increased yield strength and the potential for a longer range of action, there is a theoretical advantage in using heat-reated stainless steel wire for springs in removable appliances, but this has not found widespread use. The wire components of most functional appliances are primarily acting as connectors and 0.7 mm cold drawn stainless steel wire is usually the minimum size to use. Wire up to 1.125 mm in diameter can be used for some of the thicker connector wires.

Fixed appliances

A very wide variety of wires are used in fixed appliance treatment to deliver controlled forces to the teeth that are to be moved, and also to provide stability for the anchor teeth. No single type of wire can match these opposing demands and differing wire combinations are required throughout treatment. There are, however, commercial pressures to buy the latest, most flexible or resilient wire. These are not necessarily suitable for all stages of treatment, and to produce a satisfactory outcome of therapy with the fixed appliance technique requires the application of appropriate wires in various stages of the treatment.

Soft stainless steel wire (11.1.2)

Soft stainless steel wire which has been thoroughly annealled to relieve any work hardening is presented with a diameter of 0.009, 0.010, 0.011, 0.012 or 0.014 in, and is used for ligating archwires into brackets. Soft wire is essential as this enables the ligature to be tied tightly on to the archwire. This wire can also be used for maintaining groups of teeth together, for instance holding canines back once they have been retracted. Because of its low yield strength there may be some extension in length during use and the wire should be stretched as it is placed to reduce the amount of give in the wire.

In the 1990s stainless steel ligatures are used much less frequently than in the past in view of the difficulty of placing them when wearing rubber gloves and the simplicity of using elastic modules. They should still be used in the early stages of treatment to ligate nickel–titanium wire to teeth that are displaced from the line of the arch, for rotation ties and for secure ties when the full expression of a torquing archwire is required.

Archwires

Archwires are used to apply forces to the teeth via brackets attached to them. There are many different kinds of archwire and they differ in their composition, the method of their production, their diameter and their overall shape.

At one time stainless steel was the most commonly used material for archwires and nickel–chromium–cobalt alloys (11.3.3) have been used in the past, but they are rarely used in the 1990s. During the 1980s alloys of nickel–titanium and titanium–molybdenum–vanadium (11.4.1) were developed, and in view of their mechanical properties these alloys are now used almost exclusively in the early stages of fixed appliance treatment.

The way in which a wire is manufactured affects its physical characteristics and thereby its performance. Some are made merely by drawing through dies in the cold state, whilst another form is heat-treated to improve its properties.

Stainless steel Cold drawn stainless steel archwires are easy to form and, although the archwire work hardens during shaping, loops, coils or labial segment curves can be readily made from straight lengths of wire. However, because it possesses a low yield strength, it is readily distorted in the mouth (11.1.2).

Heat-treated stainless steel wire Largely due to the influence of the Begg technique, high tensile heat-treated stainless steel wire (Australian) is one of the best stainless steel wires available. It is difficult to form but is very resilient and is not often distorted in the mouth except in unsupported lengths. Its resilience makes it ideal, particularly when used with vertical loops for the correction of rotation or labiolingual tooth position, although it is difficult to form into loops. It is also one of the best wires for reducing the overbite by levelling the curve of Spee. However, it sometimes fractures when being formed or when in use in the mouth. The sizes most commonly used range from 0.012 to 0.020 in. The very lightest should only be used for accessory springs and the thickest wire only for the retention phase of stabilization of a treated malocclusion.

Unfortunately, wire of this quality is only available in round cross section. It is available in straight lengths, which is ideal for the construction of archwires which require vertical or closing loops. It is also available in a coil which can be constructed fairly readily to match an archform. In coil form it has the greatest resilience and is the roundwire of choice for reducing an overbite.

Braided stainless steel arch wires A variety of different types of wire made from braided stainless steel is available. These are produced by a number of different methods, including the plaiting of three elements together, or by plaiting a light wire around a single strand, i.e. a coaxial wire. They are also produced in rectangular cross-section of various dimensions for use in early stages of apical control in edgewise and straight wire techniques. The braided wires are very flexible and are good for initial alignment but they suffer from two disadvantages. One is that they are readily distorted in the mouth and require frequent replacement; the other is that the ends of the wire that protrude beyond the buccal tubes can cause trauma to the cheeks. This is because these ends are difficult to bend in the mouth and frequently become unravelled, giving rise to discomfort. This is particularly undesirable in the early stages of the treatment of a patient. However, they are cheap to produce compared with some of the titanium alloys.

Nickel–titanium alloy wire (11.4.1)

These alloys are an offshoot of the space research programme but they only became available for use in orthodontics during the 1980s. The first alloys to be used were in the *martensitic* form, but more recently an *austenitic* form has been developed for orthodontic use.

There is a wide variation in the composition of the alloys used and the manufacturers appear to be developing new alloys all the time. The method of manufacture of the wires gives rise to a range of characteristics and even wires with the same trade name may show batch variations of composition and hence mechanical properties.

The wires have low stiffness, low flexural rigidity, high range and high springback. They also possess a shape memory effect, which allows them to be deformed at, say, room temperature, and on warming to above a characteristic temperature (which is controlled by small variations in the composition of the alloy), they return to a shape which was built into them at an even higher temperature. This phenomenon occurs because the alloys exist in two different crystallographic grain structures – a low temperature martensitic phase and a high-temperature austenitic phase. As a result, they have the ability to transform from one structure to the other and back again.

The wires are thus available in three forms – martensitic stabilized alloy, martensitic active alloy, and austenitic active alloy.

1. Martensitic stabilized alloy is the original form and in the manufacturing process the shape memory effect is suppressed by work hardening. The change to the austenitic form occurs during activation and is responsible for the favourable force/deflection curve, which provides a constant force over a long working range.
2. Martensitic active alloys show *superelastic* properties, in that their stress/strain curves possess a region in which elastic deformation occurs without any significant increase in the applied load. These wires are not work-

hardened during manufacture and they have an austenitic–martensitic transformation temperature which is below mouth temperature. Any transformation that occurs in these materials is as a result of a stress-induced change in their crystallographic structure.
3. Austenitic active alloys allow the shape memory effect to take place as the wire reaches the temperature of the mouth.

Clinical points in relation to archwires

All forms of the wire are able to provide light forces over a long range of action. Nickel–titanium wires are ideal for initial alignment and correction of rotations but they are not rigid enough to be used for sliding mechanics, stabilization of anchor teeth or final stages of consolidation and retention. Because the wire is not easy to form, it cannot be used to make loops or hooks and it cannot be soldered. However, it is manufactured in both straight lengths and in archform shape. In addition, it is not easy to introduce any shape into the straight lengths, or to adjust the shape of the preformed arches, but this can be achieved by drawing the wire through triple-beak pliers.

The wires are presented in a range of sizes from 0.012 to 0.020 in and are also manufactured in rectangular cross-section. Rectangular nickel–titanium wire is also available in a variety of sizes and can be used as an intermediate archwire when changing from round wire to rectangular stainless steel wire. A rectangular braided nickel–titanium archwire is available, but whilst it is extremely flexible it is doubtful whether it has any significant advantage over the non-braided wires.

Coil springs made from nickel–titanium alloy are extremely efficient. They can be threaded on to an archwire to open a space between teeth, or they are available in different lengths and strengths for the application of intramaxillary forces.

The martensitic stabilized form of the nickel–titanium wire sometimes fractures in use. Also, the small-diameter wires tend to slide in the brackets, and either become displaced from molar tubes or protrude from their ends. This can sometimes be prevented by annealing the end of the archwire in a flame to enable the end of the wire to be turned over where it emerges from the end of the tube; however, when the teeth are irregular it is not always possible to estimate accurately the length of the archwire needed before tying it in.

The superelastic form appears to have better clinical properties for initial alignment and correction of rotations. In the mouth it can be retied over a period of several visits until full bracket engagement is obtained.

The austenitic-active alloy has the distinct advantage that it can be retied in the mouth and reactivation automatically occurs, hence the need for archwire changes is reduced. Its force/deflection curve is unique, in that there is little increase in force despite quite large alterations in deflection. This means that it can provide a physiological level of force over a long distance. Unlike the other forms of the nickel–titanium alloys, it can easily be formed and has a good shape memory, such that it always reverts to its original archform shape as soon as it reaches mouth temperature.

Studies of the frictional resistance between nickel–titanium archwires and brackets have provided contradictory results as to their comparison with stainless steel.

Beta-titanium alloy wires (11.4.1)

These alloys contain titanium, molybdenum zirconium and tin. They are similar to the nickel–titanium alloys in that they have a low elastic modulus (and they are moderately stiff) and good springback. However, unlike the nickel–titanium alloys, they can be worked to a certain extent, and it is possible to bend closing loops and other simple bends in the archwire. This is not easy to achieve, but it does give it advantage over nickel–titanium. It is also available in straight lengths, like the nickel–titanium, which can be useful particularly when using a sectional archwire. Its principal use is in the finishing stages of treatment, when it can be used as a rectangular cross-section wire with dimensions that nearly approximate to those of the archwire bracket channel. If one or two teeth require some additional torque, this can be readily built into appliances made in these wires.

Cobalt–chromium–iron–nickel wires (11.3.2)

These alloys were introduced primarily for techniques which require complex wire bending, especially in wires with rectangular cross-sections. The archwire may be constructed and shaped in a softened state and then hardened by a simple heat treatment, either by the passage of an electric current or by using an oven. This treatment gives the appliance a character similar to that of stainless steel. Classically this type of archwire has been used in the bioprogressive technique, but with modern materials it is doubtful if it now has much of a place.

Archwire form

There are two basic types of archwire – round and rectangular wire. Round wire can be used for any fixed appliance technique, whereas rectangular wire is designed for use in edgewise systems. Round wire can be readily formed into archforms and loops can be incorporated to increase its flexibility, to act as stops, or to create hooks for intraoral elastics. It is commonly available in straight lengths or in the shape of preformed arches. Whilst it can be utilized in all types of fixed appliance systems, including Begg and edgewise, if apical torque is required it necessitates the use of auxiliary springs. Rectangular wire, on the other hand, has the ability to control apical position of teeth in all three planes of space when used with edgewise brackets because of the interaction of the wire and its accurate fit in the bracket. The interaction of the archwire and the bracket is an important clinical consideration and wires with dimensions between 0.016×0.016 in and 0.019×0.025 in are commonly used. The dimensions of the wire and the size of the bracket channel determine the fit of the wire and hence provide control of the tooth position. However, this also gives a greater chance of applying excessive forces to the tooth. A detailed discussion of this topic is beyond the scope of this chapter.

Solder and fluxes (9.4)

It is possible to solder on to stainless steel archwire but it is not possible to solder to the titanium alloy archwires. Silver solder is necessary for soldering on to stainless steel and a fluoride-containing flux has to be used.

Brass wire is usually soldered to an archwire to provide hooks for the attachment of elastics and ties. Soldering is made easier by using presoldered brass wire. Whilst this is specifically designed for electric soldering, it can be used equally well with traditional soldering methods.

Directly bonded brackets and attachments

The ability to bond brackets and attachments to the surface of teeth has revolutionized the practice of orthodontics. Attachment is in most cases by means of a mechanical bond formed by an intermediate resin positioned between the bracket and the tooth. To achieve this it is necessary to prepare the surface of the tooth by acid-etching. Whilst the bond which forms must not fail during treatment, it is essential that the tooth is not damaged by the bonding process nor by the removal of the bracket at the end of treatment.

Brackets (17.1)

The selection of a particular design of bracket is dependent upon a number of choices which have to be made by the operator, and these relate to the technique that is being used. The variety of brackets is extensive and not within the scope of this chapter. However, of practical significance is the design of the bracket base as the attachment of a bracket to the tooth is by means of a mechanical lock.

Cast base

Undercuts on the surface of the bracket base can be produced by casting them in. These grooves are designed to produce a region into which the composite can flow, thus providing a mechanical lock (Fig. 8.5). In both clinical practice and in laboratory experiments the lock produced by this system does not seem to be as satisfactory as with other methods of providing retention.

Mesh base

These brackets are supplied with a fine mesh brazed

to the base and this gives a satisfactory form of mechanical lock for the composite (Fig. 8.6). The degree of lock can be enhanced either by electro-etching or by sand-blasting.

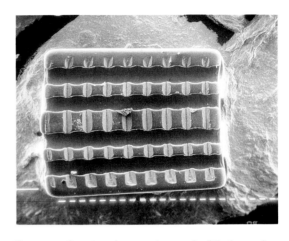

Figure 8.5 Scanning electron micrograph of the base. of a cast bracket. Courtesy of Mr D. Regan.

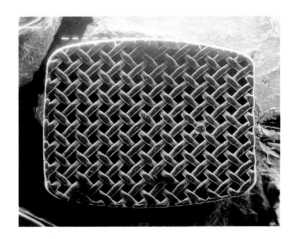

Figure 8.6 Scanning electron micrograph of the base of a mesh bracket. Courtesy of Mr D. Regan.

Aesthetic brackets

For some time a variety of brackets which are aesthetically more acceptable has been available. The earliest of these were made in polycarbonate, but these had several drawbacks. The prime disadvantage was that the bracket was not sufficiently rigid to be able to transmit forces, particularly torquing forces to the tooth. The other disadvantages were that they were prone to fracture and liable to stain. However, as they are cheap to produce, attempts have been made recently to reinforce them to give greater stiffness.

More recently ceramic brackets have been produced from alumina (aluminium oxide) in one of two forms – monocrystalline and polycrystalline. These are a considerable improvement on polymeric brackets but they are seven times as hard as stainless steel brackets and are therefore likely to give rise to enamel abrasion of the opposing teeth. Because of their stiffness, they are able to transmit torquing forces just as effectively as stainless steel brackets. However, they are much more expensive than the equivalent stainless steel brackets.

The amount of friction between ceramic brackets and the archwire is greater than that observed with stainless steel brackets. This may have clinical significance when reducing an overjet with sliding mechanics.

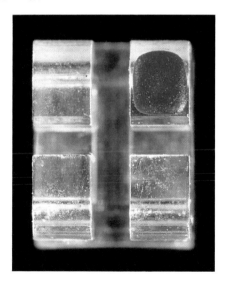

Figure 8.7 Monocrystalline bracket. Courtesy of Ms Lindsey Winchester.

Monocrystalline brackets

These brackets are made from single crystals of alumina, which are artificially grown into a shape which can be cut and milled to produce a bracket channel. With this material it is possible to produce a true Siamese bracket. The brackets are clear and have a glass-like appearance (Fig. 8.7). However, they are rather brittle and problems have been encountered with breakage of tie wings and other parts of the bracket.

Polycrystalline brackets

These brackets are produced by injection-moulding particles of aluminium oxide with a binder and heating to a high temperature, thus producing a bracket with an opalescent tooth colour (Fig. 8.8). Whilst they are less brittle than the monocrystalline brackets, they are still likely to fracture, especially on removal. Only single brackets or semi-Siamese are produced in polycrystalline alumina; as yet it has not been possible to produce twin pattern brackets. Hooks can be incorporated and brackets are available with hook attachments on their gingival aspect (Fig. 8.9). Special bracket removal pliers are required to aid their removal.

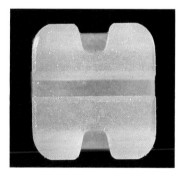

Figure 8.8 Polycrystalline bracket. Courtesy of Ms Lindsey Winchester.

Bonding and debonding aesthetic brackets

In the 1990s bracket bonding is achieved either by mechanical lock or by a chemical bond via a silane coating. When first introduced, both forms of bonding were tried by different manufacturers, and for a while the use of silane bonding became predominant. However, this gave rise to such a high bond strength that bracket removal became very difficult, and often resulted in damage to the enamel. So now there is a trend towards the use of more dilute silane solutions in an attempt to reduce the bond strength to the bracket and thus make debonding easier and safer.

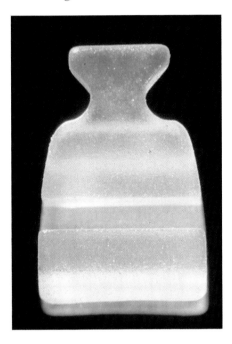

Figure 8.9 A bracket with a hook attachment on the gingival aspect. Courtesy of Ms Lindsey Winchester.

The excellent retention provided by these methods does give the advantage that loss of brackets during use is extremely uncommon and time does not have to be spent rebonding. Because of their stiff and brittle nature it is not possible to peel the bracket off the tooth as it is with the more flexible stainless steel. The bracket can shatter when attempts at removal are made, and it may be necessary to use burs to complete its removal, with water cooling to avoid overheating. It is unwise to use these brackets on lower incisors for two reasons: firstly, because they are difficult to remove it is uncomfortable for the patient and there may be a risk of damage to the crown, and secondly, due to the greater surface hardness of the bracket compared to enamel, they are likely to cause abrasion of the opposing teeth.

Future advances in materials will probably result in aesthetic brackets that are radiopaque, safe, convenient and economical to use. It is likely that in time these will replace stainless steel brackets on the upper anterior teeth.

Bonding agents

Etchant

To obtain a mechanical lock with the surface of the tooth the enamel has to be etched to a depth of about 25 μm by using phosphoric acid. This produces an etched zone with a subsurface porous zone and the bonding resin flows into this layer.

Phosphoric acid is used to etch the surface of the enamel and this is popularly supplied as a coloured gel with an acid concentration of between 30 and 50%. Although this is sometimes applied to the tooth for as much as 60 seconds, there is evidence that etching times of only 15 seconds are adequate, and similar results may also be obtained using weaker acids applied for longer times. A fluoride-containing gel is also available, which provides similar bond strengths to the fluoride-free acid gels, although the acid concentration is somewhat higher.

Bracket bonding agents (17.2)

There is a variety of adhesives available for attaching brackets to the teeth. These are usually lightly filled composites based on diacrylate resins. They fall into two categories according to their method of curing, namely those that are chemically activated and those that are light-activated.

Light-activated diacrylate

These consist of unfilled or lightly filled diacrylic resins, which are polymerized by the use of visible blue light. The use of this command setting means that there is an extended working time and a bracket may be positioned accurately on the tooth before the cure is effected by exposure to the light. However, the total cumulative time for bonding-up a complete arch is rather longer than that when using other techniques. This system requires investment in a curing light.

Chemically-activated diacrylate

These are supplied as either mix or no mix systems.

Mix system In this system the composite is activated by mixing two pastes together and placing it on the bracket base and immediately positioning the bracket on the etched surface of the tooth. This appears to produce the strongest bond strengths but surplus cement is difficult to remove from around the bracket once it has set.

No mix technique In this system the chemical initiator for the polymerization reaction is incorporated in a liquid which is painted on to the surfaces of both the tooth and the base of the bracket. The composite resin, which contains a chemical activator, is then placed on the bracket base before positioning on the tooth. One of the disadvantages of this system is that the bracket may slide on the surface of the tooth before the cement has set. Polymerization occurs most readily in the absence of oxygen and therefore the surplus cement around the edge of the bracket tends to remain unset, which makes for easy removal of the surplus. This method is currently the most popular for bracket bonding.

Glass–ionomer cements (2.1.10)

These can be used for directly bonding brackets on to teeth. The advantage of their use is that it is not necessary to etch the surface of the enamel. However, the bond strength achieved is not as high as that with composite resin cements. If ionomer cement is used, care must be taken to keep the tooth dry until the cement has set and archwires must not be tied in until at least 20 minutes after the brackets have been bonded.

Bracket removal

It is possible to aid the removal of composite-retained brackets by the use of peppermint oil. This is placed around the edge of the bracket where it partially dissolves the composite and renders bracket removal easier than hitherto. Excess adhesive must be removed with burs specifically designed for trimming composite, taking care not to damage the enamel.

Cements

Cements are used in orthodontics primarily for the fixation of bands, particularly molar bands and, where necessary, premolar bands. Glass–ionomer cements have proved to be exceptionally useful for retaining molar bands as they adhere to both the surface of the enamel and the stainless steel of the bands. As the bond to the stainless steel is slightly less than that to enamel, if the band becomes loose then there is minimal damage to the surface of the tooth under the band as the failure is at the junction between the band and the cement. The cement remains attached to the tooth with little chance of decalcification occurring. They also have the advantage that they release fluoride ions which may inhibit decalcification around the periphery of the band.

An alternative cement is zinc phosphate. However, whilst this is just as strong as glass ionomer cement, it does not adhere to either the enamel or the stainless steel. Failures thus tend to be more frequent, with a greater chance of decalcification.

Polycarboxylate cements have been found to be unsatisfactory and their use cannot be recommended.

Elastics (11.5.1)

Elastics are used to provide intra-arch and interarch forces. These are best provided by polyurethane elastics, which are available in a variety of different sizes, thicknesses and strengths. They are supplied in a range of colours to enable the patient to remember the strength of elastic being used. After about a day-and-a-half, water saturation and hysteresis plasticizes them and they become soft and less effective and must be replaced by the patient.

Bracket elastics

The use of elastics to engage the archwire into brackets is now common practice. They are quick and easy to apply, are comfortable for the patient, and they do not have the difficulty associated with the application of steel ligatures when working with rubber gloves. They are available in a range of diameters and thicknesses, and are often coloured to encourage patient motivation. To obtain an adequate force it is sometimes necessary to double the elastic over both sides of a Siamese bracket. They are particularly useful for engaging a tooth which is displaced from an archwire, as when they are stretched they apply the necessary force needed for minor tooth movements. However, full expression of the torquing values cannot be achieved with bracket elastics and it is better to use stainless steel ligatures to achieve this.

Chain elastics

Polyurethane elastic chain is commonly used in orthodontics for tooth movement along archwires and also for bringing a displaced tooth into the line of the arch. It is available in a range of sizes, which have different lengths between the rings that fit over the brackets. This allows them to be used in a variety of clinical situations such as moving lower incisors, where the interbracket distance is smaller than that used with upper incisors, and in situations where different forces are needed in various parts of an arch. This can also be useful for applying intramaxillary forces when applied directly to the brackets; however, it is difficult to measure the force applied and the force level decays fairly rapidly. Chain elastics are thus most useful for closing small spaces. To close larger spaces it is preferable to use an elastomeric module on a ligature, which is itself tied from the molar hook to a hook on the archwire mesial to the canine. Chain elastics have the disadvantage that they are difficult to keep clean and tend to accumulate food debris. If breakage occurs there is the possibility of unwanted tooth movement taking place, for example space opening at the site of the failure.

Elastic ligature

Elastic ligature or thread made from polyurethane is available in several forms, the main ones being either a solid thread or very fine tubing. Tubing has the advantage that when a knot is tied in it the tubing is compressed and the knot remains tight, thus overcoming the problem of the knot untying in the mouth. Elastic ligature has three main functions:

1. to assist in the correction of rotations;
2. to bring a displaced tooth into the arch; and
3. to promote space closure.

When used to correct rotations, especially of premolars, elastic thread is tied to a cleat on the palatal aspect of the rotated premolar, and attached to the buccal archwire. Care must be taken to ensure that the thread does not cross the occlusal surface of the rotated tooth. However, it is extremely strong and is not usually broken by occlusal forces. It has a long range of action but it is difficult to gauge the force being applied.

It is used in a similar way for bringing a displaced tooth such as a canine into the arch with a cleat or attachment bonded to the tooth and the elastic thread coupled to the archwire.

Care must be taken to ensure that the direction of force is appropriate and a hook or a loop in the archwire may be necessary to achieve this. The thread has a relatively long range of action but will require replacement at each visit. It is, however, a most efficient way of bringing a tooth into the line of the arch.

Space closure

Elastic thread may also be used to close space between incisors, in which case the thread is tied in a figure of eight around the incisors, taking precautions, such as applying a temporary lump of composite, to prevent the thread slipping into the gingival sulcus, causing damage. The end of the elastic thread must be cut and the spare end tucked away, otherwise it may obtrude into the lip. A disadvantage is that it is difficult to gauge the force being applied in this manner. The elastic thread may also be used for space closure in the buccal segments, or for intramaxillary traction.

Polymeric bases and materials

Acrylic (12.1)

Acrylic resin is used extensively in the construction of removable and functional appliances. For removable appliances a self-activated material is generally used as the thickness of the acrylic can be carefully controlled, especially where it covers the tags of springs and clasps. It is not as strong as heat-activated acrylic but is generally considered to be satisfactory for most removable appliances. A clear base is preferable to pink or other colours for the construction of appliances as this enables the tissues under the appliance to be examined for areas of displacement when it is in the mouth.

Heat-activated acrylic

This is stronger than self-activated acrylic and is the material of choice for functional appliances where high strength is required, for example the functional regulator of Frankel.

Self-activated higher acrylics, such as those used in temporary crowns or border-moulding, are used for adding to appliances which are going to be replaced immediately in the mouth. These resins are most useful for additions to removable and functional orthodontic appliances. They are thixotropic and can be readily managed as they start to set. They are especially useful for building up bite planes on removable appliances.

Thermoformed sheet

Rigid sheets of co-polymers such as poly(butadiene-styrene), may be shaped when warm using vacuum or pressure-forming techniques. These sheets are supplied in various thicknesses and are useful for the construction of splints and retainers. Flexible splints may also be formed in this way from sheets of poly(vinyl acetate). However, because of their softness they can be readily destroyed in the mouth and have only a limited lifespan.

Further reading

General

Gottlieb, E.L. and Vogels, D.S. (1984) 1983 JCO Orthodontic practice study. Part 1: Trends, Part 2: Practice success. *Journal of Clinical Orthodontics*, 18, 167–173, 247–253

Wires

Kapila, S. and Sachdeva, R. (1980) Mechanical properties and clinical applications of orthodontic wires. *American Journal of Orthodontic and Dentofacial Orthopedics*, 96, 100–109

Khier, S.E., Brantley, W.A. and Fournelle, R.A. (1988) Structure and mechanical properties of as-received and heat-treated stainless steel orthodontic wires. *American Journal of Orthodontic and Dentofacial Orthopedics*, 93, 206–212

Khier, S.E., Brantley, W.A. and Fournelle, R.A. (1991) Bending properties of superelastic and non-superelastic nickel-titanium orthodontic wires. *American Journal of Orthodontic and Dentofacial Orthopedics*, 99, 310–318

Kusy, R.P. and Whitley, J.Q. (1990) Dynamic mechanical properties of straight titanium alloy archwires. *Dental Materials*, 6, 228–236

Tidy, D.C. (1989) New wires for old. *Dental Update*, 16, 137–145.

Waters, N.E., Houston, W.J.B. and Stephens, C.D. (1976) The heat-treatment of wires: a preliminary report. *British Journal of Orthodontics*, 3, 217–222

Brackets and bonding

Garcia-Godoy, F. Hubbard, G.W. and Storey, A.T. (1991) Effect of fluoridated etching gel on enamel morphology and shear bond strength of orthodontic brackets. *American Journal of Orthodontics and Dentofacial Orthopedics*, 100, 163–170

Sadowsky, P.L., Retief, D.H., Cox, P.R. *et al.* (1990) Effect of etchant concentration on the retention of orthodontic brackets: an *in vivo* study. *American Journal of Orthodontics and Dentofacial Orthopedics*, 98, 417–421

Smith, N.R. and Reynolds, I.R. (1991) A comparison of three bracket bases. An *in vitro* study. British Journal of Orthodontics, 18, 15-20.

Waldron N. (1991) An alternative method for debonding ceramic brackets. *American Journal of Orthodontics*, 18, 370–371

Bracket–wire friction

Angolkar, P.V., Kapila, S., Duncanson, M.G. Jr. and Nanda, R.S. (1990) Evaluation of friction between ceramic brackets and orthodontic wires of four alloys. *American Journal of Orthodontics and Dentofacial Orthopedics*, 98, 499–506.

Ireland, A.J., Sherriff, M. and McDonald, F. (1991) Effect of bracket wire composition on frictional forces *European Journal of Orthodontics*, 13, 322–328

Kusy, R.P. and Whitley, J.Q. (1990) Coefficients of friction for arch wires in stainless steel and polycrystalline alumina bracket slots. I. The dry state. *American Journal of Orthodontics and Dentofacial Orthopedics*, 98, 300–312

Tidy, D.C. (1989) Frictional forces in fixed appliances. *American Journal of Orthodontics and Dentofacial Orthopedics*, 96, 249–254

Bracket wear of enamel

Douglass, J.B. (1989) Enamel wear caused by ceramic brackets. *American Journal of Orthodontics and Dentofacial Orthopedics*, 95, 96–98

Viazis, A.D., DeLong, R., Bevis, R.R. *et al.* (1990) Enamel abrasion from ceramic orthodontic brackets under an artificial environment. *American Journal of Orthodontics and Dentofacial Orthopedics*, 98, 103–109

Banding cements

Stirrups, D.R. (1991) A comparative clinical trial of a glass-ionomer and a zinc phosphate cement for securing orthodontic bands. *British Journal of Orthodontics*, **18**, 15-20

Elastics

Ferriter, J.P., Meyers, C.E. Jr and Lorton, L. (1990) The effect of hydrogen ion concentration on the force-degradation rate of orthodontic polyurethane chain elastics. *American Journal of Orthodontics and Dentofacial Orthopedics*, **98**, 404–410

Part Three

Properties of dental materials

A classified list of the materials referred to in Part Two with further details of their properties

1 Instruments, burs, abrasives and polishes

1.1 Straight hand instruments

Types

Carvers, chisels, condensers, excavators, plastics, probes, scalers, mouth mirrors, spatulas.

Presentation

These can be either one-piece, medium-carbon stainless steel (0.4–0.6% carbon; 12% chromium) or they can have steel or anodized (black) aluminium tips with either chromium-plated brass or ceramic handles. Composites and polyalkenoate cements tend to stick less readily to anodized aluminium. Instruments for handling composites are also available made completely out of polymer or with polymer-coated tips. Scalers and chisels often have a shaped tungsten carbide–cobalt composite tip brazed to the steel. Reusable dental mirrors are either silvered on the front surface of glass, which gives a clearer image, or are silvered on the rear of the glass, which makes them less vulnerable to damage. Disposable mirrors are made from a metal-coated polymer film.

1.2 Surgical instruments

1.2.1 Forceps

Constructed out of stainless steel, which is heat-treated to give them the strength needed to withstand the high stresses encountered in use.

1.2.2 Elevators and chisels

These have tempered steel tips and often have hollow stainless steel handles.

1.3 Orthodontic instruments

To resist indentation and deformation, orthodontic pliers are made out of tough, extra-hard stainless steel.

1.4 Maintenance of instruments

Instruments can be sharpened with stones or abrasive discs at the chairside. However, as the steel is heat-treated during the manufacture of the instrument to obtain the optimum springiness (temper), instruments should not be allowed to reach red heat, otherwise they will lose their springiness.

Tungsten carbide instruments are usually sharpened by specialists.

1.5 Sterilization of instruments

The following methods are suitable for sterilizing steel instruments, except where indicated:-

1.5.1 Autoclaving

Distilled water should be used without any kind of additives.

1.5.2 Dry heat

The temperature must not exceed 160°C, as this can cause loss of the temper of the steel which could cause failure in a stress-bearing area under load. Instruments with hollow handles, such as elevators, should not be sterilized in this way.

1.5.3 Cold disinfectants

Solutions which contain chlorine or iodophors should be avoided, because, although they are effective disinfectants, they are corrosive. Quaternary ammonium compounds and phenols are safe for metals but ineffective against many viruses. The optimum agent is a 2% alkaline solution of glutaraldehyde together with sodium phenate, e.g. Cidex; Sporicidin; Totacide.

After sterilization, all instruments should be dried with a sterile towel and stored dry.

1.6 Rotary instruments (burs)

Types

Round, fissure (cylindrical or tapered, cross-cut or plain), inverted cone and other shapes for special purposes.

Presentation

1. *Steel:* single piece of tempered tungsten–vanadium alloy steel with machined cutting edges.
2. *Tungsten carbide:* a stainless steel shank to which is brazed or welded a tungsten carbide–cobalt composite tip, which is then ground with diamond to produce the cutting edges.
3. *Diamond:* a steel shape (former) to which graded industrial diamonds are bonded by an electroplated metallic layer.
   (*Common brands:* D&Z; GC Smooth Cut; HiDi; Jico-Max; Komet; Meisinger; Premier; TDA Diamonds; U.S.A.)

International Organization for Standardization (ISO) bur numbering system This was introduced in 1986 and identifies completely any bur in terms of the material of its working part (steel, tungsten carbide or diamond), the sort of handpiece fitting (friction, ratchet or laboratory), the shape and length (if appropriate) of the working part and its surface characteristics, e.g. grain of the abrasive or pattern of the cutting surface and, finally, the diameter of the largest section of the working part.

As an example, here is a medium-grain, diamond fissure bur suitable for use in a friction grip handpiece.

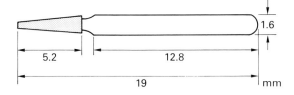

Its ISO number is

806	314	173	524	014
A	B	C	D	E

A refers to the material of the head. The choices are:-

Steel	310
Tungsten carbide	500
Diamond	806

B indicates what sort of handpiece is needed. The choices are:-

	Shank diameter (mm)	length (mm)
Standard laboratory handpiece	104 2.35	44.5
3 mm laboratory handpiece	124 3.00	44.5
Right-angle (ratchet)	204 2.35	22.0
Short friction grip (FG)	313 1.60	16.5
Standard friction grip (FG)	314 1.60	19.0

C indicates the shape and size of the working part and how the cutting surface is distributed. For example, some diamond-coated fissure burs bear the numbers 197 and 198 according to the height of the cone. However, similar burs without diamond at their tips bear the numbers 218 and 219.

The complete list is too extensive to include here, and reference should be made to the data sheets of each manufacturer. However, the shape ranges are as follows:

Round shapes	001–002
Inverted cones	010–020
Diablo/double cones	030–039
Wheels	040–099
Cylinders	100–150
Cones	160–229
Pears/flames	230–299
Discs	320–399

D represents the surface finish. For diamond-coated burs the possibilities are:

Ultra-fine	494
Super-fine	504
Fine	514
Medium	524
Coarse	534

Some manufacturers place coloured rings on the bur shank to identify the surface finish, e.g.

Super-fine	Yellow
Fine	Red
Medium	No colour
Coarse	Green

For machine-cut burs in tungsten carbide or steel the designations include:

Straight tooth	001
Right-hand, twist	006
Cross-cut, twist	007
Double diagonal	019
Coarse flute	071
Fine flute	072
Fine diamond cut	140
Medium tooth lab.	175
Coarse diamond cut	190
Coarse tooth lab.	215
Medium coarse diamond cut	220

E indicates the maximum diameter of the working part and varies as follows:-

Round burs	008–033
Inverted cones	008–060
Wheels	008–100
Cylinders	008–027
Cones	009–040
Pears/flames	010–025
Discs	200–220

where 008 is equivalent to 0.8 mm and 220 is equivalent to 22 mm.

Handling

Relative hardness values (Vickers pyramid number):

Dentine	60
Enamel	300
Steel	750
Tungsten carbide	1500
Diamond	Hardest known material

The cutting efficiency increases with the difference in the hardness values. Water cooling protects the pulp and the bur from overheating and removes debris from the cutting edges.

Sterilization

Diamond and tungsten carbide burs After use burs should be placed in a holding solution of 0.2% glutaraldehyde and sodium phenate (e.g. ID 220 or

Sporicidin) for at least 10 minutes. Cleaning with either a bur brush or in an ultrasonic bath containing a neutral solution should follow. Sterilization in an autoclave or dry heat sterilizer will complete the cleaning cycle.

Steel burs The warm, moist environment of an autoclave allows steel burs to corrode. Therefore it is not recommended. Steel burs should be sterilized by dry heat or by immersion in a concentrated cold sterilant for 10 minutes prior to ultrasonic cleaning.

1.7 Abrasives

Types and composition

Graded by hardness and by size of the abrasive particles
1. Hard abrasives:

Diamond	
borides	Chromium
Carbides	Boron, tungsten, silicon (carborundum)
Oxides	Silicon (silica, sand, quartz); aluminium (alumina) aluminium/iron (emery-natural, impure aluminium oxide, also known as corundum)

2. Medium abrasives:

Silicates	Magnesium/aluminium (garnet); pumice, tripoli
Zircates	Zirconium silicate
Kieselguhr	Diatomaceous silica: also used as an inert filler in impression materials.

Action

By definition, abrasives must be harder than the substance to which they are applied so that surface layers are removed by the action of the abrasive.

Handling

Presented for use in the form of:

1. Powders of various particle sizes stuck to, or extruded as part of, flexible strips or discs made of paper, cloth, polymer, metal or metallic glass (e.g. Enhance; Microflex; Soflex)

2. Powders of various particle sizes bound together in a soft matrix and presented as cutting discs, rubber wheels, points and cups (e.g. Identoflex).
3. Pastes and soap bricks, including flavoured prophylaxis paste (prophy paste) free from oil (e.g. Oraproph; Proxyl (coarse, medium and fine); Zircate Prophy).
4. Pastes containing finely divided abrasives such as alumina in a glycerine base are designed to produce a smooth finish on composite surfaces (e.g. Compafin; Prisma Gloss).
5. Baker-Curzon burs, consisting of a steel shank to which is brazed a *bladeless* tungsten carbide–cobalt composite tip for finishing preparations and restorations.

1.8 Polishing materials

Composition

Calcium carbonate (whiting: precipitated chalk). Oxides: zinc, tin, iron (rouge), chromium. Sodium bicarbonate (used in air-polishing). Dentifrices: calcium phosphate, magnesium oxide, acrylic spheres.

Action

Involves the flow of surface layers to produce a smooth (smeared) finish. Although little material is removed, polishes are really mild abrasives. In metals the smeared surface is known as a Beilby layer.

Handling

Presented in the form of:

1. Powders: used as a slurry, i.e. suspension in water or alcohol.
2. Powders bound in a soft matrix, e.g. pastes and soap bricks.
3. Oil- and fluoride-free pastes for use prior to acid-etching, e.g. Nupro (fine, medium, coarse); Orapol.
4. Silicone rubber polishing cups, webbed and ribbed (soft, medium, hard); flame-shaped points and lens-shaped discs (coarse, medium, fine).

Further reading

Bloxham, G.P., Dennison, J.D. and Charbeneau, G.T. (1990) A clinical scanning electron microscope study of tooth surface preparation and bonding. *Australian Dental Journal*, **35**, 345–351

Brockman, S.L., Scott, R.L. and Eick, J.D. (1990) A scanning electron microscopic study of the effect of air polishing on the enamel-sealant surface. *Quintessence International*, **21**, 201–206

Lester, K.S. and Mitchell, P.T. (1990) An evaluation by scanning electron microscopy of small dental cutting instruments through use and cleaning. *Australian Dental Journal*, **35**, 1–13

Whitehead, S.A., Wilson, N.H.F. and Watts, D.C. (1990) The effects of approximal finishing strips. *Restorative Dentistry*, **6**, 20–30

Wilson, F., Heath, J.R. and Watts, D.C. (1990) Finishing composite restorative materials. *Journal of Oral Rehabilitation*, **17**, 79–87

2 Cements and varnishes

2.1 Cements

These are used for:

1. Cavity linings: thermal/chemical/electrical protection of pulp.
2. Luting: sealing the gap between castings and prepared teeth.
3. Temporary fillings.
4. Pulp capping.
5. Root canal sealing (*see also* section 4.10.2.1).
6. Retention of orthodontic brackets.
7. Bonding of Maryland bridges.
8. Retention and luting of veneers made of composite resin or ceramic.

2.1.1 Zinc oxide–eugenol (unmodified)

Presentation   White powder (zinc oxide) with yellow liquid (eugenol–oil of cloves).

Manipulation   Mixed to a thick paste in about 1 minute, powder : liquid ratio 3 : 1.

Properties   Takes more than 24 hours to harden; reaction accelerated in moist atmosphere.

Applications   Limited to temporary fillings where the obtundent effect of the eugenol deadens the pain which accompanies a carious exposure.

2.1.2 Accelerated zinc oxide–eugenol

Presentation   White powder (zinc and magnesium oxides and zinc acetate (accelerator)) with yellow liquid (eugenol), also available as two pastes.

Common brands   Cavinol (two pastes); Sedanol; Templin; Temrex.

Manipulation   Mixed to a thick paste in about 1 minute, powder : liquid ratio 3 : 1.

Properties   Sets within 5 minutes to form zinc eugenolate. Compressive strength 15 MN/m^2.

Applications
1. Cavity lining, but not under polymer-based fillings which soften and discolour.
2. Temporary fillings.

2.1.3 Resin-bonded zinc oxide–eugenol

Presentation   White powder (90% zinc and magnesium oxides, 10% hydrogenated rosin) with yellow liquid (90% eugenol, 10% polystyrene).

Common brands   Aristonol; Kalzinol; Kalsogen; Temp D; Zinroc.

Manipulation   Mixed to a thick paste in about 1 minute, power/liquid ratio 4 : 1.

Properties   Sets within 5 minutes. Compressive strength 40 MN/m^2.

Applications
1. Cavity lining, but not under polymer-based fillings.
2. Endodontic applications.

2.1.4 Polymer-reinforced zinc oxide–eugenol

Presentation   White powder (80% zinc oxide and

zinc acetate (accelerator) and 20% poly(methyl methacrylate beads) with yellow liquid (eugenol).

Common brand IRM (Intermediate Restorative Material).

Manipulation Mixed to a thick paste in about 1 minute. Powder : liquid ratio 5 : 1.

Properties Sets within 5 minutes to produce a cement which is harder and less soluble than other eugenol-based materials.

Applications Temporary restorations.

2.1.5 Ethoxybenzoic acid (EBA) cement

Presentation White powder (65% zinc oxide, 30% quartz, 5% hydrogenated resin) with pink liquid (37.5% eugenol, 62.5% *o*-ethoxybenzoic acid).

Common Brands Fynal; Opotow; Staline.

Manipulation Mixed with a stellite (cobalt–chromium) spatula to a thixotropic (flows under stress) paste in about 1 minute. Powder : liquid ratio 7 : 1.

Properties Sets within 5 minutes. Compressive strength 90 MN/m^2.

Applications
1. Luting of inlays, crowns and bridges (see also 4.8).
2. Cavity lining (not under polymer-based fillings).

2.1.6 Zinc phosphate

Presentation White powder (zinc and magnesium oxides); the powder of one brand also contains calcium and aluminium hydroxides: with clear liquid (50% aqueous solution of phosphoric acid, buffered with some zinc and aluminium ions). In one brand there is up to 8% aluminium hydroxide.

Common brands Often just called zinc cement,

e.g. De Trey's Zinc; Dropsin (with calcium and aluminium hydroxides); Elite Cement; Harvard Cement; Lumicon; Ortho-Gold (with yellow pigment); Phosphacap (encapsulated); Tenet.

Manipulation To avoid overheating and too rapid a set it is mixed by *slowly* incorporating the powder into the liquid to produce a thick paste for lining or a thin, creamy paste for luting. Time required, 30–60 seconds for normal use. Extended manipulation prolongs the working time, as does the use of a cold, glass mixing slab. The liquid bottle must be kept stoppered to prevent loss or gain of water.

Properties Sets within 5 minutes to form zinc phosphate. Compressive strength 100 MN/m^2. Low pH at early stages of setting is a potential hazard to the pulp. Can be placed over calcium hydroxide in double-lining technique.

Applications
1. Cavity lining, under all filling materials.
2. Luting of inlays, crowns and bridges.

2.1.7 Copper phosphate

Many other metallic oxides (e.g. cupric, cuprous and silver) react in a similar way to zinc oxide with phosphoric acid to produce setting cements. Amongst those still in use, black copper cement is the most widespread.

Presentation Black powder (cupric, oxide) with clear liquid (50% aqueous solution of phosphoric acid buffered with some zinc and aluminium ions).

Common brand Ames Copper.

Manipulation Must be mixed very rapidly on a glass slab which has been chilled. It is then used instantly. Protect patient's lips with petroleum jelly.

Properties Very fluid and has a very low pH when first mixed. Copper may have bactericidal effect.

Applications The retention of silver cap splints in oral surgery procedures.

2.1.8 Zinc silicophosphate

Presentation A pigmented opalescent powder comprising a mixture of zinc and magnesium oxides and fluoroaluminosilicate glass, sometimes fused together, and in some cases containing small amounts of mercuric ammonium chloride as a potent bactericidal agent; with a clear liquid, 50% aqueous solution of phosphoric acid containing zinc and aluminium ions.

Common brands Fluoro Thin; Kryptex (germicidal, with 2% mercuric ammonium chloride); Petralit.

Manipulation The powder is incorporated into the liquid in increments to produce a thick paste for fillings or a thin paste for luting, in about a minute.

Properties More translucent than zinc phosphate but more soluble. Can cause pulpal irritation. Sometimes contains bactericidal or bacteriostatic heavy metal salts. Fluoride leaches out to form fluorapatite.

Applications Superseded by more recent materials such as glass-ionomer cements (2.1.10), which have superior properties and are less irritant.
   However, it may be used for:
1. The cementation of porcelain jacket crowns.
2. Filling of deciduous teeth.
3. The production of dies.
4. Cementation of orthodontic bands.

2.1.9 Zinc polycarboxylate

Presentation
1. *Type A:* White powder (zinc and magnesium oxides) with a clear, syrupy liquid (40% aqueous solution of poly(acrylic acid), or an acrylic acid co-polymer with other unsaturated carboxylic acids).
2. *Type B:* White powder (zinc and magnesium oxides plus dehydrated poly(acrylic acid) or acrylic acid co-polymer) mixed with water only.

Common brands
1. *Type A:* Bayer; Bondalcap (encapsulated); Carboco; Durelon.

2. *Type B:* AquaBoxyl; Aqualox; Opus PCF; Poly F Plus.

Manipulation Mixed thickly for linings or to a creamy paste for luting. Time required: 1 minute.

Properties Sets within 5 minutes to form zinc polycarboxylate. Compressive strength 90 MN/m^2. Adheres to clean dry enamel and to stainless steel.

Applications
1. Cavity lining, under all filling materials.
2. Luting of inlays, crowns and bridges.
3. Temporary fillings.
4. Cementation of stainless steel orthodontic brackets and bands.

2.1.10 Glass-ionomer (glass polyalkenoate)

Presentation
1. *Form A:* Pigmented, opalescent powder (fluorocalcium aluminosilicate glass) with clear, viscous liquid (50% aqueous solution of poly(acrylic acid) or poly(maleic acid), poly(alkenyl carboxylic acids) and tartaric acid).
2. *Form B:* Pigmented, opalescent powder fluorocalcium aluminosilicate glass plus dehydrated (freeze-dried) poly(acrylic acid) or poly(maleic acid) and poly(alkenyl carboxylic acids). This is mixed with clean water or a solution of tartaric acid.
3. *Form C:* Photosensitive, radiopaque powder (fluorocalcium aluminosilicate glass plus photoinitiator) with a clear, viscous liquid (a solution of poly(carboxylic acid) with pendant methacryloxy groups, together with hydroxyethyl methacrylate (HEMA) and water). These are often designated LC (light-cured) or VLC (visible light-cured).

Forms A and B may also contain finely divided metal powder (see section 3.4.3), and both forms are available as either bulk constituents or encapsulated.

Classification
Glass-ionomer cements can be classified according to the applications for which they are intended, as follows:

1. *Type I:* Luting cements. These flow readily to form a thin film.

2. *Type II:* Restorative materials:
   (a) Aesthetic filling materials. These are viscous pastes which have good colour and translucency.
   (b) Reinforced (including silver cermets). These metal-filled pastes are radiopaque and somewhat more wear-resistant than the unfilled cements.
3. *Type III:* Fast-setting lining cements. These flow readily and are opaque to both light and X-rays.
4. *Type IV:* Fissure-sealing cements. These have good flow.
5. *Type V:* Orthodontic cements. These are viscous and set rapidly.
6. *Type VI:* Core build-up cements. These are viscous, radiopaque pastes which set rapidly. Some contain finely divided metal powders (see section 3.4.3).

The properties of each type are targeted by their manufacturers to appeal to users in the various applications. Note the variations of viscosity and flow, setting speed, translucency and radiopacity. With an awareness of these properties in mind, these materials can often be used in more than one advertised application

Common brands

1. *Type I:* Aquacem; Aqua Meron; Ceramcem; Fuji Ionomer I; Gem-Cem; Ketac-Cem; Kromoglass3; Meron.
2. *Type II:* (see section 3.4.2).
3. *Type III:* Alpha-Bond; Aqua Ionobond; BaseLine; BaseLine VLC (light-cured); Ceramlin; Ceramlite; Core-Shade; Fuji Lining LC (light-cured); GC Dentin Cement; Gem-Base; Ioline; Ionobond; Ketac-Bond; Kromoglass 1; LCL 8 (light-cured); Photo-Bond Aplicap (light-cured/encapsulated); VariGlass VLC; Vitrebond (light-cured); XR Ionomer (light-cured); Zenith Alpha Base; Zionomer.
4. *Type IV:* CeramSave; Fuji Ionomer III; Gem-Seal.
5. *Type V:* Intact; Orthocem B; Precedent; Sumo.
6. *Type VI:* Ceram-Core; Chelon-Silver; Gem-Core; Ion S; Ketac-Silver; Legend Silver; Miracle Mix; Opus-Silver; Hi-Dense; Zenith Alpha Silver.

Manipulation Mixed thickly for cores, or to creamy pastes for luting, fissure sealing and orthodontic applications. The optimum viscosity for each application is obtained by using the powder to liquid ratio which is produced by using the measuring scoops and dropper bottles supplied with each product. The time required for manual mixing is about a minute. For those products which are presented in capsules, mixing time is between 5 and 10 seconds.

Properties Forms A and B have setting times between 3 and 6 minutes. Form C can be light-cured to produce a semirigid mass within 20 seconds. Chemical setting continues after this. Low solubility once set. Adheres to clean, dry enamel and to dentine, particularly if it has been cleaned with pumice powder and water, and the smear layer has been removed with a dilute solution of poly(acrylic acid) or tannic acid. All forms release fluoride ions throughout their lifetime.

Applications

1. *Type I:* Luting of inlays, crowns and bridges (glass-ionomer will form a chemical bond to gold if the fitting surface of the restoration has been tin-plated).
2. *Type II:* As a filling material (see section 3.4.2).
3. *Type III:* As a cavity lining (on top of a calcium hydroxide base) especially in the replacement dentine technique.
4. *Type IV:* The sealing of fissures in permanent teeth.
5. *Type V:* The retention of stainless steel orthodontic brackets and the stabilization of bands.
6. *Type VI:* The build-up of cores where retention does not require the use of dentine pins.

2.1.11 Calcium hydroxide

Presentation Either:

1. *Form A:* Two white or cream pastes in tubes or chlorofluorocarbon-free pressure packs:
   (a) *Tube a:* Calcium hydroxide plus diluent inert fillers such as zinc and titanium oxides plus barium sulphate as radiopacifier, all in a fluid, non-reacting carrier containing ethylene toluene sulphonamide.
   (b) *Tube b:* Reactive polysalicylate fluid plus

diluent inert fillers and radiopacifiers

or:

2. *Form B:* A single paste consisting of a calcium hydroxide-filled, light-curing dimethacrylate resin and photoinitiator, plus radiopacifier.

Common brands

1. *Form A:* Alka-Liner; Calcimol; Care; Dycal; Life; Nu-Cap; Procal; Recal.
2. *Form B:* Prisma VLC Dycal.

Manipulation

1. *Form A:* Equal volumes mixed together for about 10 seconds.
2. *Form B:* A thin layer is applied to the cavity floor and light-cured for at least 20 seconds.

Properties   Form A sets by an acid–base reaction to produce an amorphous calcium disalicylate complex which contains an excess of calcium hydroxide. Setting occurs from the outside inwards and takes from 3 to 3.5 minutes. Setting is accelerated by moisture. Compressive strength 15 MN/m^2 (this is adequate for most applications). pH = 11, even when set. Induces mineralization in the adjacent pulp but the mechanism is not clear.

Applications

1. Cavity lining. The cement is intended for use in thin films only. It can be used under all filling materials, especially as the first layer (close to the pulp) in the double-lining technique.
2. Pulp capping (only the two-paste version).
3. Protection of freshly cut dentine during acid-etching of enamel for resin retention. Reline cavity if acid destroys the integrity of the cement film.

2.1.11.1 Non-setting paste for pulp capping

Calcium hydroxide for pulp capping is also available as a paste which does not react and set.

Common brands   Calxyl; Reogan.

Presentation   Glass syringe cartridge or jar of a paste containing calcium and magnesium hydroxide plus barium sulphate (to make it radiopaque), held together with casein.

Manipulation   The paste can be syringed so as to produce a thin layer at the base of the cavity.

Properties   No structural strength. Any effects are entirely biological.

Applications   Pulp capping, particularly in deciduous teeth; ossification and apexification.

2.1.12 Acrylic resin (poly(methyl methacrylate))

Presentation   A colourless powder (spheres of poly(methyl methacrylate) plus dibenzoyl peroxide as initiator) with a clear liquid (methyl methacrylate monomer plus a tertiary amine activator). Some also contain reagents which promote the formation of a chemical bond to clean metal surfaces. One of these is 4-methacryloxyethyl-trimellitate anhydride (4-META).

Common brands   Sevriton; Super-Bond C & B (with 4-META); Surgical Simplex.

Manipulation   Powder and liquid are mixed to a thin paste and used instantly on clean dry surfaces.

Properties   Exothermic setting reaction accompanied by considerable shrinkage on polymerization. Absorbs water; can become unhygienic.

Applications

1. Luting.
2. Retention of orthodontic brackets.
3. Surgical implant and splint fixation.
4. Temporary crown and bridge material.
5. Retention of Maryland bridges.

2.1.13 Dimethacrylate (Bowen's) resin

Cements based on this are similar to the resins used as the matrices of composites and they have an equally complex chemistry. However, they all set by cross-linking polymerization reactions involving methacrylate groups at the end of molecules with high molecular weights. Setting can be brought about as follows:

2.1.13.1 Self-curing (chemically activated)

Presentation   Either as two low-viscosity, lightly filled pastes, one containing dimethacrylate resin and dibenzoyl peroxide as initiator and the other an activator such as a tertiary amine, or as a powder and a liquid. Some also contain components which promote the formation of an adhesive bond to metal surfaces. One contains titanium as a reinforcing filler.

Common brands   A.B.C. (with adhesive monomer); Biomer; Cemper; Comspan; Den-Mat Crown Reline and Cementation system; Flexi-Flow (with titanium filler); Indirect Porcelain System; Microfill Pontic; Microjoin; Mirage ABC (with adhesive monomer); Nimetic Grip; Panavia Ex (with adhesive monomer); Resiment; Sticky Post; Until.

Manipulation   Equal volumes of each component are mixed for about 30 seconds and instantly applied to the surfaces to be bonded, which must be clean and dry.

Properties   Lower exotherm and less polymerization shrinkage than acrylic; neutral pH.

Applications
1. Luting inlays, crowns and bridges.
2. Retention of polymeric and metallic orthodontic bands and brackets.
3. Retention by flow into the etch-pits formed on enamel and the base metal framework of a Maryland bridge (see section 4.4.3).
4. Retention of endodontic posts.

2.1.13.2 Light-activated

Presentation   Single syringe or plastic, light-proof bottle of lightly filled paste containing a light-sensitive initiator and pigments. Often supplied with a bifunctional primer (silane) to promote bond formation with ceramics.

Common brands   Durafill Bond; Heliolink; Porcelite; V-Bond.

Manipulation   The fluid paste is applied to the surfaces to be bonded and activated by visible blue light.

Properties   Lower exotherm and a greater modulus than acrylic.

Applications   Retention of veneers made of composite, porcelain or glass-ceramic.

2.1.13.3 Dual-cure (self- and light-activated)

Presentation   Two pastes. One which contains resin and two sorts of initiator – one (such as dibenzoyl peroxide) can be chemically activated, and the other (such as camphorquinone) can be activated by intense blue light. The other paste contains resin and a chemical activator. Both may contain small amounts of filler and pigments. Some also contain fluorides.

Common brands   ABC Dual; Adherence M5; Bifix; Compa Adhasiv; CuRay-Dual Match; Dicor MGC Luting Composite; Dual Cement; Duo Cement; Gem-Bond; Infinity; Kulzer Adhesive Cement; Mirage FLC; Porcelite Dual Cure; Sono-Cem; Twinlook; Ultra-Bond.

Manipulation   The bonding surfaces are coated with light-curing resin before the two pastes of the dual-cure cement are mixed in equal volumes and applied to the precoated surfaces, which are then mated. Excess is removed, the exposed composite covered with a gel such as Airblock, to prevent oxygen inhibition, and the edges are exposed to intense blue light. One is thixotropic and made free-flowing by ultrasonic energy.

Properties   The first few millimetres cross-link via the light-curing mechanism in about 30 seconds. Cement which has not received enough light to start the cross-linking reaction slowly sets via chemically-activated polymerization.

Applications   The retention of laboratory-constructed composite or ceramic inlays and onlays.

2.1.14 Light-cured cavity liners

Presentation   Single-paste materials based on dimethacrylate resins and containing HEMA to facilitate wetting of the dentine; camphorquinone as a light-sensitive initiator; barium sulphate as a radiopacifier; and one or more fillers, such as synthetic hydroxyapatite or glass-ionomer cement powder. May also contain phosphates to promote adhesion to dentine.

Common brands   Basic (also presented as a two-paste, self-curing system); Cavalite; Fluoroseal; Interface; Ionoseal; New Era; Timeline.

Manipulation   Fluid paste is applied over dentine (but *not* close to the pulp) and light-cured.

Properties   Acid-resistant, radiopaque film has low solubility, which can hinder the leaching of fluoride ions if present. pH varies from 6.5 to 12, according to which fillers are present.

Applications   Linings in *shallow* cavities under amalgam or composite.

2.1.15 Polyester resin

Presentation ˙Powder consisting of zinc oxide filler and peroxide initiator, and a liquid polyester.

Common brand   F 21.

Manipulation   A scoop of powder is mixed with two drops of liquid to produce a smooth paste.

Properties   The working time out of the mouth is about 6 minutes and within the mouth about 3 minutes. The set cement is strong, bonds well to metals (better to base metals than gold alloys) and has a very low solubility. Care is needed to keep it away from sensitive dentine.

Applications   The luting of inlays, crowns, bridges and posts.

2.2 Varnishes

Used in dentistry for:
1. Barriers to the movement of chemical irritants down the dentinal tubules, e.g. under acid or polymer-based fillings.
2. Temporary barriers to reduce the loss of moisture into and out of the surface of fillings, e.g. glass-ionomer cements.
3. Protection of calcium hydroxide cements during acid-etch procedures.
4. Aids to marginal sealing, e.g. amalgam.
5. Temporary protection of sensitive dentine and exposed cementum.
6. One method of applying topical fluoride.

Presentation   Clear or opaque, colourless or yellow liquids consisting of natural or synthetic resins dissolved in an organic solvent, sometimes with solids in suspension.

Resins

Natural: copal (from tropical trees), colophony (from turpentine residues) sandarac (from North African conifers).
Synthetic: polystyrene.

Solvents

Ether, chloroform, alcohols.

Optional additives

Zinc oxide, calcium hydroxide, fluorides, antiseptics (e.g. thymol di-iodide); one brand contains finely powdered amalgam alloy and silver.

Common brands   Amalgam Liner; Bifluorid 12 (with sodium and calcium fluoride); Cavisol II (with fluoride); Copalite; Duraphat (with topical fluoride); Hydroxyline; Ketac Varnish; Tubilitec.

Manipulation   Applied with a pledget of cotton wool; the solvent should be evaporated with gently applied warm air. Single layers tend to be porous and multilayers (2–3) are required for adequate sealing. Allow each layer to dry and harden before applying the next.

Properties   The thin layers produced by varnishes (20 μm thick) are not an adequate barrier to thermal trauma. Use a cement on top if thermal protection of the pulp is necessary.

Further reading

Liners

Arcoria, C.J., Vitasek, B.A., Dewald, J.P. and Wagner, M.J. (1990) Microleakage in restorations with glass ionomer liners after thermocycling. *Journal of Dentistry*, **18**, 107–112

Brannstrom, M., Mattson, B. and Torstenson, B. (1991) Materials techniques for lining composite resin restorations: a critical approach. *Journal of Dentistry*, **19**, 71–79

Fuss, J., Mount, G.J. & Makinson, O.F. (1990) The effect of etching on a number of glass ionomer cements. *Australian Dental Journal*, **35**, 338–344

Holtan, J.R., Nystrom, G.P., Olin, P.S., Rudney, J. and Douglas, W.H. (1990) Bond strength of a light-cured and two auto-cured glass ionomer liners. *Journal of Dentistry*, **18**, 271–275

Hume, W.R. and Massey, W.L. (1990) Keeping the pulp alive: the pharmacology and toxicology of agents applied to dentine. *Australian Dental Journal*, **53**, 32–37

Kanca J. III. (1990) An alternative hypothesis to the cause of pulpal inflammation in teeth treated with phosphoric acid on dentin. *Quintessence International*, **21**, 83–86

Kingsford Smith, E.D. and Martin, F.E. (1990) Acid etching of a glass ionomer cement base: SEM study. *Australian Dental Journal*, **35**, 236–240

McCourt, J.W., Cooley, R.L. and Huddleston, A.M. (1990) Fluoride release from fluoride-containing liners/ bases. *Quintessence International*, **21**, 41–45

Meeker, H.G., Kaim, J.M., Linke, H.A.B. and Scherer, W.J. (1990) Antibacterial properties of Dycal and visible-light-cured Dycal (Prisma VLC Dycal). *General Dentistry*, **38**, 121–124

Mitra, S.B. (1991) Adhesion to dentin and physical properties of a light-cured glass ionomer liner/ base. *Journal of Dental Research*, **70**, 72–74

Mount, G.J. (1990) Esthetics with glass ionomer cements and the 'sandwich' technique. *Quintessence International*, **21**, 93–101

Mutter, J., Horz, W., Bruckner, G. and Kraft, E. (1990) An experimental study on the biocompatibility of lining cements based on glass ionomer as compared with calcium hydroxide. *Dental Materials*, **6**, 35–40

Papadakou, M., Barnes, I.E., Wassell, R.W. and McCabe, J.F. (1990) Adaption of two different calcium hydroxide bases under a composite restoration. *Journal of Dentistry*, **18**, 276–280

Papagiannoulis, L., Eliades, G. and Lekka, M. (1990) Etched glass ionomer liners: surface properties and interfacial profile with composite resins. *Journal of Oral Rehabilitation*, **17**, 25–36

Pashley, E.L., Galloway, S.E., Pashley, D.H. (1990) Protective effects of cavity liners on dentine. *Operative Dentistry*, **15**, 10–17

Tjan, A.H.L. and Dunn, J.R. (1990) Microleakage at gingival dentine margins of Class V composite restorations lined with light-cured glass ionomer cement. *Journal of the American Dental Association*, **121**, 706–710

Welbury, R.R. and Murray, J.J. (1990) A clinical trial of the glass ionomer cement-composite resin sandwich technique in Class II cavities in permanent premolar and molar teeth. *Quintessence International*, **21**, 507–512

Luting

Black, S.M. and Charlton, G. (1990) Survival of crowns and bridges related to luting cements. *Restorative Dentistry*, **6**, 26–30

Christensen, G.J. (1990) Glass ionomer as a luting cement. *Journal of the American Dental Association*, **120**, 59–62

Graver, H., Trowbridge, H. and Alperstern, K. (1990) Microleakage of castings cemented with glass ionomer cements. *Operative Dentistry*, **15**, 2–9

3 Filling materials

3.1 Amalgam

Dental amalgam is the oldest of the filling materials in use today and can trace its origins to M. Taveau's *pâté d'argent* of 1850. After a turbulent adolescence it became stabilized as a result of the work of Black, Flagg and Tomes as an alloy of silver and tin (with small amounts of copper and zinc), which was mixed with mercury to produce an amalgam. Modern dental amalgam alloys now have several complex formulations, in many of which much of the silver is replaced with copper.

Presentation   Silvery (or silvery-pink) powder. Triple-distilled liquid metal (mercury, Hg).

Types of powder: composition and morphology (shape)

1. *Type A:* Irregular, lathe-cut particles of the gamma-phase of silver–tin alloy, Ag_3Sn, may contain 0–6% copper and 0–2% zinc (added to scavenge for oxygen during manufacture).
2. *Type B:* Spherical particles of the same composition as A.
3. *Type C:* A mixture or blend of irregular, lathe-cut particles of Ag_3Sn plus spherical particles of the eutectic composition of the silver–copper binary alloy (epsilon-phase). This is termed a high-copper dispersant or admix system.
4. *Type D:* Spherical particles of a ternary alloy silver–tin–copper (Ag–Sn–Cu) with a copper content of 12–30%. This is termed a high-copper unicompositional alloy.
5. *Type E:* Lathe-cut particles of the same composition as D.
6. *Type F:* Irregular, lathe-cut Ag–Sn–Cu or Ag_3Sn

particles plus spherical Ag–Sn–Cu particles. This has been called a hybrid system.

Any of the above alloys may contain up to 2% of mercury, in which case they are termed pre-amalgamated alloys. All types of alloy can be presented as bulk powder, as tablets of alloy, or with both alloy powder and mercury contained in some type of disposable capsule.

Common brands

1. *Type A:* Aristaloy; DSD Autofine, Fine grain; Lumicon; Mattiloy; Regel Star; Standalloy; Veraloy.

2. *Type B:* Amalcap Plus; Shofu; Spheralloy; Starburst (with lathe-cut particles).

3. *Type C:* Aristaloy 21; Cupraloy; Dispersalloy; Luxalloy; Nu Alloy DP; Phasealloy; Optaloy II; SDI Permite.

4. *Type D:* Flint Edge; Indiloy (5% In); SDI Lojic (with Pt); Sybraloy; Tytin; Valiant (0.5% Pd).

5. *Type E:* ANA 2000; Mattiloy Plus 43; Minargent; Solila Nova.

6. *Type F:* Arjalloy; Artalloy (80% Ag); Contour; Duralloy; Oralloy; Panorama; Permite C; Starburst Non-Gamma II; Vivalloy HR.

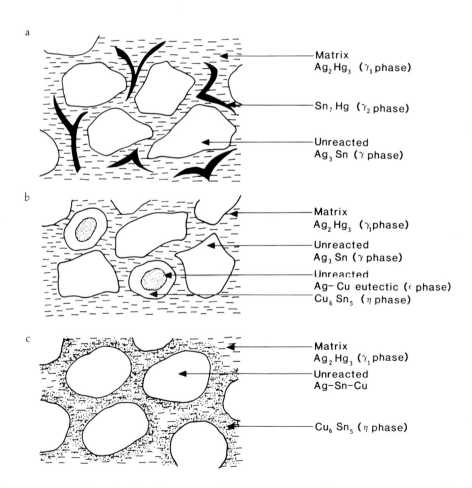

Figure 1 The microstructure of set dental amalgam prepared from: (a) conventional low-copper composition alloy; (b) dispersion-phase (admix) high-copper alloy; (c) single-composition, high-copper alloy.

Setting reaction (Fig. 1)

Using type A or B powder (conventional, low-copper alloy):

$$Ag_3Sn \ + \ Hg \ = \ Ag_3Sn \ + \ Ag_2Hg_3 \ + \ Sn_7Hg \ + \ voids$$

γ-phase $\qquad\qquad$ γ-phase $\quad$ γ_1-phase $\quad$ γ_2-phase

powder $\quad$ *liquid* $\quad$ *unreacted* $\quad$ *solid amalgam matrix*

Using type C powder (high-copper, dispersant alloy):

$$Ag_3Sn \ + \ Cu\text{-}Ag \ + \ Hg \ = \ Ag_3Sn \ + \ Cu\text{-}Ag \ + \ Ag_2Hg_3 \ + \ Cu_6Sn_5 \ + \ voids$$

γ-phase $\quad$ ϵ-phase $\qquad\qquad$ γ-phase $\quad$ ϵ-phase $\quad$ γ_1-phase $\quad$ η-phase

powder $\quad$ *eutectic* $\quad$ *liquid* $\quad$ *unreacted* $\qquad\qquad$ *amalgam* $\quad$ *forms*

$\qquad\qquad$ *spheres* $\qquad\qquad\qquad\qquad\qquad\qquad\qquad$ *matrix* $\qquad$ *around*

$\qquad\qquad\qquad\qquad\qquad\qquad\qquad\qquad\qquad\qquad\qquad\qquad\qquad\qquad\qquad\qquad$ *spheres*

Using type D powder (high-copper, single composition alloy):

$$Ag\text{-}Sn\text{-}Cu \ + \ Hg \ = \ Ag\text{-}Sn\text{-}Cu \ + \ Ag_2Hg_3 \ + \ Cu_6Sn_5 \ + \ voids$$

ternary $\qquad\qquad\qquad$ ternary $\qquad$ γ_1-phase $\quad$ η-phase

alloy $\qquad\qquad\qquad\quad$ alloy

powder $\quad$ *liquid* $\quad$ *unreacted* $\qquad$ *amalgam* $\quad$ *forms near*

$\qquad\qquad\qquad\qquad\qquad\qquad\qquad\qquad$ *matrix* $\qquad$ *alloy particles*

Manipulation The aim is to produce a void or pore-free amalgam with a minimum final mercury content (less than 55% Hg in lathe-cut alloy and less than 45% Hg in spherical alloy amalgams of any composition). Stages are as follows:
1. Proportioning: by weight or volume.
2. Trituration: by hand or mechanically *(see below)*.
3. Dispensing: transfer to the cavity without contamination.
4. Condensing: packing with pluggers, burnishers, plastic instruments or mechanical vibrators.
5. Carving: various sharp instruments may be used.
   After at least 24 hours:
6. Polishing: burs, abrasives, polishes.

Trituration
1. Hand methods: by mortar and pestle, finger stall or surgical glove finger. *Note:* excess mercury is required for trituration and once the amalgam is triturated, the excess must be squeezed from the amalgam within a dental napkin.

Caution: Mercury is very reactive towards other metals.

Mercury *vapour* is toxic and chronic exposure to even small amounts should be avoided. The threshold limit value (TLV) of a substance which emits a toxic vapour is said to represent the concentration to which it is generally believed workers may be exposed throughout their working life without being in danger of suffering adverse effects to their health. The TLV for mercury is currently set at 0.05 mg/m^3 in the UK.

Symptoms of chronic poisoning: erethism, tremors, gingivitis, nephrosis and mercurialentis, severe headaches, irritability, fatigue, insomnia. The pregnant woman should be particularly mindful of the potential hazard of exposure to mercury vapour during pregnancy. Although no symptoms are generally noticed by the woman, mercury can be transferred across the placenta and can cause fetal harm.

The TLV for pregnant employees is 0.01 mg/m^3, and those members of the dental team in this condition should avoid removing or placing amalgam restorations whenever possible.

Thus: Do *not* let spills go uncollected, especially if they are in danger of being heated.

Do *not* allow mercury to come into contact with gold and silver jewellery, lead or copper sink pipes.

2. Mechanical methods:

(a) The Dentomat, Duomat and Dentomat 2 or 3: automatic proportioning into a screw-on, reusable capsule followed by mechanical trituration. A maximum of three double actions (3 alloy + 3 mercury) should be triturated at one mix. The amalgam produced does not need squeezing to remove excess mercury as the ratio of alloy powder to mercury is 1:1 or less.

(b) Reusable or disposable capsules. The reusable capsule is filled by the dental surgery assistant from volume dispensers, and the disposable capsule already contains the correct ratio of constituents. Both types are triturated on a mechanical vibrator. The disposable capsules are not suitable for refilling. After removing the mixed amalgam from disposable capsules, they should be reassembled and stored in a sealed container ready for incineration.

Properties

1. *General to all compositions and morphologies*

   (a) Optimum properties reached after 24 hours.

   (b) High coefficient of thermal conductivity usually requires that a low conductivity cement lining is placed to protect the pulp.

   (c) A slight expansion should occur on setting.

   (d) If the alloy contains zinc, particular care should be taken to avoid contamination with water during manipulation as this can produce excess expansion due to the production of hydrogen.

2. *Related to the particle morphology*

   (a) Lathe-cut alloys take 6 hours or so to reach their occlusal strength, whereas spherical alloys take 3 hours. The occlusal strength is that needed to cope with soft foods without breaking.

   (b) Lathe-cut particles require more mercury to cover their greater surface area than spherical

particles do.

3. *Related to composition*

   (a) Conventional, low-copper amalgam suffers from creep and corrosion. Both are factors which have been associated with the manifestation of marginal failure.

   (b) High-copper amalgams do not corrode or creep to any significant degree and they show much less tendency to marginal failure. This is due to the absence of the $\gamma_2(Sn_7Hg)$ phase.

Applications

1. Long-term posterior filling material.
2. Pinned cores for cast restorations.
3. Retrograde root filling.
4. Historically: dies from rigid impressions.

3.2 Composites

Dental composites consist of a matrix of organic polymer filled with inert ceramic particles.

Whilst historically many different sorts of filler particles have been used, including regular particle shapes such as rods and spheres, by the 1970s most composites were using irregular particles of hard, strong and, frequently, radiopaque glass or ceramic. These inert particles are coated by the manufacturer with a vinyl silane such as γ-methacryloxypropyl trimethoxysilane. This bifunctional primer creates a bond between the filler particle and the set polymer matrix.

Three filler categories (Fig. 2) have evolved during the 35 years of composite development:

1. *Conventional filler.* This was an irregular glass or ceramic material, whose particles ranged in size from 4 to 40 μm. Fillers used included quartz, aluminosilicate or borosilicate glass, tricalcium phosphate, hydroxyapatite or lithium aluminium silicate. The composites of the 1960s and 1970s contained only conventional filler and today they would be called conventional or traditional. Composites of that era — Adaptic; Blendant; Cavex-Clearfil; Concise; Cosmic; HL72; and Smile — were all examples of these traditional materials. Composites of the 1990s with the same or similar names are all examples of the *hybrid* systems.

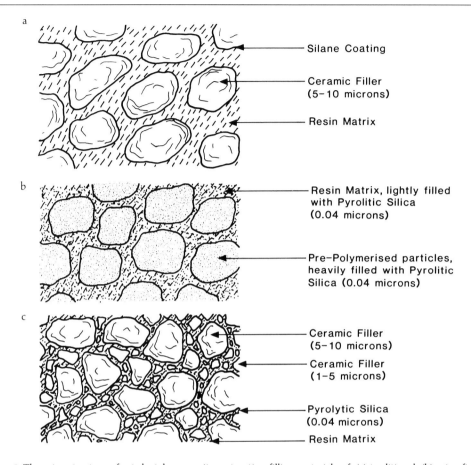

Figure 2 The microstructure of set dental composite restorative filling materials of: (a) traditional; (b) microfine and (c) hybrid filler loading.

2. *Microfine filler.* This consists of pyrogenic silica having a particle size between 0.01 and 0.1 μm with a mean of 0.04 μm. This is distributed by the manufacturer into dilute diacrylate resin, which is then heat-polymerized. The set, filled resin is broken into lumps with an average size of about 50 μm. These lumps are used as a filler instead of the large particles of glass or ceramic which were employed as fillers in the conventionally filled materials. The silica particles are *not* radiopaque and neither are the composites which employ them exclusively as a filler. To overcome this, several utilize rare-earth metal compounds to make them opaque to X-rays. The silica in the microfilled composite represents 30–60% of the weight of the set material.

3. *Hybrid filler.* This is a blend of conventional glass or ceramic filler particles, such as zirconia or silica, which range in size from 0.5 to 10 μm, together with pyrogenic silica whose particles are between 0.01 and 0.1 μm. In those hybrid systems which are advocated by their manufacturers for use in posterior teeth, the filler particles are graded into several distinct size groups with the aim of filling the available space with as much inorganic material as possible. As the hybrid composites contain particles made from glasses which contain barium aluminoborate or strontium glasses, they are radiopaque. The filler particles in the hybrid systems represent 78–85% of the weight of the set material.

Presentation

1. *Form A:* Chemically-cured: base paste + activator paste in syringes or pots.
2. *Form B:* Light-cured: single, light-proof syringe or 'compule' containing a light-sensitive paste.

Either form is a variation on the basic system which consists of:

1. A fluid monomer: historically methyl methacrylate was used in composites such as Palakav, Polycap and TD71, but now some type of diacrylate is employed. Many composites contain bis-GMA, which is formed by the reaction between bis-phenol A and glycidyl methacrylate. This is often known as Bowen's resin. Other composites use either aliphatic or aromatic diacrylates as their monomer. All these resins are very viscous and have to be diluted with about 25% triethylene glycol dimethacrylate to increase their fluidity. These additives also help in cross-linking reactions.
2. An initiator to start the polymerization reaction. In chemically activated systems this is usually 0.5% by weight of dibenzoyl peroxide. In light-activated systems the initiator depends on the wavelength of light being used.
3. An activator to stimulate the initiator – either a chemical such as dimethyl-*p*-toluidine or 2-hydroxyethyl-*p*-toluidine or visible light.

    The visible light-activated systems were preceded by those which were activated by ultraviolet light. These contained benzoin methyl ether to absorb the ultraviolet light (wavelength 365 nm) and create the free radicals necessary to initiate polymerization.

    The visible light-activated system, which has replaced it, contains an α-diketone, such as camphorquinone, and an amine which, under the influence of blue light (wavelength 440–480 nm), produces the necessary free radicals. These light-activated materials are sometimes called command setting resins.
4. Pigments to create a colour match with enamel and dentine, and fluorescers to produce a natural response to intense natural and artificial light, which has an ultraviolet component.
5. Minor additions to inhibit premature polymerization, and ultraviolet stabilizers which increase the shelf-life of the material.
6. An inert filler, which occupies 50–75% of volume of the set composite.

Common brands

Microfine filler

Chemically activated (two-paste system) – Isomolar; Isopast; Silar.
Light-activated (single-paste system) – Adaptic LCM; Aristofil DP; Aristolux; Bis-Fil-M; Degufill-M; Durafill; Estilux; Heliomolar; HelioProgress; Perfection; Silux Plus; Topaz; Visio-Dispers.

Hybrid filler

Chemically activated (two-paste system) – Adaptic Universal; Cavex-Clearfil; Compolite; Concise; Delphic; Finesse; Gem-CC1; Miradapt; P 10; Profile; SpectraBond.
Light-activated (single-paste system) – Adaptic II; Aurafil; Bis-Fil-I; Brilliant; Cavex Clearfil Ray-Posterior; Certain; Charisma; Command Ultrafine; CompaFill-MH; CompaMolar; Compolite II; Degufill H; Ful-Fil; Gem-Lite 1; Herculite; Lite-Fil II; Lumifor; Lux-a-fill; Occlusin; Opalux; Pekafill; Pekalux; Pertac Hybrid; P 30; P 50; Polofil; Polofil Molar; Prisma AP.H; Prisma TPH; Prisma-Fil; Restolux SP2; Restolux SP4; Schein 20/20; Tetric; Valux; Visio-Fil; Visio-Molar; XRV; Z100.
Dual-cure–Geristore; Marathon.

Setting reaction   The initiator is stimulated either by the chemical or light activator. Once adequately stimulated, the initiator picks up molecules of monomer one by one, forming long and cross-linked polymer chains and thus setting.

Manipulation

Chemically activated   The constituents are mixed with an abrasion-resistant spatula as recommended by the manufacturers to a uniform consistency in about 30–40 seconds.

Light-activated   Light of the correct wavelength and intensity is applied for the recommended time; range 10–60 seconds.

Note: All visible light-cured composites can be cured by any blue light source, but these vary in intensity of light output, area of light guide tip and sensitivity to age of the bulb.

Light-cured composites cannot be overcured, but for optimum results:

1. Do not exceed the composite manufacturers' recommended thickness for curing at one exposure.
2. Place the tip of the light guide as close and as near to perpendicular to the surface of the composite as possible.
3. Remember that dark shades need a longer exposure than light shades, and the composites straight from the refrigerator take longer to cure than those at room temperature.
4. Do not spatulate the composite as this introduces air which will both inhibit polymerization and create voids. Voids are a source of weakness.
5. To minimize the effects of polymerization shrinkage, fillings should be built up as a series of wedges, alternating the position of the thick and thin parts of each wedge.

Caution: Conventional fillers in particular can abrade steel instruments and produce grey stains. Celluloid matrix strips and crown formers can be softened by the resins and diluents, hence polyester (Mylar) strips are recommended.

Hazards from visible light-curing units

Staring at the intense blue light used to activate modern composites, fissure sealants and orthodontic cements can cause spots before the eyes. These *may* be the forerunners of chronic, permanent degenerative damage, *hence* do not stare at the light when it is in contact with the teeth. Position the light guide and look away before switching on the light source. If you feel that it is necessary to watch the light, use a pair of spectacles with orange filters which will absorb wavelengths up to about 510 nm (common brands: Guardian Protection Glasses; Healthco Protective Glasses; Topaz Glasses).

Finishing Contour with water-cooled, straight-cut, tungsten carbide burs or fine diamond points in a slow-speed handpiece. Smooth with lubricated stones, flexible discs (e.g. Soflex; Rainbow, various grades) and finishing strips. A glaze coat of unfilled resin produces a temporary gloss finish on hybrid composites.

Properties The chemically activated materials set throughout their bulk within 5 minutes. The command set materials set from the surface downwards, and a suitable thickness, well-activated by an appropriate light source (as described above), will cure within 20–60 seconds according to brand. High compressive and tensile strengths. Insoluble but slightly absorbent. Inferior abrasion resistance to amalgam *in vivo* such that they can only be recommended for use in occlusal cavities when aesthetics is the prime concern. In small cavities the microfine composites show somewhat superior wear resistance to the hybrid materials.

Applications

Hybrid and microfine composites

1. Class III and V anterior restorations.
2. Class IV incisal edge restorations, bonded to enamel etched with 40–50% phosphoric acid, washed and dried.
3. Facings (veneers) for stained teeth.
4. Pinned cores for cast restorations.
5. Splints and the retention of Rochette bridges to etched enamel.
6. Class I and II restorations where aesthetics is of prime concern and which do not involve cusp replacement.

3.2.1 Dimethacrylate resin-based products

Presentation and Applications

Dimethacrylate resins, which are either activated by chemicals contained in their two components or are single-component, light-activated systems, are available in several marketing variations, which contain various amounts of filler, including titanium powder and pigment powders for use specifically as:

1. *Core materials*, e.g. Alpha-Core; Aristocore; Blue Core Build-up; Clearfil Core; Concise Crown Build-up; Coradent; Corelite; Den-Mat Core

Paste; Coreform; Prosthodent VL-2 (with cure indicator); Resilient; Ti-Core (with titanium filler). *Applications:* The build-up of cores in and from endodontically prepared roots and the cementation of pins and posts.

2. *Opaquing and laminating materials,* e.g. Den-Mat Tetra Paque (a single- or two-paste system); Den-Mat Paste Laminate (a single-paste system); Estilux Color (a single-paste system); Helio-colour (a single-paste system). *Applications:* The covering of tetracycline-stained teeth or fluorosis. The laminates can also be used to close diastemas.

3. *Colouring resins,* e.g. Command Ultrafine Color; CompaColor; Den-Mat Rembrandt (a paint-on, light-cured, microfilled composite); Estilux Colour; Heliocolour. *Applications:* Accurate colour matching of restorations to teeth and shading of acrylic facings and transparent laminates.

4. *Metal-masking agents,* e.g. Den-Mat Gingival Margin Repair Kit (a light-cured, shaded paste with a porcelain-bonding agent). *Applications:* The masking of the gingival metal margins of porcelain-fused-to-metal crowns.

3.2.2 Composite inlays and onlays (see also 13.8.1)

Composite resins placed in posterior teeth suffer from the following drawbacks:

1. Contact points are difficult to make.
2. Adequate curing is a problem.
3. Curing of composite bonded to the tooth can distort it and cause pain.
4. Occlusal wear and marginal fracture occur, in part due to inadequate curing.

In an attempt to overcome these drawbacks manufacturers now supply composites for creating inlays outside the mouth, and the equipment to polymerize them extraorally.

Presentation   Kits of composite resin in various shades. The composites contain either hybrid or microfine fillers and are generally supplied with units variously known as curing chambers, tempering ovens and light boxes.

Common brands   Charisma Inlay (with Translux

Lightbox or Dentacolour XS curing unit); Coltene Brilliant (with DI 500 heat- and light- tempering oven); Kulzer Inlay System (with Translux Light-box' or Dentalcolour XS curing unit); Prisma AP.H Inlay System (utilizing any heat- and light-tempering unit, an oven at 120°C or boiling water); TrueVitality (a tri-cured resin system for direct and indirect inlays, heat-, light- or self-curable); Vivadent S.R. Isosit Inlay/Onlay (with Ivomat heat and steam pressure chamber); 'Vivadent E.O.S. System' (utilizing a normal light-curing source and wand).

Manipulation   Each product has its own manipulative sequence, which involves an impression, one or two dies, coating a die with separating medium, creating the inlay or onlay, partially curing it, fully curing or tempering it, relieving and roughening the fitting surface, and cementing it into place with a dual-cure cement (see section 2.1.13.3). The E.O.S. system uses one silicone elastomer (Redphase P) for impressions and another (Bluephase P) to produce a die. The Prisma AP.H System employs a similar silicone elastomer (Model Silicone) for the same purpose.

3.2.3 Composite inserts

Presentation   Preformed shapes and sizes of glass–ceramic whose surfaces have been silane-treated.

Common brand   Beta-Quartz.

Manipulation   These inserts are pressed into a cavity preparation that is already filled with unpolymerized composite. The composite which is extruded during the insertion is removed and that which remains is allowed or caused to cure according to type. The restoration is then contoured using diamond rotary instruments and polished.

Properties   The inserts have a low coefficient of thermal expansion and are wear-resistant. Their presence is said to reduce polymerization shrinkage by up to 75% and to increase the stiffness of the filling. They are radiopaque.

Applications Used to minimize the marginal-contraction gaps in composite fillings.

3.3 Unfilled resins

Presentation A pigmented powder (microspheres of poly(methyl methacrylate) containing up to 0.5% by weight of dibenzoyl peroxide as an initiator) with a clear, colourless liquid (methyl methacrylate monomer containing up to 2% tertiary amine chemical activator (typically dimethyl-*p*-toluidine) and a small amount (0.01% maximum) of hydroquinone as a stabilizer).

Common brand Sevriton.

Manipulation Polymer powder is added to two drops of monomer in a Dappens dish until excess powder remains. The pot is inverted to allow any dry powder to fall away and one drop more of monomer is added. The thin paste thus produced is stirred and used instantly. Celluloid matrices should not be employed, neither should acrylic of this type come into contact with zinc oxide–eugenol cements, which plasticize the acrylic, softening and discolouring it.

Properties A high polymerization shrinkage, low modulus of elasticity and low compressing strength are all factors which can contribute to severe marginal leakage. Good initial aesthetics, but they wear rapidly and can discolour when the amine activator dissociates under the ultraviolet light present in sunlight.

Applications
1. Temporary crowns and bridges (see section 4.6).
2. Splints and splint cementation (see section 2.1.12).
3. Formerly used for class III and V anterior fillings.
4. Formerly used for class IV incisal edge restorations (acid-etch retention).

3.4 Acid-leachable glasses

The first of these was silicate cement, which appeared in 1904. This was followed in 1920 by the silicophosphate cement (see section 2.1.8) which was much less soluble. Following the development of polycarboxylate cements by Smith in the 1960s, the Laboratory of the Government Chemist under Wilson developed the glass-ionomer cements in the 1970s. Both silicate and glass-ionomer cements are formed when hydrogen ions in the acids react with a special type of glass to displace aluminium ions. These combine with the acid to form a salt. This causes the material to set.

3.4.1 Silicate cements

Presentation Opalescent powder (fluoroaluminosilicate glass) with a clear fluid (50% aqueous solution of phosphoric acid, containing zinc and aluminium ions).

Common brands Achatit-Biochromatic; Biotrey; M.Q.; Silicap (encapsulated).

Setting reaction (Fig. 3)
1. *Initial ion exchange:*
Fluoroaluminosilicate glass $+ H_3PO_4 \rightarrow H^+ + H_2PO_4^-$

accompanied by the release of Al^{3+}, Ca^{2+}, Na^+ and F^- ions

2. *Formation of matrix*

$$Al^{3+} + H_2PO_4^- \rightarrow AlPO_4$$

$$Na^+ + H_2PO_4^- \rightarrow NaH_2PO_4$$

$$Ca^2 + F^- \rightarrow CaF_2$$

The hardening reaction follows the sequence:

$$H_3PO_4 + Al^{3+} \rightarrow Al(H_2PO_4)_3 + Al^{3+} \rightarrow Al_2(HPO_4)_3 + Al^{3+} \rightarrow AlPO_4$$

$Al(H_2PO_4)_3$ is very soluble and acidic
$Al_2(HPO_4)_3$ is a soluble and acidic gel
$AlPO_4$ is a relatively insoluble and neutral solid

Manipulation The cement must be mixed within a minute into a thick paste with either a cobalt–chromium (stellite) or agate spatula on a cool, dry

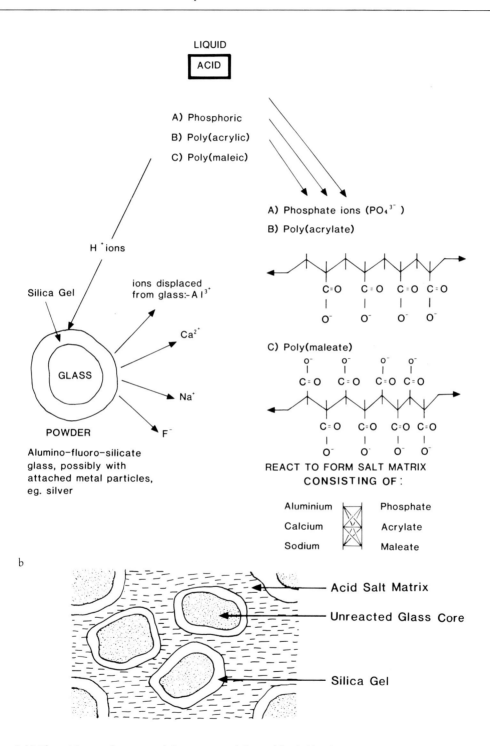

Figure 3 (a) The setting mechanisms and (b) structure of the acid-leachable glass cements.

slab. The powder is divided into two parts and one of these is subdivided into four parts. The *largest* portion is added to the liquid first and mixed with a rolling action. The remainder of the powder is then added, as necessary, to produce a stiff paste which looks dry on the slab but shows as moist when pressed with the spatula.

The cavity must be as dry as possible and the cement must be kept dry and undisturbed under a polymeric matrix strip until set. After finishing and polishing with abrasive strips, the restoration should be coated with varnish. Keep the liquid bottle stoppered to prevent water loss or gain.

Properties   Good translucency and colour match. Dissolves in stagnation areas (low pH). Loss of water from the structure causes crazing. Fluoride leaches out to form calcium fluorapatite.

Applications   Class III and V anterior restorations, especially if secondary caries is anticipated. Contraindicated for mouth-breathers.

3.4.2 Glass-ionomer cements (type II; see also 2.1.10)

Presentation   Opalescent powder (fluorocalcium aluminosilicate glass) with either:
1. *Form A:* A clear, viscous liquid consisting of a 50% aqueous solution of a co-polymer of poly(acrylic acid) and itaconic acid, together with tartaric acid as a hardening agent. (Light-cured systems have similar acids with pendant vinyl groups, in which case the powder also contains a light-sensitive initiator; these cements are designated LC or VLC)

or:

2. *Form B:* The same acids in powder form (freeze-dried) or an alternative powdered co-polymer of acrylic and maleic acids. These dry powder acids are supplied *blended* with the glass powder and only require clean water or a dilute solution of tartaric acid to activate them. They are often termed anhydrous.

Form B is sometimes supplied with its ingredients encapsulated.

Common brands
1. *Form A:* (powder + liquid); Fuji II LC; Gem-Fil; Glasionomer II; Hi-Fi; Ionofil-U; VariGlass VLC.

2. *Form B:* (anhydrous: bulk and capsules): Aqua-Fil; Aqua Ionofil; Ceram-Fil B; Chelon-Fil; ChemFil Superior; Discovery; FujiCap II (LC); Ketac-Fil; Kromoglass 2; Legend; New-Era; OpusFil W; Photac-Fil Aplicap (LC); Rexodent RGI.

Setting reaction   The acids act as proton donors which extract Al^{3+} and Ca^{2+} ions from the glass and these react with the carboxylate groups on the acids, causing ionic cross-linking of the polymer chains. The calcium ions are responsible for the initial precipitation and gelation of the subsequent hardening stage. The tartaric acid aids the extraction of the cations from the glass and this sharpens the set. Once set, the material increases in strength and becomes more translucent due to the formation of hydrated silicates within the structure. These reduce the sensitivity of the cement to water.

Manipulation   Areas of cavity close to the pulp should receive a little calcium hydroxide cement. The remainder of the dentine should be treated with a 10% solution of poly(acrylic acid) to remove the smear layer. Bulk constituents are mixed for about a minute into a thick paste using the proportions recommended by the manufacturer, who always provides a powder scoop and liquid dropper bottle. An abrasion-resistant spatula (cobalt–chromium or agate) should be used. Materials in capsules require insertion into a press to free the liquid component, followed by vigorous oscillation in a high-speed mixer (e.g. Silamat).

Mixed cement is then extruded through nozzle on capsule into the cavity under dry conditions. It must be covered with a close-fitting, flexible matrix until the first stage of setting is complete (about 3 minutes).

On removal of the matrix the cement should be covered with a layer of unfilled, light-activated, diacrylate cement. This should not be cured as it acts as both a lubricant for the finishing stages and as a barrier to reduce the loss or gain of moisture. Trimming at this stage should be performed using sharp hand instruments only. A second layer of resin should then be applied and activated with the curing light.

Properties   Unique adhesion to the apatite of both enamel and dentine via a dynamic (self-repairing) bond, which forms when the carboxylate groups of the various carboxylic acids are involved in an ion-exchange reaction with the calcium and phosphate ions of the apatite. The poly-acids are also absorbed on to the collagen of dentine and this also contributes to the formation of a bond. Attachment to both enamel and dentine is increased by conditioning with poly(acrylic acid) or tannic acid. Citric acid conditioners are not recommended.

Good degree of translucency. Soluble until completely hardened (needs protective layer of varnish or unfilled resin). Carvable with sharp hand instruments. Fluoride leaches out to form fluorapatite.

Applications

1. Erosion cavities, class III and class V cavities where minimum preparation is desirable.
2. For applications other than as a filling material see sections 2.1.10, 15.3.2 and 17.2.1.

3.4.3 Glass-ionomer cements with metal additives (cermets)

Presentation Either encapsulated, or as bulk powder, to which clean water or a solution of tartaric acid is added.

The powder may be either an intimate mixture of fluoroaluminosilicate glass and metal powder (silver or silver amalgam alloy), or the same sort of glass powder to which pure metallic silver has been fused. In some cases the powders are supplied ready-mixed, in others the dentist mixes the glass and metal powders as required.

The liquid is either pure water or a solution of tartaric acid. In the encapsulated material this liquid is contained within a foil envelope within the capsule.

Common brands Chelon-Silver; Hi-Dense; Ion S; Ketac-Silver; Legend Silver; Miracle Mix; New-Era Silver; OpusSilver; RGI Reinforced.

Manipulation Bulk materials are mixed using the proportions recommended by the manufacturer, who supplies a powder scoop and a liquid dropper bottle. Mixing time is about 1 minute.

Capsules are activated by bursting the water envelope and rehydrating the acid during mixing on a high-speed vibrator. The acid reacts with the glass to form a paste which is extruded as required. The cement sets to produce a structure consisting of unreacted glass particles and metal particles (which may or may not be fused to the glass according to type), held together by a metal–salt matrix.

Surfaces exposed to saliva should be protected with a layer of light-activated, unfilled diacrylate resin.

Properties Adheres to enamel and dentine. Radiopaque.

Fluoride leaches out to form fluorapatite. Metal provides increased abrasion resistance. Light metallic appearance.

Applications

1. Small class I restorations.
2. Build-up of cores (without pins).
3. Replacement dentine technique, including tunnel preparations from the occlusal surface to remove proximal caries.

Further reading

Amalgam

Black, G.V. (1896) The physical properties of the silver-tin amalgams. *Dental Cosmos*, **38**, 965–992

Boyer, D.B. and Edie, J.W. (1990) Composition of clinically aged amalgam restorations. *Dental Materials*, **6**, 146–150

Curtis, R.V. and Brown, D. (1992) The use of dental amalgam – an art or a science? *Dental Update*, **19**, 239–245

Flagg, J.F. (1891) in *Plastics and plastic fillings*, 4th edn, The Author, Philadelphia, pp. 37–92

Jagadish, S. and Yogesh, B.G. (1990) Fracture resistance of teeth with Class II silver amalgam, posterior composite and glass ionomer cement restorations. *Operative Dentistry*, **15**, 42–47

Mahler, D.B., Engle, J.H. and Adey, J.D. (1990) Effect of Pd on the clinical performance of amalgam. *Journal of Dental Research*, **69**, 1759–1761

Marek, M. (1990) The effect of tin on the corrosion behaviour of the Ag-Hg phase of dental amalgam and the dissolution of mercury. *Journal of Dental Research*, **69**, 1786–1790

Masaka, N. (1990) Restoring the severely compromised molar through adhesive bonding of amalgam to dentin. *Compendium of Continuing Education in Dentistry*, **12**, 90–98

Mjör, I. A., Jokstad, A. and Qvist, V. (1990) Longevity of posterior restorations. *International Dental Journal*, **40**, 11–17

Osborne, J.W. (1990) Clinical assessment of 14 amalgam alloys. *General Dentistry*, **38**, 206–208

Osborne, J.W. (1990) Five-year clinical assessment of 14 amalgam alloys. *Operative Dentistry*, **15**, 202–206

Osborne, J.W. and Gale, E.N. (1990) Relationship of restoration width, tooth position and alloy to fracture at the margins of 13- to 14-year-old amalgams. *Journal of Dental Research*, **69**, 1599–1601

Osborne, J.W. and Norman, R.D. (1990) 13-year clinical assessment of 10 amalgam alloys. *Dental Material*, **6**, 189–194

Taveau, L.A.O. (1837) *Notice sur un ciment oblitérique pour arrêter et guérir la carie de dent offrant un mode nouveau de traitement pour conserver celles qui en sont atteintes sans avoir recours a l'extraction de ces précieux organes.* L'auteur, Paris, p. 16

Tomes, C.S. (1872) On the chemical and physical properties of amalgams. *Transactions of the Odontological Society of Great Britain*, **4**, 135–159

Mercury

Berglund, A. (1990) Estimation by a 24-hour study of the daily dose of intra-oral mercury vapour inhaled after release from dental amalgam. *Journal of Dental Research*, **69**, 1646–1651

Fung, Y.K., Molvar, M.P., Strom, A., Schneider, N.R. and Carlson, M.P. (1990) *In vivo* mercury and methyl mercury levels in patients at different intervals after amalgam restorations. *General Dentistry*, **39**, 89—92

Haikel, Y., Jaeger, A., Livardjani, F. and Alleman, C. (1990) Intra-oral air mercury vapour released from dental amalgam, before and after restorative procedures: a preliminary study. *Clinical Materials*, **5**, 265–270

Marek, M. (1990) The release of mercury from dental amalgam: the mechanism and *in vitro* testing. *Journal of Dental Research*, **69**, 1167–1174

Smales, R.J., Gerke, D.C. and Hume, W.R. (1990) Clinical behaviour of high-copper amalgams with time, site, size and class of cavity preparation. *Journal of Dentistry*, **18**, 49–53

Composites

Atmadja, G. and Bryant, R.W. (1990) Some factors influencing the depth of cure of visible light-activated composite resins. *Australian Dental Journal*, **35**, 213–218

Chung, K-H. and Greener, E.H. (1990) Correlation of conversion, filler concentration and mechanical properties of posterior composite resins. *Journal of Oral Rehabilitation*, **17**, 487–494

Dietschi, D. and Holz, J. (1990) A clinical trial of four light-curing posterior composite resins: two-year report. *Quintessence International*, **21**, 965–975

Dionysopoulos, P. and Watts, D.C. (1990) Sensitivity to ambient light of visible light-cured composites. *Journal of Oral Rehabilitation*, **17**, 9–13

Donly, K.J., Dowell, A., Anixiadas, C, and Croll, T.P. (1990) Relationship among visible light source, composite resin polymerization shrinkage and hygroscopic expansion. *Quintessence International*, **21**, 883–886

Feilzer, A.J., De Gee, A.J. and Davidson, C.L. (1990) Quantitative determination of stress reduction by flow in composite restorations. *Dental Materials*, **6**, 167–171

Koike, T., Hasegawa, T., Manabe, A., Itoh, K. and Wakumoto, S.

(1990) Effect of water sorption and thermal stress on cavity adaptation of dental composites. *Dental Materials*, **6**, 178–180

Osborne, L.W., Norman, R.D. and Gale E.N. (1990) A 12-year clinical evaluation of two composite resins. *Quintessence International*, **21**, 111–114

Pintado, M.R. (1990) Characterization of two small-particle composite resins. *Quintessence International*, **21**, 843–847

Rees, J.S. and Jacobsen, P.H. (1989) The current status of composite materials and adhesive systems. Part 1: composite resins – review and recent developments. *Restorative Dentistry*, **5**, 91–93

Rueggeberg, F.A. and Margeson, D.H. (1990) The effect of oxygen inhibition on an unfilled/filled composite system. *Journal of Dental Research*, **69**, 1652–1658

Saunders, W.P. (1990) Effect of fatigue upon the interfacial bond strength of repaired composite resins, *Journal of Dentistry*, **18**, 151–157

Soderholm, K-J. M. and Roberts, M.J. (1990) Influence of water exposure on the tensile strength of composites. *Journal of Dental Research*, **69**, 1812–1816

Warren, K. (1990) An investigation into the microhardness of a light-cured composite when cured through varying thicknesses of porcelain. *Journal of Oral Rehabilitation*, **17**, 327–334

Acid-leachable glasses

Smith, D.C. (1968) A new dental cement. *British Dental Journal*, **125**, 381–384

Wilson, A.D. and Kent, B.E. (1977) A new translucent cement for dentistry. The glass-ionomer cement. *British Dental Journal*, **132**, 133–135

Glass-ionomer cements

Billington, R.W., Williams, J.A. and Pearson, G.J. (1990) Variation in powder/liquid ratio of a restorative glass ionomer cement used in dental practice. *British Dental Journal*, **169**, 164–167

Burke, F.M., Hamlin, P.D. and Lynch, E.J. (1990) Depth of cure of light-cured glass ionomer cements. *Quintessence International*, **21**, 977–981

Council on Dental Materials, Instruments and Equipment (1990) Using glass ionomers. *Journal of the American Dental Association*, **120**, 181–188

Knibbs, P.J. and Plant, C.G. (1990) An evaluation of a rapid setting glass ionomer cement used by general dental practitioners to restore deciduous teeth. *Journal of Oral Rehabilitation*, **17**, 1–7

McLean, J.W. (1990) Cermet cements. *Journal of the American Dental Association*, **120**, 20–22

Robbins, J.W., Cooley, R.L. and Barnwell, S. (1990) Fracture resistance of reinforced glass ionomer as a build-up material. *Operative Dentistry*, **15**, 23–26

Robinson, P.B. and Brackett, W.W. (1990) Composite resin and glass ionomer cement: current status for use in cervical restorations. *Quintessence International*, **21**, 445–447

Smith, D.C. (1990) Composition and characteristics of glass ionomer cements. *Journal of the American Dental Association*, **120**, 20–22

Watson, T.F. (1990) A confocal microscopic study of some of the factors affecting the adaptation of a light-cured glass ionomer to tooth tissue. *Journal of Dental Research*, **69**, 1531–1538

Williams, J.A. and Billington, R.W. (1990) The radiopacity of glass ionomer dental materials. *Journal of Oral Rehabilitation*, **17**, 245–248

4 Concomitant conservation materials

4.1 Dentine pins

Use   The purpose of these devices is to aid retention in those cases where little or none exists, so that amalgam or composite cores or restorations may be formed. They do *not* provide any degree of reinforcement and may act as stress-raisers.

Materials   They are made from type 316L (medical-grade) stainless steel, gold-plated base metal alloys, titanium, titanium–aluminium–vanadium alloys or gold–platinum alloys.

Construction   Most of these particular preformed devices have either a screw thread or a roughened surface which enables them to be retained either in specially cut holes in the dentine or down suitably reamed root canals. In some cases the head of the pin or post is shaped to aid both insertion and the retention of either amalgam or composite. Several have smooth surfaces intended for use with cements, such as polycarboxylate or cyanoacrylate, which bond to them and to dentine.

Retention   The pins are retained by the elastic recoil of dentine, by the use of cements, or by a thread cut in the dentine before the pin is inserted.

Insertion   Some pins have to be inserted and driven in with small, manually rotated drivers, whilst others can be placed in a handpiece and rotated in the hole until a section of the pin (which is thinner than the rest) shears, leaving the pin *in situ*.

Commercial types   Ceramicor (Au-Pt); Denlok; Dentatus; Filpin Nova; FO-Pin; Max Pin; Microdontic Pin System; Parapin; PCR-Pin; Penpin;

Precious Pin; Securipin; Stabilok; TMS Link.

4.2 Crown posts

Uses   The purpose of these devices is to act as an alternative to cast posts for the support of metal, ceramic or metal–ceramic crowns.

Materials   They are made from stainless steel, titanium, platinized gold, platinum–iridium, cobalt–chromium–nickel alloy wire, or epoxy-bonded pyrolitic carbon.

Construction   One type has a threaded stainless steel post fitted with an aluminium–bronze core. In other cases cores are either built-up in amalgam or composite or a gold core is cast on to a wrought post or wire, but not on to titanium or stainless steel, whose oxide films prevent the formation of a reliable bond. The epoxy-bonded carbon post is constructed from anisotropic fibres.

Retention   Most of these crown posts are retained by micromechanical retention with cement but at least one is held in threaded dentine. The epoxy-bonded carbon fibre post forms a chemical bond with the composite used to construct the core and the resin-based cement used to retain it.

Commercial types
1. *Preformed posts:* Anchorex; Anchorextra; Composipost (epoxy-bonded carbon fibres); Cytco; Dentorama; Exatec; Filpost; Flexi-Anterior; Flexi Cast; Flexi-Post; GT Root-Post; Kerr Endo-Post; Kurer Crown Anchor; Mooser RC Post; MP Pirec; OP-PO; Para-Post Plus; Para-Post Unity; Radix Anker; Safix-Anker; Titancor; Titronic-K; Tri-Flex Root Pin; Velva.
2. *Wires:* Irido-Platinum (Pt-10Ir); Wiptam (Co-30Cr-25Ni).

4.3 Retentive Meshes

Use   The idea behind these shaped pieces of metallic mesh is to provide a means by which mechanical retention can be effected between the components of a Rochette-type bridge and etched dental enamel, via an intermediate layer of composite restorative resin.

Materials Meshes can be made from either precious or base metal alloys.

Manipulation Supplied either as pieces of mesh which have to be cut to size and carefully adapted to the tooth surface, or as preshaped components intended as fitting surface inserts to cast frameworks. In each case retention to etched enamel is via a layer of composite restorative resin.

Commercial types
1. Bulk mesh for cutting and adaption.
2. Pre-shaped mesh for casting fitting surfaces: e.g. Klett-O-Bond-Renfert.

4.4 Retention to enamel and dentine

4.4.1 Retention to enamel

4.4.1.1 Mechanical attachment This can be achieved by etching the enamel with phosphoric acid. The best results are obtained using an aqueous solution which contains 30–50% phosphoric acid. Supplied either as a liquid or a gel, the latter is easier to control *in vivo* and is just as effective in causing the selective dissolution of the enamel structure.

Presentation and common brands Each manufacturer of resin or composite tends to supply acid in the form of either liquid or gel, often in syringes fitted with blunt needles, and in a concentration considered suitable for the product being used. There are thus no brand names, although the acid is sometimes referred to as a surface conditioner. Those manufacturers who supply unfilled diacrylate resins for applying to etched enamel prior to the addition of the composite material often refer to these resins as bonding agents or enamel bond.

Manipulation The acid is applied to lightly ground and (pumice- and water-) cleaned enamel with a brush, sponge or pledget of cotton wool. Recommended etching periods vary between 5 and 120 seconds but, whatever time is used, etching should be followed by thorough water-rinsing and drying with oil-free air, after which the enamel should have a frosty appearance. The etched surface must *not* be contaminated with salivary proteins prior to the application of the resin or composite.

Applications Whilst the acid-etch procedure is part of many routine treatments, specific applications include:
1. The retention of orthodontic brackets via diacrylate resins.
2. The retention of non-preparation (or minimal preparation) bridges and splints.
3. The retention of porcelain and glass–ceramic, laboratory-made veneers to anterior teeth.

4.4.1.2 Chemical attachment *Glass-ionomer cements* form a unique adhesive bond to enamel via an intermediate layer formed when calcium and phosphate ions are displaced from the apatite by the carboxylate groups of the poly(acrylic-) or poly(maleic acid). To achieve a bond the enamel needs to be free from salivary pellicle.

4.4.2 Attachment to dentine

Vital dentine is a porous, sensitive and wet tissue which, when prepared during operative procedures, becomes covered with a loosely attached *smear layer*. This is composed of the detritus of cavity preparation and is a mixture of apatite crystals from enamel and dentine, dentinal collagen (which has been denatured by the heat generated by the bur), a complex cocktail of oral bacteria and water. Much of this smear layer is in the form of plugs within the dentinal tubules. It is to this unpromising layer and damp substrate that it is hoped to form a durable bond. As materials such as composites contain hydrophobic resins, some method is needed to create a link between the hydrophilic dentine and smear layer and the hydrophobic resin. The successful agents penetrate the intertubular dentine and create a resin-reinforced dentine surface.

Presentation The options available are:
1 Remove the smear layer completely with acid (opening up the tubules in the process), and form a bond which is chemical, mechanical (involving the infiltration of the tubules with resin which polymerizes *in situ*) or a combination of both.

2. Modify the smear layer in some way with suitable chemical agents, such as special resins, which have an affinity for both hydrophilic and hydrophobic surfaces. These may combine with it to produce a retentive surface, and may even pass through the smear layer to form chemical bonds with the underlying components of the dentine.

3. Merely wet the smear layer without modifying it, thus allowing hydrophilic resins to penetrate it and create a surface which is sympathetic to the attachment of the hydrophobic molecules used in the resin matrices of all composites.

Utilizing option 1:

(a) *Glass-ionomer cements:* These form chemical bonds to dentine. Their presentation, manipulation, properties and applications are indicated in sections 2.1.10 and 3.4.2. As they are hydrophilic in nature, once the loose smear layer has been removed, they have no difficulty in forming durable, self-repairing bonds with the apatite of dentine.

(b) *Resin-based systems:* Two systems which have utilized acids to remove completely the smear layer before seeking to form a bond with the exposed dentine are Clearfil Bond and Gluma.

Clearfil Bond became available in the late 1970s. It contained a mixture of phosphonated monomer and the water-soluble monomer known as HEMA. This latter acted as a wetting agent and allowed the resin to penetrate the dentinal tubules once the smear layer had been removed with phosphoric acid. It was said that the phosphate groups produced a form of polar interaction, and this contributed to the formation of a chemical bond. In the late 1980s Clearfil New Bond and Clearfil Photo Bond were introduced. These contained more sophisticated phosphonated monomers and HEMA, but they still required the smear layer to be dissolved away to obtain the best bond. In the 1990s a new concept was added – the addition of an intermediate *elastic* layer between the smear-layer free, primed dentine and the composite filling material. The dentine was conditioned with a mixture of citric acid and calcium chloride (CA Agent) and primed with N-methacryloyl 5-aminosalicylic acid (SA Primer). This neutral-pH

monomer restores the spatial structure of the collagen fibres of the dentine and allows a dual-curing agent (Photo Bond) to penetrate and form a bond. To this is added the elastic liner (Protect Liner). This is a light-curing microfine composite, which is intended to absorb the stresses generated by the shrinkage of the composite.

Gluma became available in the mid 1980s as a three-component system. The first component is a 17% solution of ethylene diamine tetra-acetic acid (EDTA), which is used to dissolve the smear layer. However, unlike phosphoric acid, which opens up the tubules and appears to destroy their organic contents, the EDTA removes the smear layer and some of the apatite, but leaves the collagen fibres intact. On to this surface an aqueous solution of 5% glutaraldehyde/35% HEMA is applied and left *in situ*. To this layer is added one of unfilled resins, and this is followed by the composite. This was the first system to utilize an aqueous primer.

Utilizing option 2:

(a) *Phosphate ester systems:* The early 1980s saw the arrival of many systems based on the phosphate esters of bis-GMA, which are hydrophobic.

Scotchbond was the first of these and, like many of the materials which followed it on to the market, consisted of two components which were mixed together prior to use to start the polymerization reaction. One component was water-based and contained an acid salt which softened the smear layer and allowed resins within the other component (which were dissolved in ethanol) to penetrate the smear layer and effect a bond. In later presentations light-activated initiators were used to enable the resin to be light-cured.

Similar chemistry was employed in systems such as Bondlite; Creation Bond; Dentin Bonding Agent and Prisma Universal Bond.

(b) *Phenyl glycine-based systems:* The complex bifunctional molecule N-phenyl glycine-glycidyl methacrylate (NPG-GMA) was tried as a dentine-bonding agent back in the 1960s, and was the basis of the material sold as Cervident. However, the durability of bonds formed between dentine and composite using this agent was very low, probably because, although it wet the surface of the dentine, it lacked any means of controlling the smear layer − at that time there was little awareness of its significance.

NPG-GMA is incorporated in several systems available in the 1990s:

Tenure is presented as three components. The first is an aqueous conditioner, which contains 2.5% nitric acid, 3.5% aluminium oxalate, and which nowadays contains NPG-GMA to assist in wetting the dentine. The dentine adhesive is presented as two solutions − solution A, which contains N-tolyl glycidyl methacrylate (NTG-GMA) in acetone, and solution B, which contains pyromellitic acid dimethacrylate (PMDM), also in acetone.

The acid conditioner dissolves the smear layer and the calcium and phosphate ions are believed to combine with the aluminium oxalate to produce insoluble aluminium phosphate and calcium oxalate. The compounds act like a mordant to the collagen fibres.

In later variations on this formulation, the oxalate has been omitted. Two products of the 1990s which utilize 2.5% nitric acid to remove the smear layer and partially demineralize the dentine surface whilst at the same time etching any enamel it meets, are Mirage Bond and Restobond 3. Both systems use similar monomers to those found in Tenure.

(c) *Dentine softening systems:* Milder agents to prime the dentine and soften it (so that resins may impregnate the smear layer and thus reinforce it prior to attaching it to the composite) are employed in several systems of the 1990s.

Scotchbond 2 is presented as a two component system, as are many of these agents. The first is Scotchprep, which is an aqueous *primer* based on maleic acid and HEMA. This is acidic enough to soften and modify the smear layer and allow the second component to penetrate it. This is the adhesive, and consists of a 2 : 1 mixture of bis-GMA and HEMA.

Scotchbond Multi-Purpose has three components, the first of which is an etching gel containing 10% maleic acid. This is strong enough to etch the enamel, but only softens the dentine and prepares it for the primer. This

contains HEMA and the light-sensitive polymer found in light-cured glass-ionomer cements. The third component, the adhesive, contains a mixture of bis-GMA and HEMA, together with a photoinitiator. It is advocated not only for bonding composite to tooth, but also for bonding porcelain veneers to teeth, composite to old amalgam, and for the repair of both porcelain and composite restorations.

XR Bond uses a primer (XR Primer) consisting of a dilute solution of phosphonated ester in alcohol and water to soften the smear layer before adding the adhesive mixture of dimethacrylates. This resin mixture saturates the smear layer and is then light-cured to create a bond which is mainly mechanical.

Prisma Universal Bond 2 employs a primer based on a more complex phosphonated ester together with HEMA in ethanol. In this system the adhesive resin mixture contains the diluent resin triethylene glycol dimethacrylate (TEG-DMA) and a small amount of glutaraldehyde, which may provide additional retention via the collagen.

Utilizing option C:

Wetting the smear layer without altering it so that resins may penetrate it and create attachment is the philosophy behind several of the dentine bonding systems of the 1990s.

Tripton was the first of the acid-free systems and uses a primer based on a polyhexanide to wet the smear layer. This allows a bonding agent based on urethane dimethacrylate, TEG-DMA diluent and an organic monophosphate to penetrate the layer and form bonds with both the organic and inorganic constituents of the dentine.

Syntac uses a primer consisting of maleic acid and poly(ethylene glycol dimethacrylate) in acetone. This provides a combination of good wetting and penetration of the smear layer and allows the adhesive, which is an aqueous solution of poly(ethylene glycol dimethacrylate) and glutaraldehyde, to enter the tubules and create attachment. A.R.T. Bond, Imperva Bond and Topaz L.C. Dentine Adhesive are similar.

Denthesive uses a primer which acts in the same way, allowing a two-component adhesive mixture to react with both the organic and inorganic parts of the dentine and creating a substantial bond in a very short time.

All-Bond and All-Bond 2 are further variants on the same theme, in which a dentine conditioner acts as a wetting agent and a co-polymerizable monomer. This penetrates the smear layer prior to the use of a two-part primer which enters the tubules. An adhesive resin is then applied to link the impregnated smear layer to the composite. All-Bond 2 also forms bonds with a range of synthetic dental materials.

Pertac Universal Bond employs the same principles of wetting the smear layer, thus allowing the penetration of a mixture of hydrophilic and hydrophobic dimethacrylate resins which are light-cured. However, in this case all the constituents are incorporated into a single container.

Gluma 2000 and Prisma Universal Bond 3 encourage firstly the dimineralization of dentine and then precipitation of calcium oxalate and aluminium phosphate. Glycine is then absorbed on to the surface and the dentine is infiltrated with a dual-curing version of HEMA.

Manipulation The diversity of the presentation of these systems is such that *it is essential* that the manufacturer's instructions are followed to the letter. The systems are all technique-sensitive and unforgiving. If the appropriate handling sequence is not followed, the optimum bond will not be produced. Curing of the bonding resin prior to the application of the composite is recommended, as it is unlikely to cure via the composite. Also, as the curing of this resin layer is inhibited by the presence of air, it must be at least 15 μm thick if it is to cure. Thus, it should not be air-thinned.

Composite restorations bonded to these agents should be built up in increments in order to reduce the effects of polymerization shrinkage and thus limit the stress placed on the bond to the dentine.

Properties Bond strength values to non-vital dentine determined under laboratory conditions are often quoted and compared. Values reported in manufacturers' literature vary from 5 MPa (theirs) to 20 MPa (ours); in some cases these values increase with time. Limited shelf-life, extendable if kept refrigerated. Solvents will evaporate if caps are not replaced.

Applications
1. Sealing of margins and the retention of composite restorations in class V cavities.
2. Dentine coverage under ceramic veneers or inlays, and composite inlays or onlays retained with resin-based cements.
3. Bonding directly placed composite to dentine to reinforce a posterior tooth with a class II cavity.

4.4.3 Mechanical attachment to enamel and retention to metal

Used in the retention of bridges to sound abutment teeth which require a minimum of preparation. The enamel is etched to provide retentive etch pits into which lightly filled, self-curing resins flow and set.

The metal surface can be made similarly retentive either by creating features at the wax-up stage (*macromechanical attachment*) or by treating the surface after casting so as to produce retentive etch pits (*microretentive attachment*).

The cast metal surface may also be treated with agents so that chemical bonds will form via one of several bifunctional primers (*adhesive attachment*).

4.4.3.1 Mechanical attachment to metal
4.4.3.1.1 Macromechanical attachment: Techniques using polymeric meshes (Duralingual) or beads (Micro-Retentive), which are applied to the fitting surface of the wax pattern, are available. The fitting surface can also be given retentive features at the wax-up stage by applying one of the following:
(a) 200 μm, cubic salt grains to the pattern (Virginia Salt). These are dissolved out in boiling water after casting to produce cubic retentive pores.
(b) Large particles of porcelain powder (Ceramco II) to the pattern. After casting, the porcelain is dissolved away using hydrofluoric acid, leaving retentive pores.
(c) A mixture of salt grains and spherical acrylic beads (Crystal Bond) to the pattern. The beads burn away during heating of the invested pattern and the salt can be dissolved away with boiling water to produce a multifaceted retentive surface.

Applications and limitations

(a) Can be used with any alloy, noble or base metal.
(b) Provides consistent bond strengths, which tend to be lower than other techniques.
(c) Framework needs to be thick to accommodate the retentive surface.
(d) Sensitive to casting technique and conditions.

4.4.3.1.2 Micromechanical attachment: The fitting surface of the cast metal bridge can be etched using one of the following:

(a) An *electrolytic technique* in which those areas not to be etched are protected with sticky wax. The bridge is made the anode in an electrolytic cell containing acid. Etching current and time are critical and unique for each alloy. A black surface is produced and the ultrasonic cleaning in hydrochloric acid which follows produces a matte grey surface full of retentive etch pits 30–50 μm deep.
(b) A *chemical etch* based on strong acids and presented as a gel. This is applied to the fitting surface of heated metal, which is then ultrasonically cleaned. This method is less technique-sensitive than the electrolytic procedure

Applications and limitations

(a) Only suitable for certain nickel–chromium alloys. However, these have a high modulus, which allows the use of very thin sections. Compared with the chemical etch procedure, the electrolytic technique requires special equipment, is more time-consuming and requires greater skill to produce consistently good etch patterns.
(b) An alternative form of micromechanical attachment, which can be used with either noble or base metal alloys applies a porous metal coating of 25 μm metal particles to the surface (Inzoma P990) and bonds it to the surface by sintering during firing at 970°C.

4.4.3.2 Chemical attachment to metal This allows the attachment of a bridge to etched enamel using chemical adhesives incorporated in resin-based cements. The metal surface requires a minimum of surface preparation. Whilst the technique is limited to alloys which form surface oxides, other alloys can receive surface coatings which promote chemical bonding.

4.4.3.2.1 4-META resin cements: This system employs the reactive monomer 4-META, which forms a chemical bond to both *oxidized* precious and base metal alloys. (4-META is also a component of Orthomite Super-Bond (orthodontic bonding resin) and Meta-Dent (metal-bonding denture base resin).)

Common brands Amalgambond; C & B Metabond; Cover-Up II; Super-Bond C & B.

Presentation Polymer (generally poly(methyl methacrylate)), monomer (methyl methacrylate) and a catalyst such as tri-N-butyl borane oxide (TBB-O), together with 4-META.

Manipulation The enamel is etched with phosphoric acid and the metal framework (which may be either precious or base metal) is sand-blasted and then oxidized. The monomer, polymer and catalyst are mixed and applied to the metal substrate which is then seated on the etched enamel.

Setting reaction The mixed components polymerize and retention is achieved by mechanical interlock with the etched enamel and chemical bonding via the oxide on the metal substrate.

Applications and limitations Good initial bond strength but it deteriorates with time, particularly in water. Suitable only for alloys that produce a good surface oxide. Noble metal alloys which contain substantial amounts of base metal such as copper can be oxidized. Other noble metal alloys can be tin-plated or exposed to low-fusing gallium–tin alloy to provide a surface to which the 4-META will bond. Amalgambond and Cover-Up II are marketed as metal repair systems.

4.4.3.2.2 Phosphonated resin cements: This system utilizes a phosphate ester monomer to form a chemical bond to base metal alloys and to tin-plated noble alloys.

Common brands Clearfil Photo Bond; Panavia Ex.

Presentation Filled or unfilled powders (some radiopaque), a mixture of aromatic and aliphatic methacrylates and phosphate ester monomer, together with activators, plus 10-methacryloxy-decyl dihydrogen phosphate (MDP) adhesive phosphate.

Manipulation The powders and liquids are mixed and applied to the sand-blasted and oxidized fitting surface of the metal, which is then seated on the etched enamel. The setting of the monomers is severely inhibited by oxygen, and any exposed cement must be protected either with a layer of Oxyguard (polyethylene glycol gel) or unfilled, light-cured resin.

Setting reaction The metal primer forms an ionic bond with the sandblasted metal surface and its methacrylate end-group bonds with the resin of the cement.

Applications and limitations Forms a strong, durable bond to sand-blasted base metal or tin-plated noble metal alloys. Thin films are produced and the bond formed is water-resistant. The cement must be applied only to dry surfaces and the use of rubber dam is recommended where possible. Can also be used for repairs.

4.4.3.2.3 Biphenyl dimethacrylate (BPDM) cements: This system contains many different components, which enable it to form bonds with many different surfaces. It contains BPDM, which forms an adhesive bond with metals.

Common brand GoldLink 2.

Presentation The system consists of a combination of surface conditioners and primers, together with a range of filled and unfilled, self-cured or dual-cured resins for various applications.

Manipulation Surfaces to be bonded should be sand-blasted and coated with a thin layer of the BPDM primer. This is followed by dual-cure opaque resin or self-cured dimethacrylate cement.

Applications and limitations Strong, durable bonds to many types of surface. No tin-plating is needed on noble metal alloys.

4.4.3.2.4 Bonding via ceramic surface coatings: Noble metal alloy surfaces, which will not form adequate bonds with 4-META or MDP, can be coated with ceramic layers. To these, bifunctional primers known as silanes can be applied, and these will form bonds between the ceramic and any resin-based cement. The methods available for producing ceramic layers include:

(a) *Heat decomposition of alkyl silicate*

Technique A sand-blasted metal surface is solvent-cleaned and either exposed to a stream of silica, which forms in a Silicoater as alkyl silicate decomposes in a propane gas flame, or it is painted with a layer of Sililink, which is fired in a Silicoater MD oven. Either procedure produces a 0.5 μm thick layer of silica on the surface, which must be rapidly coated with a silane bonding agent (p. 149) followed by a layer of unfilled resin.

Applications and limitations Strong, durable bonds can be provided to either noble or basemetal alloys. Requires space for the resin layer. Technique sensitive and high capital cost.

(b) *Surface impregnation with silicon compounds*

Technique The metal is firstly sand-blasted with corundum to clean and activate the surface. It is then blasted with ceramic silicate (Rotatec-Plus) applied at 90° to the surface to produce a matte black finish. This is immediately treated with a silane bonding agent and covered with a layer of unfilled resin.

Applications and limitations Strong, durable bonds can be provided for either noble or base metal alloys. Care is needed not to destroy delicate sections by aggressive sand-blasting.

4.5 Occlusal registration materials and indicators

4.5.1 Occlusal registration materials

Any material which is self-supporting, which will flow when the teeth come together, which sets to produce a localized impression of the occlusal relationship and which can be removed without permanent distortion can be used for bite registration. Traditionally, materials such as wax and quick-setting plaster have been used; however, several materials are now marketed which are claimed to have superior properties. Two basic types of these are now available.

4.5.1.1 Zinc oxide pastes These are presented

as two pastes, one of which contains zinc oxide and the other a carboxylic acid such as eugenol. The mixed pastes set rapidly in the mouth to produce a rigid impression.

Common brands: Kerr's Bite Registration Paste; Nogenol (eugenol-free).

Manipulation: Equal lengths are mixed to produce a homogeneous paste and applied directly to the teeth on a gauze mesh held in a plastic frame.

Properties: The mixed pastes harden by a chemical reaction which is accelerated by moisture. Stable on storage. Compatible with dental stone.

Applications: Occlusal surfaces where there is no possibility of the material getting caught in undercuts or interproximal areas.

4.5.1.2 Elastomeric materials These are presented as two viscous or putty-like pastes based on either addition-curing silicone or polyether impression materials.

Common brands: Detail; Memosil C.D. (transparent); Regisil; Stat-BR (addition-curing silicones); Ramitec (polyether).

Manipulation: Equal lengths of base and reactor paste are mixed and either transferred to the mouth on a bite registration tray or syringed directly on to the teeth.

Properties: Fast setting. Elastic when set. Dimensionally stable and compatible with dental stone.

Applications: Occlusal surfaces, particularly if there is the possibility of the material entering undercut or interproximal areas.

4.5.2 *Indicators*

Apart from a variety of papers and foils covered in thin layers of coloured wax on one or both sides, several aerosol sprays, creams and wax pastes are available, together with a zinc oxide–eugenol paste.

Presentation The aerosol sprays consist of finely powdered wax/chalk mixture propelled by a non-toxic fluorocarbon gas. The creams and pastes consist of white or yellow pigments in inert oils and wax mixtures respectively. The zinc oxide and eugenol are mixed together prior to use.

Common brands
1. *Aerosol powders:* Hydent; Occlude; Quick Check.
2. *Creams and pastes:* Pressure Relief Cream; Disclosing Wax.
3. *Zinc oxide–eugenol:* Multiform.

Manipulation For identifying high spots the powder is sprayed on to the occlusal surface (or, if two colours are used, on to two surfaces). Gentle articulation then reveals the contact points. For showing up high spots in cast restorations the powder is sprayed, or the cream is painted, inside the crown. To indicate the pressure points on poorly fitting dentures the powder is sprayed on or the wax paste is applied to the fitting surface of the denture which is seated on to *moist* oral tissues. The zinc oxide–eugenol paste is placed inside crowns in order to indicate areas needing relief.

Properties The powder can be washed off with water. The waxes adhere to dry surfaces and are easily displaced at mouth temperature.

Applications
1. Locating high spots in the natural or restored dentition.
2. Seating cast restorations.
3. Identifying pressure points and determining the fit of full and partial dentures.

4.6 Temporary crown and bridge materials

Presentation Either two tubes of paste or a powder and a liquid.
System include the following types:
1. *Type A:* Methyl methacrylate (liquid monomer) with poly(methyl methacrylate).
2. *Type B:* Co-monomer of methyl methacrylate and urethane dimethacrylate with poly(methyl methacrylate).
3. *Type C:* Butyl methacrylate with poly(ethyl methacrylate).
4. *Type D:* A chemically activated, filled ethoxylated bis-phenol A (bis-acryl) resin with two activator pastes, one containing dibenzoyl peroxide, the other malonyl sulphamide.

Each system contains suitable initiators, activators or catalysts to make them self-curing.

Common brands
1. *Type A:* Alike; Sevriton; Snap; Tab 2000.
2. *Type B:* Ceri-Temp; TemDent.
3. *Type C:* Crobrit; Trim.
4. *Type D:* Protemp II.

Manipulation The pastes or powder and liquid are mixed to a homogeneous consistency. The resulting paste is inserted into either a cellulose acetate crown-forming matrix or into an alginate impression taken prior to cutting the preparations. The materials self-cure *in situ* and are then removed, trimmed and temporarily cemented.

Properties Types B, C and D have lower exotherms and contain less irritant monomers than type A. Type C has a lower glass-transition temperature than either type A or B. All have poor mechanical properties, including low strength and resistance to wear.

Applications The temporary replacement of crowns or missing teeth on bridge preparations during the period of manufacture of the permanent restorations.

Note: Preformed anatomical crowns of polycarbonate and stainless steel are also available, and both aluminium and tin thimbles can be used on molar and premolar teeth.

4.7 Temporary filling materials

Whilst most cements can be used as temporary filling materials, those based on zinc oxide–eugenol (particularly the accelerated and resin-bonded varieties) are popular for their ease of removal. Zinc polycarboxylate is also employed. Two materials which do not require mixing are also available.

4.7.1 Self-curing mixtures

Common brands Cavit; Cavit-G; Cavit-W; Cavitemp; Cimpat; Coltosol; GC Caviton; Interval; Provipast; Tempit.

Presentation A single jar or syringe of ready-mixed paste which may contain zinc oxide, calcium hydroxide, titanium dioxide, calcium, barium and zinc sulphate, triethylene glycol diacetate, poly(vinyl acetate), poly(vinyl chloride acetate), triethanolamine and pigments.

Manipulation A suitable quantity of the paste is packed into the cavity where it sets due to the action of saliva in about 15 minutes.

Properties Hardens within the cavity (Cavit and Cavit-W are harder than Cavit-G). Reasonable strength; will resist masticatory loads for short periods. Impermeable to medicaments. Can be easily removed when required. Jar must be kept closed to prevent moisture access.

Applications
1. Temporary sealing of cavities.
2. Sealing in of pulpal medicaments.

4.7.2 Gutta-percha

Common brands De Trey Gutta-Percha; Kemdent Black GP; Kemdent Temporary Stopping.

Presentation Sticks containing gutta-percha (the transisomer of polyisoprene) together with zinc oxide or wax and sometimes cellulose. A black pigmented sheet form is available for maxillofacial applications, and tapered points are used to fill root canals. The points contain heavy metal salts to make them radiopaque.

Manipulation It is warmed over a flame and, being thermoplastic, softens between 60 and 65°C. It is used whilst it is soft.

Properties It flows under pressure at mouth temperature, but as a temporary filling material it does not adapt well to the cavity and marginal leakage is excessive.

Applications
1. Root canal filling material.
2. Emergency temporary filling material.

3. Pulp vitality tester (at 65°C).
4. Functional impression material (cleft palate).

4.7.3 Flexible polymers

Common brands   Clip; Fermit.

Presentation   Single tubes of light-activated polyester/urethane dimethacrylate resin containing 16% by weight of microfine silica and 33% by weight of splintered, prepolymerized, microfilled resin.

Manipulation   Moulded to the cavity and light-activated to cure. Removed in one piece without damaging prepared borders.

Properties   Elastic when set. Absorbs water during its time in the mouth and seals cavity margins.

Applications   Temporary protection of teeth which have been prepared for inlays or onlays. Temporary fillings of all types.

4.8 Temporary luting cements

For the temporary cementation of crowns and bridges a paste–paste presentation of a zinc oxide–eugenol type of cement is available:.

Common brands   Nogenol (eugenol-free); Provicol (with calcium hydroxide); Temp Bond; ZOE Plus.

Presentation   Two tubes of paste, one containing eugenol or a carboxylic acid and inert filler and the other zinc oxide in a non-reactive oily base; the latter also contains zinc acetate as an accelerator. A third paste (modifier) is sometimes provided and this contains no active ingredients and thus has no effect on the rate of set. Instead, when added to the reactive pastes in various proportions the modifier weakens the set cement by interfering with the development of a coherent structural matrix. Calcium hydroxide may be included as a promoter of tooth vitality.

Manipulation   The two (or three) pastes are spatulated to produce a homogeneous mix in 20–30 seconds. The cement is added to a restoration which is seated under positive pressure.

Properties   Rapid setting possible. Moderate strength (weakened by the modifier). Separates cleanly from preparations when crowns are removed prior to permanent cementation.

Applications   The temporary cementation of crowns and bridges.

4.9 Dentine isolation materials

Dentine which has become exposed to the oral environment by either wear or gingival recession can be very sensitive during dental treatment and a number of agents can be used to provide protection. These include the usual dental varnishes and several materials which polymerize in the presence of moisture to produce a hydrophobic film on the dentine:

Common brands   Barrier; Dentin Protector; Protect; Tresiolan.

Presentation   *Either:* Bottles or ampoules of clear, liquid siloxane ester or polyol/isocyanate mixtures, or liquids which form a polyamide layer when they polymerize in the presence of moisture to produce a thin, retentive and protective film *or:* Solutions which deposit calcium oxalate in the tubules.

Manipulation   The liquids are applied with a pledget of cotton wool to the surface of dried dentine or are expressed through a wick directly from the ampoule. The application can be repeated after a few minutes to increase the durability of the film. When used on soft, carious dentine the cavity should be sealed with a temporary filling and further applications should be applied at subsequent visits. Once the carious dentine has hardened it can be removed with an excavator.

Properties   Rapidly form a hydrophobic layer on the surface of the tooth without adversely affecting the pulp or irritating the gingiva. May be left *in situ* for long periods.

Applications The desensitization of tooth necks (and in the case of Tresiolan) the hardening of soft, carious dentine by silicification.

4.10 Endodontic filling materials

These are employed in the hope of achieving a hermetic seal. More realistically, they aim to fill the empty space left after pulpal extirpation. Although over 250 materials have been tried for root canal obturation, two types of filling are currently employed, either singly or together – points or cones and setting pastes.

4.10.1 Points or cones

4.10.1.1 Gutta-percha points

Presentation Thermoplastic points based on gutta-percha, the transisomer of polyisoprene (which comes from the sap of a Taban tree). There are two crystalline forms, α and β. α is the natural form and melts at 65°C. However, unless it is cooled very slowly, the β form develops and this melts at 56°C. Commercial gutta-percha is in the β form. The points are available in various sizes and tapers. Zinc oxide is present as a filler and heavy metal salts are used to make the points radiopaque. They also contain wax or resin.

Manipulation and properties Sterilized in alcohol, 1–5% sodium hypochlorite or 5% chloramine and then applied to the clean root canal by lateral condensation, either by the use of warm instruments or after the points have been softened in chloroform. Gutta-percha oxidizes in air or when exposed to bright light and becomes brittle.

Gutta-percha is also available for hot injection into the root canal.

Common Brand: Ultrafil. Another brand, SuccessFil, contains a solid core made from titanium.

4.10.1.2 Silver cones

Presentation Various sizes and tapers of cones made of silver containing 0.1–0.2% of copper and nickel.

Manipulation and properties Adaptation to the geometry of the root canal is not easy and a cement

is needed to create a seal. In such a crevice the silver tends to corrode and release cytotoxic reaction products.

4.10.1.3 Titanium points

Presentation Various sizes and tapers of cones made of commercially pure titanium.

Manipulation and properties Used in a similar manner to silver cones. However, they do not seem to undergo the same degree of corrosion.

4.10.2 Setting pastes

These are intended to be used either on their own or for sealing the gap between the canal wall and cones or points such as silver or gutta-percha. Each material is a variant of one of the basic systems listed below. However, to achieve the radiopacity necessary in these materials they may contain:

1. Powdered metallic silver.
2. Heavy metal salts, e.g. barium sulphate; bismuth phosphate, carbonate, iodide, nitrate or trioxide; lead tetraoxide; zirconium oxide or various combinations of these compounds.

Most contain one or more of the following antibacterial compounds: camphor; disclorophene; iodoform; nitrofurazone; paraformaldehyde; phenylmercuric-borate; thymol iodide. Several contain pharmacologically active steroids such as: dexamethasone; hydrocortisone acetate; prednisolone or mixtures of these.

4.10.2.1 Zinc oxide–eugenol cements (see section 2.1) These are modified with inert fillers such as titanium dioxide and Staybelite resin so that they set slowly by the formation of zinc eugenolate.

Unbranded Materials The names of Grossman and Rickert have been associated with several of these cements which can be made up as follows:

Grossman's sealer

Powder:	Zinc oxide	42 parts
	Staybelite resin	27 parts
	barium sulphate	15 parts
	Bismuth carbonate	15 parts
	Anhydrous sodium borate	1 part

Liquid: Eugenol   85 parts
        Aracus oil   15 parts

Rickert's paste
Powder: Zinc oxide   38 parts
        Powdered silver 25 parts
        Oleoresins   25 parts
        Thymol diiodide 12 parts
Liquid: Oil of cloves   80 parts
        Canada balsam   20 parts

Common brands With steroids: Endomethazone; Hermetic; Propylor. Without steroids: Kerr's Sealer; Mynol; Proco-Sol; Tubli-Seal; N 2 may or may not contain steroids in its frequently altered formulation. The components listed below may thus not always be present in any one presentation:

Powder: Zinc oxide   62–69 parts
        Lead tetroxide   11–12 parts
        Paraformaldehyde   6.5 parts
        Bismuth carbonate   5–9 parts
        Bismuth nitrate   2–4 parts
        Titanium dioxide   2–3 parts
        Barium sulphate   2–3 parts
        Phenylmercuric borate 0.16 parts
        Hydrocortisone   1.2 parts
        Prednisolone   0.2 parts
Liquid: Eugenol   92–100 parts
        Geraniol   8 parts

Properties Setting is accelerated by moisture. Free eugenol always remains as a potential tissue irritant.

4.10.2.2 Calcium hydroxide cements These are based on the reaction between calcium hydroxide and a salicylate ester-aldehyde condensate. They also contain zinc oxide, zinc stearate and *o-p* N-ethyl toluene sulphonamide.

Common brand Sealapex.

Properties Setting accelerated by moisture. Excess calcium hydroxide present when set.

4.10.2.3 Thick solutions These are basically gutta-percha dissolved in chloroform. One variant contains a considerable amount of zinc oxide as a filler and Canada balsam as a binder. The chloroform evaporates leaving behind a coherent layer of (filled) resin.

Common brands Without filler: Chloropercha. With filler: Kloroperka N-O.

Properties Chloroform toxic to tissues when present. Forms a thin layer of film. Volume is reduced when solvent evaporates, reducing the sealing efficiency.

4.10.2.4 Resorcinol–formaldehyde cements These are based on one of the oldest synthetic polymer reactions in which a phenol (resorcinol) forms cross-links with formaldehyde in the presence of an acid to form a solid polymer. In practice, a zinc oxide-rich powder is mixed with two liquids, one containing formaldehyde and glycerine, and the other containing resorcinol, glycerine and hydrochloric acid.

Common brand Traitement SPAD (with steroid).

4.10.2.5 Polyketone–metal complex cements These set when zinc ocide reacts with propionylacetophenone to form water-insoluble polyketones.

Common brand Diaket.

Properties Toxic when first mixed. Low flow and high film thickness. Good volume stability.

4.10.2.6 Epoxy resins Based on the hardening of bis-phenol-diglycidyl ether with hexamethylene tetramine.

Common brand AH 26.

Properties Long setting time (24–48 hours). Forms a good seal with good volume stability. Almost insoluble. Can cause patient sensitization if used frequently.

4.10.2.7 Calcium phosphate cements These are based on the reaction that takes place in a 0.2% aqueous solution of phosphoric acid between tetracalcium phosphate and dicalcium pyrophosphate dihydrate. The result is the precipitation of hydroxyapatite. No commercial brands are available.

Properties The set material is biocompatible and osteoconductive. It develops a good seal when used as an endodontic sealer–filler.

Further reading

Attachment to dentine

Cheung, G.S.P. (1990) An *in vitro* evaluation of five dentinal adhesives in posterior restorations. *Quintessence International*, **21**, 513–516

Diaz-Arnold, A.M., Williams, V.D. and Aquilino, S.A. (1990) A review of dentinal boding *in vitro:* the substrate. *Operative Dentistry*, **15**, 71–75

Hegarty, S.M. and Pearson, G.J. (1990) The effectiveness of dentine adhesives as demonstrated by dye penetration and SEM investigations. *Journal of Oral Rehabilitation*, **17**, 351–357

Munksgaard, E.C. (1990) Amine-induced polymerization of aqueous HEMA/aldehyde during action as a dentine bonding agent. *Journal of Dental Research*, **69**, 1236–1239

Paterson, R.C. and Watts, A. (1990) The dentine smear layer and bonding agents. *Restorative Dentistry*, **6**, 19–25

Prati, C., Nucci, C., Davidson, C.L. and Montanari, G. (1990) Early marginal leakage and shear bond strength of adhesive restorative systems. *Dental Materials*, **6**, 195–200

Rees, J.S. and Jacobsen, P.H. (1990) The current state of composite materials and adhesive systems: Part 4. Some clinically related research. *Restorative Dentistry*, **6**, 4–8

Tsai, Y.H., Swartz, M.L., Phillips, R.W. and Moore, B. K. (1990) A comparative study: bond strength and microleakage with dentine bonding systems. *Operative Dentistry*, **15**, 53–60

Wendt, S.L., Jebeles, C.A. and Leinfelder, K.F. (1990) The effect of two smear layer cleansers on the shear bond strength to dentine. *Dental Materials*, **6**, 1–4

Youngson, C.C., Grey, N.J.A. and Martin, D.M. (1990) *In vitro* marginal microleakage associated with five dentine bonding systems and associated composite restorations. *Journal of Dentistry*, **18**, 203–208

Zidan, O. and Al Jabab, A. (1990) Evaluation of the bond mediated by eight dentine bonding agents to enamel and dentine. *Dental Materials*, **6**, 158–161

Attachment to metal

Hansson, O. (1990) Strength of bond with Comspan opaque to three silicoated alloys and titanium. *Scandinavian Journal of Dental Research*, **98**, 248–256

Matsumura, H., Yoshida, K., Tanaka, T. and Atsuta, M. (1990) Adhesive bonding of titanium with a titanate coupler and 4-META/-TBB opaque resin. *Journal of Dental Research*, **69**, 1614–1616

Ohno, H., Araki, Y. and Endo K. (1992) A new method for promoting adhesion between precious metal alloys and dental adhesives. *Journal of Dental Research*, **71**, 1326–1331

Endodontic filling materials

Sugawara, A., Chow, L.C., Takagi, S. and Chohayeb, H. (1990) *In vitro* evaluation of the sealing ability of calcium phosphate cement when used as a root canal sealer-filler. *Journal of Endodontics*, **16**, 162–165

Sugawara, A., Nishiyama, M., Kusama, K., Moro, S., Nishimura, S., Kudo, I., Chow, L.C. and Takagi, S. (1992) Histopathological reactions of calcium phosphate cement. *Dental Material Journal*, **11**, 11–16

Pins and posts

King, P.A. and Setchell, D.J. (1990) An *in vitro* evaluation of a prototype CFRC prefabricated post developed for the restoration of pulpless teeth. *Journal of Oral Rehabilitation*, **17**, 599–609

Lloyd, C.M. and Butchart, D.G.M. (1990) The retention of core composites, glass ionomers and cermets by a self-threading dentine pin: the influence of fracture toughness upon failure. *Dental Materials*, **6**, 185–188

Peutzfeldt, A. and Asmussen, E. (1990) Flexural and fatigue strength of root canal posts. *Scandanavian Journal of Dental Research*, **98**, 550–557

Retention to enamel

Schvermer, E.S., Burgess, J.O. and Matis, B.E. (1990) Strength of bond of composite resin to enamel cleaned with a paste containing fluoride. *General Dentistry*, **38**, 381–383

Temporary luting cements

Olin, P.S., Rodney, J.D. and Hill, E.M.E. (1990) Retentive strength of six temporary dental cements. *Quintessence International*, **21**, 197–200

5 Impression materials

5.1 Rigid (when set)

Used for recording the details of dental tissues either where no undercuts are present, or where undercuts are present and the sectional removal of the set impression material is acceptable.

5.1.1 Impression and inlay waxes

Presentation

1. For impressions: cakes of pigmented mixtures of paraffin and beeswaxes.

2. For inlays: hexagonal blue sticks of mixtures of paraffin, ceresin carnauba and beeswaxes.

Common brands
1. Impression wax: Kerr's Impression Wax; Korecta.
2. Inlay waxes: Kem-Dent; Kerr's Inlay; Pinnacle.

Manipulation   Impression wax is melted on a water bath and applied to the saddle areas of partial denture frameworks prior to their insertion into the mouth. Inlay wax is flame-softened and, when plastic, inserted into the cavity under finger pressure. Carved when rigid before being removed for investing.

Properties   Both materials are thermoplastic but, whilst inlay wax softens at about 42°C and becomes rigid at 37°C (mouth temperature), impression wax flows at mouth temperature under occlusal load. The resulting impression is poured immediately. Inlay wax carves without chipping or flaking and 'burns out', leaving no residue.

Applications
1. Impression wax: functional impressions of denture support areas.
2. Inlay wax: inlay patterns in the mouth (direct technique) or on a model or die (indirect technique).

5.1.2 Impression compound

Presentation   Sheets or sticks of thermoplastic mixtures of resin, fillers and lubricants.

Common brands   Exact; Kerr's Compo; Paribar; Replica; Stents.

Manipulation   Sheets are softened in a water bath at 55–60°C, sticks are flame-softened; avoid overheating.

Properties   Thermoplastic; softens at high temperature and becomes rigid at 37°C.

Applications
1. Sheets: primary impressions of edentulous mouths.
2. Sticks: copper band impressions; modification of impression tray peripheries.

5.1.3 Impression plaster

Presentation   Pink powder containing calcium sulphate β-hemihydrate 4% potassium sulphate to reduce expansion and 0.4% borax to slow down the setting reaction (which is accelerated by the potassium sulphate).

Common brands   Calspar; Gypsogum; laboratory plaster mixed with antiexpansion solution (4% K_2SO_4 + 0.4% borax in water).

Manipulation   The plaster is added to the water and spatulated gently to produce a smooth paste.

Properties   Sets by a precipitation reaction in a few minutes and accurately reproduces surface detail. Little shrinkage occurs on storage of set plaster. A separating agent is needed when gypsum is used to produce a model from a plaster impression.

Applications   Used in a special tray for impressions of the edentulous mouth.

5.1.4 Impression paste

Presentation   Two pastes:
1. Zinc oxide in a non-reactive oily base.
2. Either eugenol or a carboxylic acid plus inert filler and zinc acetate (accelerator).

Common brands   Coe-Flo; Kelly's Paste; Luralite; S. S. White Paste; Nogenol (eugenol-free).

Manipulation   Equal lengths are mixed to a homogeneous paste.

Properties   Hardens by a chemical reaction which is accelerated in the presence of water. Records fine detail. Stable on storage. Compatible with dental stone; separated by softening the set paste (which is thermoplastic) in water at 60°C.

Applications   Used in thin section as a wash impression in either a special tray or existing denture.

5.2 Elastic (when set)

Used for recording the details of dental tissues when undercuts are present.

5.2.1 Reversible hydrocolloids (agar-agar)

Presentation A gel of agar-agar in water containing borax and potassium sulphate is supplied in collapsible plastic tubes and syringe packs.

Common brands Acculoid; Agarloid; Lactona-Surgident and Lactona-Thompson; Rubberoid; Van R.

Manipulation Tubes of agar are conditioned in boiling water (to form a sol) and then stored at 55–60°C. Impressions are taken in water-cooled trays and poured in dental stone after a short soak in a solution containing potassium aluminium sulphate (alum).

Properties High temperature fluid sol cools to become an elastic gel at 37°C. A hydrophilic material giving good surface detail but having a poor dimensional stability. Contains 80% of water when set and this can evaporate to produce shrinkage. Syneresis or imbibition can occur on standing in dry or wet environments respectively. Low strength; tears around severe undercuts. Disinfection possible in 2% solution of aldehydes and quaternary ammonium salts (e.g. ID 210) for maximum of 20 minutes.

Applications
1. Impressions of the dentate and edentulous.
2. Model and denture duplication in the laboratory (the material is reusable because of the reversible nature of the sol–gel transformation).
3. Used as denture mould in the pour-and-cure technique for self-curing acrylic.
4. Excellent for inlay, crown and bridge impressions, provided laboratory facilities are instantly available.

5.2.2 Irreversible hydrocolloids (alginate)

Presentation Powder containing 12% soluble alginate salt (e.g. sodium, potassium or ammonium alginate), 12% calcium sulphate, 3% trisodium phosphate, 70% inert diatomaceous earth or microcrystalline filler, plus various combinations of dust suppressors (Duomeen and zinc stearate), modifiers to improve the elasticity (triethanolamine or silicone), chromatic indicators, flavourings and antipathogenic antiseptics. Available as type I – fast setting – or type II – normal setting.

Common brands Alginoplast; Aroma Fine; Blend-a-print; Blueprint Asept (antiseptic); Blueprint Cremix; Blueprint Plus Antibac (antiseptic); CA 37; Coe Alginate; D.S.A.; Elastigel; Empress; Exact; Fidelity; Hydrogum; Jeltrate; Kromogel; Neocolloid; Orthalgenat; Orthoprint; Palain Star; Phase; S.S. White Alginate; Supreme (germicidal); Ultrafine (silicone modified); Xantalgin select; Zelgan; 1st Impression.

Manipulation A measure of water at 20°C is added to a corresponding measure of powder which is gently incorporated and then *mixed vigorously* to produce a smooth creamy paste in about 1 minute. The impression is often taken in a perforated stock tray coated with a methyl cellulose-based adhesive such as Fix, Hold, Redifix or Stick. The set impression must be kept in a damp humidor bag and ideally poured in dental stone within the hour. Disinfection is possible in 2% solution of aldehydes and quaternary ammonium salts (e.g. ID 210) for a maximum of 20 minutes.

Properties Sodium, potassium or ammonium alginate dissolves to form a sol and this is cross-linked by calcium ions to become calcium alginate gel. The material thus sets – a process which takes between 1 and 3 minutes at mouth temperature. This is an irreversible reaction whose rate is controlled by the trisodium phosphate. A hydrophilic material giving good surface detail but poor dimensional stability. Contains 70% of water when set and this can evaporate to produce shrinkage. Syneresis and imbibition can occur on standing in dry or wet environments respectively. The silicone-modified alginates have a higher tear strength. Several are produced as dust-free materials to reduce the potential hazard of inhalation by the dentist and assistants during the proportioning and mixing stages.

Application Impressions of the dentate and edentulous mouth.

5.2.3 Agar-alginate hydrocolloid system

Presentation Syringes of reversible hydrocolloid (agar-agar) and any alginate powder.

Common brands Cohere; Duoloid; Verilloid.

Manipulation The agar-agar syringes are boiled to form a sol and stored at 55–60°C until required. The alginate is mixed to a creamy paste. The agar is then syringed around the prepared teeth and the mixed alginate is loaded into an adhesive-coated and perforated tray and seated over the agar. The set impression is removed with a snap action and poured in dental stone immediately.

Properties Both materials set in the mouth in 2–3 minutes, the agar by turning physically into a gel and the alginate by chemical cross-linking. A bond is formed between the two hydrocolloids. Hydrophilic and stronger than normal agar-agar impressions, hence a greater resistance to tearing. No water-cooled trays are required.

Applications Crown and bridge preparations where severe undercuts might cause tearing of agar-agar on its own. Immediate access to laboratory facilities is needed for optimum accuracy.

5.2.4 Elastomeric polysulphide rubbers

Also known as mercaptan or thiokol rubbers, or just rubber-base materials.

Presentation Two tubes of paste:
1. Base paste: fluid polysulphide plus inert filler.
2. Activator paste: e.g. lead dioxide or copper oxysulphate, together with sulphur in a non-reactive oily base.

Common brands Permlastic; Surflex F; Unilastic (PbO_2 activator); Omniflex (copper oxysulphate activator).

Manipulation Equal lengths of base and activator pastes are thoroughly mixed to produce a homogeneous, streak-free mix. The mixed material

is used in a special tray coated with adhesive. It is also injected around the preparations. For maximum adhesion the adhesive should be thinly applied well in advance of taking the impression. The tray should be lightly supported whilst setting occurs. The set impression can be electroplated to make a shell die, which is then filled with self-curing acrylic. Silver is the material best suited for plating polysulphides because it occurs in an alkaline electrolyte (see also 6.2.1). May be disinfected in a 2% solution of aldehydes and quaternary ammonium salts (e.g. ID 210) for a maximum of 20 minutes.

Properties Cross-linking and chain-lengthening cause the material to become an elastic solid in 5–8 minutes. Water is produced as a by-product of the condensation cross-linking reaction. Acceleration is possible by adding a drop of water to the mix. Despite being hydrophobic, excellent surface detail is possible. Good tear resistance but rocking on removal from the mouth (which can produce permanent distortion) should be avoided.

Dimensional stability: Lead dioxide- and copper oxysulphate-activated materials show fair stability; only the water produced on setting can evaporate, producing a small amount of shrinkage.

Recommended maximum storage time of the set impression: For lead dioxide- and copper oxysulphate-activated materials, 48 hours.

Applications Detailed impressions of hard tissues. Good for inlay, crown and bridge impressions.

5.2.5 Elastomeric siloxane (silicone) polymers

Presentation Two components:
1. Base: siloxane fluid plus various amounts of inert filler, e.g.
   Putty: about 60–70% filler (high viscosity)
   Paste: about 30–50% filler
   Wash : about 5–15% filler (low viscosity).
   Combinations of various viscosity materials *(multiphase)* are used according to choice. Alternatively, material of a single viscosity *(monophase)* may be used.
   Additives such as flavourings, hydrophilic promoters and gingival retraction agents may also be present.

2. Activator: liquid or paste containing a cross-linking agent and/or an activator. The paste contains an inert filler.

Types of cross-linking Two types are possible:

1. Condensation-curing (alkoxy-silanol system): cross-linking occurs via alkyl silicates in the presence of an organo–tin compound. Ethyl alcohol is produced as a byproduct when ethyl *o*-silicate is used as the cross-linking agent.
2. Addition-curing (hydrosilylation system): setting occurs as part of an addition polymerization reaction in which vinyl siloxane cross-links with other siloxane chains in the presence of a platinum compound (chloroplatinic acid) as activator. No byproducts are produced.

Common brands

1. *Condensation-curing: Multiphase materials* (putty + wash)–Acusil + Acupren; Blend-a-scon; Citricon; Coltoflax + Coltex; Lasticomp + Tewesil; Optosil Plus + Xantopren VL; Rapid; Rex-Sil + Corex; Silaplast + Silasoft; Verone; Zetaplus + Oranwash and Thixoflex.

   Condensation-curing: Monophase materials (single viscosity) – Lastic; Siccoform; Xantopren H or M.
2. *Addition-curing: Multiphase materials* (putty, paste, wash) – Absolute; Doric; Elite; Exaflex; Express; Extrude; Omnisil; Panasil; Permagum; President; Provil; Reprosil HF; Rexprint; VPS.

   Addition-curing: Monophase materials (single viscosity) – Baysilex; Blend-a-gum; Blu-Mousse; Detaseal E; Extrude Extra; Green-Mousse; Hydrosil; Impex; Imprint; Panapren; Precise; Reflect; Unosil S.

Manipulation *Pastes:* Equal lengths or volumes of base and activator paste are mixed to produce a homogeneous, streak-free mix in about a minute. Putties may be kneaded with the fingers. Several addition-curing silicones are presented as a dual syringe and are mixed automatically through a disposable static mixer tip.

Paste plus liquid: The appropriate number of drops of liquid activator are added to the corresponding length or volume of base paste and mixed to produce a homogeneous mix in about a minute. Putties may be kneaded with the fingers once the material has been spatulated.

Techniques for using putty and wash materials

1. Twin mix: both materials are mixed consecutively, the wash is syringed around the preparations and the freshly mixed putty is added to the tray, which is seated over the wash and both are allowed to set in the mouth. This is the best technique when using addition-curing silicones.
2. Two-stage, no spacer: the putty is mixed, placed in a tray, seated over the preparation and allowed to set. It is removed, trimmed from undercuts and freshly mixed wash is added to the putty impression and the whole is reseated. The wash is allowed to set. This technique works well with condensation-curing silicones but should not be used for addition-curing materials.
3. Two-stage, with spacer: the putty is mixed, placed in a tray and seated over the teeth (which may or may not have been prepared) which are covered by a thin polythene sheet. The tray is rocked to produce a considerable space and removed to set out of the mouth. The teeth can then be prepared and the wash is added to the putty and syringed around the preparation. The filled tray is reseated and the wash is allowed to set. In all cases the tray should be lightly supported once it is seated. The putty and wash bond chemically. Whilst impressions in either type of silicone are usually cast in dental stone, they may be copper- or silver-plated to produce a die.

Properties Rapid setting (about 5 minutes) to form an elastic solid. Produces excellent surface detail despite being inherently hydrophobic. Some are presented with wetting agents consisting of micronized absorbent silica in a volatile propellant (Hydrosystem). The mousse-like materials are thixotropic fluids and when set have hardness values similar to set dental plaster, hence severe undercuts need blocking out and the set impression material should be cut away from the stone model to prevent damage.

Dimensional stability

1. Condensation-curing: fair stability, but the alcohol produced as a byproduct of the cross-linking reaction can evaporate. Should be poured or plated within 6 hours for maximum accuracy.
2. Addition-curing: excellent stability, no volatile

byproducts to evaporate hence no shrinkage; as a result dies may need relieving with varnish if cast restorations are to allow room for the cement film. Impressions can be poured or plated at leisure. Porosity caused by hydrogen gas can sometimes be produced in the surface of dental stone models poured in less than 1 hour. Silicone impression materials can be safely disinfected for up to 2 hours in a 2% solution of aldehydes and quaternary ammonium salts (e.g. ID 210).

Applications Detailed impressions of hard tissues; excellent for inlay, crown, bridge and partial denture impressions. Medium-viscosity paste is suitable for impressions of the edentulous mouth.

5.2.6 Elastomeric imine-terminated polyether polymers

Presentation Two tubes of paste (or a dual syringe with a static mixer tip).
1. Base paste: unsaturated, fluid polyether with imine end groups plus plasticizer and inert filler.
2. Activator paste: aromatic sulphonate catalyst plus plasticizer and inert filler.

Common brands Impregum F; Permadyne (two-viscosity system).

Manipulation Equal lengths of each paste are mixed to produce homogeneous colour.

The mixed single-viscosity material can be syringed around the preparations and used in a tray coated with adhesive.

The tray should be lightly supported once it is seated until the impression material sets. The set impression can be silver-plated to produce a die.

The two-viscosity system is used by syringing the light-bodied paste around the preparation and, whilst it is still fluid, covering it with freshly mixed, fluid, heavy-bodied paste in the twin mix or single-stage impression technique.

Can be disinfected in a 2% solution of aldehydes and quaternary ammonium salts for 20 minutes.

Properties Cross-linking of the imine groups causes the material to set within 5 minutes without the elimination of any byproducts. Excellent surface detail is reproduced, even though the material is inherently hydrophobic. This is facilitated by additives which allow wetting of the surface of the impression by water-based model materials.

Caution: The activator paste can produce an allergic reaction in those such as dental surgery assistants who handle it frequently.

Dimensional stability: Excellent when stored dry. Ideally pour or plate within 48 hours. Do not store the impression under water or in direct sunlight.

Applications Detailed impressions and hard tissues. Excellent for inlay, crown and bridge impressions.

5.2.7 Polyether urethane dimethacrylate polymers

Presentation A heavy- and light-bodied system, whose pastes are activated by exposure to visible, blue light. The pastes contain a polyether urethane dimethacrylate resin with a diketone initiator. They contain 40–60% of filler according to their intended viscosity. The filler is a transparent silica, which has a similar refractive index to the resin.

Common brand Genesis.

Manipulation Severe undercuts need blocking out with wax. Transparent stock trays are coated with a thin layer of transparent adhesive. Light-bodied material is syringed around the preparations and the tray is filled with the heavy-bodied material and seated. It must be held in place whilst the impression material is light-cured. This procedure starts at the posterior border and moves via the lingual edge towards the occlusal surface. Exposure of the buccal surfaces follows. Each zone requires about 30 seconds' exposure, with the light wand being moved continuously. After removal any imperfections may be corrected by adding material, reseating and re-exposing to the light.

Properties Oxygen inhibition of the polymerization reaction makes areas exposed to air tacky. The set material can be very firm and unyielding. Care is thus needed to avoid severe undercuts. Should not be used on patients who are sensitive to urethanes, acrylics or methacrylates. Can be disinfected in 2% solution of aldehydes and quaternary ammonium salts for 20 minutes.

Applications Impressions of hard tissues.

5.3 Laboratory duplicating materials

These are bulk variants of the materials used in the surgery for taking impressions.

5.3.1 Hydrocolloids

Presentation Tubs of agar-agar gel containing agents such as potassium sulphate to prevent the creation of duplicated models with a chalky surface.

Common brands Cruta-Gel; Dublikat; Dupliplast; Econo-Gel; Geloform; Organa II; Vidur.

Most laboratory suppliers provide them often without a brand name, in which case they are known as duplicating gel.

Manipulation Laboratory agar is kept stirred in thermostatically controlled, lidded containers, fitted with a tap to allow controlled withdrawal of the fluid material.

Properties The material is water-based and evaporation from the poured material can result in shrinkage. Duplicates should be poured as soon as the gel has cooled.

Applications The duplication of models, especially in refractory materials on to which wax is built up prior to the casting of partial denture frameworks.

5.3.2 Silicones

Presentation Two fluid pastes or putties (base and reactor) of either addition or condensation-curing silicones, or of polyether elastomer.

Common brands Deguform; Degupress; Doric MDS; Dublisil; Flexistone; Formasil; Gi-Mask; Lab-Putty; Lab-Sil; Profisil; Quick-Pour; Vestogum (polyether); Zetalabor.

Manipulation and applications Equal lengths of the pastes (or measured quantities of the two components) are mixed and either adapted to the appropriate surfaces with a brush or spatula to provide insulating layers or reproductions of the gingivae, or they are injected or poured into impressions in order to create duplicate dies and models.

Further reading

Bagnall, R.D., Davies, C.M., Foley, J. and McCord, J.F. (1990) pH studies in modern dental alginates. *Clinical Materials*, **5**, 47–51

Chia, W.K., Stevens, L. and Basford, K.E. (1990) Dimensional change of impressions on sterilization. *Australian Dental Journal*, **35**, 23–26

Chong, Y.H., Soh, G. and Setchell, D.J. (1990) Wettability of elastomeric impression materials: a comparative study of two measures. *Clinical Materials*, **6**, 239–249

Council on Dental Materials, Instruments and Equipment (1990) Vinyl polysiloxane impression materials: a status report. *Journal of the American Dental Association*, **120**, 595–600

Lewinstein, I. and Craig, R.G. (1990) Accuracy of impression materials measured with a vertical height gauge. *Journal of Oral Rehabilitation*, **17**, 303–310

Munoz, C.A. Goodacre, C.J., Schnell, R. and Harris, R.K. (1988) Laboratory and clinical study of a visible-light-polymerized elastomeric impression material. *International Journal of Prosthodontics*, **1**, 59–66

Ralph, W.J., Ginn S.S.L., Cheadle, D.A. and Harcourt, J.K. (1990) The effects of disinfectants on the dimensional stability of alginate impression materials. *Australian Dental Journal*, **35**, 514–517

Reed, H.V. (1990) Reversible agar-agar hydrocolloid. *Quintessence International*, **21**, 225–229

Salem, N. and Combe, E.C. (1990) The effects of chemical sterilization on the dimensional stability of some elastomeric impression materials. *Clinical Materials*, **6**, 75–82

6 Model and die materials

Used for the preparation of accurate reproductions of the oral tissues from impressions of those tissues, in order that restorations and appliances can be constructed using laboratory techniques and cannot be used in the mouth.

6.1 Gypsum products

Basic reversible dehydration/hydration reaction:

Hydration
(exothermic: gives off heat)
$$CaSO_4 \cdot 2H_2O \xleftarrow{\hspace{2cm}} CaSo_4 \cdot \tfrac{1}{2}H_2O + 1\tfrac{1}{2}H_2O$$
dihydrate $\xrightarrow{\hspace{2cm}}$ hemihydrate
Dehydration
(endothermic: requires heat)
Theoretical water:powder ratio for hydration 0.186:1.00
(100 g hemihydrate requires 18.6 g water)

6.1.1 Dental plaster

Presentation A white powder consisting of large, irregular and porous particles of the β-hemihydrate of calcium sulphate. Prepared by heating dihydrate (gypsum) in an open 'kettle' at 120°C. Contains some dihydrate to accelerate setting.

Common brands Plaster is usually sold without a trade name.

Manipulation The powder is added to water (approximate proportions, 50–60 ml water/100 g plaster) by sifting to avoid the incorporation of air into the mix. It is gently but positively spatulated to a smooth mix in about a minute.

Properties
1. Sets by an exothermic hydration reaction. Setting is accelerated by:
   (a) Heat, but only up to 45°C.
   (b) Nuclei, e.g. dihydrate particles, dust, etc.
   (c) Chemical additives, e.g. K_2SO_4, NaCl.
   Setting is retarded by:
   (a) High temperatures – above 50°C.
   (b) Chemical additives, e.g. borax, potassium citrate.
2. Expands on setting by 0.3–0.4%.
3. Compressive strength after 1 hour: 10 MN/m^2 (water:plaster = 0.6). Strength doubles once the excess water needed for mixing has evaporated, but porosity remains and plaster is thus always weaker than stone.

Applications.
1. Mounting models.
2. Flasking of dentures; often mixed with stone to increase strength but retain easy deflasking.
3. As impression material, with modifying chemicals (K_2SO_4 and borax).
4. Oral study models (orthodontics, oral surgery).

6.1.2 Dental stone

Presentation A light-yellow powder consisting of small, regular particles of low porosity (the α-hemihydrate of calcium sulphate, coloured yellow with an inert dye). Prepared by heating gypsum in an autoclave under steam pressure at 120–130°C. Contains a retarder such as potassium citrate to control the setting time. When gypsum is heated under pressure in a solution of calcium or magnesium chloride an even smaller and less porous crystal of hemihydrate is produced. This is called modified α, densite or die stone. Die stones of the 1990s often contain finely divided silica filler to increase their hardness and make them resistant to wear during handling in the laboratory.

Common brands
Model stones (α-hemihydrate): Flask-Stone; Hydrocal; Kaffir D; Kemcal; Plastone L; Rapid Stone.

Hard, coloured die stones (modified α-hemihydrate): Alphadur 700; Advastone; Beta-Dur 700; Bitestone (for occlusal records); Bluejey; Crystacal R and D; Denstone; Die-Keen; Duralit; Dycron; Fujirock; Herculite; Hinriplast; Jeyrock; Kaffir HXD; Kemrock; Labstone; Micromod; Microwhite; Moldasynt; Orthodon; Rapidur; Tewerock; Topstone; Tru-Stone; Vel-Mix; Zeus Magic White.

Extra-hard, coloured die stones (modified α-hemihydrate + silica filler): Azure; Doric Dy-Rok; Duralit S; Jadestone; Prima Rock; Silky Rock; Supra-Stone; Widarock; Zeusuperock.

Manipulation The powder is added to the water (approximate ratios: model stones 23–30 ml water/100 g stone; die stones 22–24 ml water, even less for those containing inert, non-absorbent filler/100 g stone), by sifting to avoid the incorporation of air into the mix. It is gently but positively spatulated, preferably under vacuum, to a smooth mix in about 1 minute.

Properties Sets by an exothermic hydration reaction. Setting is accelerated by limited heat, nuclei and chemical additives as for plaster. Setting is retarded to give a usable material by additions such as borax, citric acid and potassium citrate. Expansion on setting: model stone 0.1–0.2%, die stone 0.05–0.1%. Compressive strength after 1 hour: model stone 30 MN/m^2; die stone 35 MN/m^2. Both materials double their strength when the excess water needed for mixing has evaporated. Separating agents are needed to facilitate the removal of wax patterns.

Applications

1. Model and dies.
2. Binder for investment materials suitable for casting alloys at temperatures below 200°C.
3. Occlusal records.

6.2 Metallic dies

6.2.1 Electroplating

Presentation A metal anode in a suitable electrolyte; the coated impression is the cathode. The anodes may be either copper or silver:

1. *Copper anode:* Electrolyte: acid solution of copper sulphate and potassium aluminium sulphate in distilled water, formula: (212 g $CuSO_4$; 12 g $K_2SO_4 \cdot Al_2(SO_4)_3 \cdot 24H_2O$; 31 ml H_2SO_4; water to 1 litre). May contain phenol or alcohol to harden the deposit. Coating for impression: colloidal graphite or metal dust. Plating conditions: 10–15 hours, 2–12 V, up to 100 mA.
2. *Silver anode:* Electrolyte: *alkaline* solution of silver cyanide and potassium cyanide, formula: (36 g $Ag(CN)_2$; 60 g KCN; 40 g K_2CO_3; water to 1 litre).

Beware! Acid added to this solution will liberate highly toxic hydrogen cyanide gas. All silver plating should be done in a fume cupboard with positive extraction.

Coating for impression: fine silver dust. Plating conditions 4–8 hours, 10 mA/tooth.

Manipulation The impression is made conductive with the coating powder and used as the cathode in the plating bath. The metal shell produced is filled with self-curing acrylic resin or die stone, together with a prefabricated die stump or dowel pin.

Properties Time-consuming process. Good abrasion resistance and accuracy.

Applications

1. Copper: electroplating of impression compound

or silicones, but *not* polysulphide, which reacts with the acidic electrolyte.
2. Silver: electroplating of all types of elastomeric impressions.

6.3 Polymeric dies

General advantages: rapid set and abrasion-resistant.
General disadvantage: shrinks on setting.

Presentation Some combination of liquids, pastes and powders, one of which is either liquid monomer (methyl methacrylate) or unsaturated polymer (epimine, epoxy, polyester or polyurethane resin). The other component may contain powdered polymer particles and a suitable initiator or activator for polymerizing or cross-linking the fluid phase to produce a solid. Either or both components may contain an inert metallic or ceramic filler (e.g. copper, silver, bronze, quartz or porcelain.)

Common brands Diemet; Goldex; Impredur; Polyroqq.

Manipulation The constituents are mixed according to the manufacturer's recommendations into a homogeneous paste in about a minute. The paste is then vibrated into the impression. Some elastomers require coating with a separating medium, often finely powdered metal.

Properties Set within an hour to become rigid, abrasion-resistant solids. All show some shrinkage on polymerization; the most heavily filled shrink the least. Epoxy resins react with polysulphide impression materials.

Application The production of dies from those impression materials with which they are compatible, generally elastomers coated with a separating medium.

6.4 Heat-hardened ceramic dies

General advantages Very hard and abrasion-resistant surfaces, which can withstand multiple firings.

Presentation Ceramic powder with binding liquid (two systems).

Common brands Ceramite H and V; Cosmotech Vest; Ducera-Lay; Doric HT2; DVP Investment; V.H.T. Investment; Vitadurvest.

Manipulation In either system the powder and liquid are mixed to a thick paste and vibrated into the impression. After standing for an hour (during which an initial set takes place) each is hardened according to type, either 600°C for 10 minutes followed by quenching in oil, or preheating followed by heating from 650 to 1015°C at 20°C per minute and then slow bench-cooling. Porcelain or glass–ceramic is built up, fired and glazed. The die material can be cut away with a tungsten carbide bur and the inner surface of the restoration cleaned by blasting with glass beads or alumina.

Properties Extremely abrasion-resistant; some shrinkage on firing; the material fired at 1015°C can be used in the fabrication of porcelain jacket crowns without the use of an intermediary platinum foil.

Application The production of dies for porcelain inlays, onlays and veneers.

6.5 Model and die surface treatment agents

Before wax patterns are built up on models and dies, it is often necessary to add something to their surfaces, either to increase their dimensions or to prevent the wax from bonding to them.

6.5.1 Die spacers

These are added to the die to increase its dimensions and thus create space for the finite thickness of luting cement that will eventually be needed when restorations made on the dies are finally seated on the preparations.

Presentation Bottles of resins dissolved in volatile solvents, often with suspended pigments to identify the film thickness each produces, together with thinners.

Common brands
For gypsum dies: Adapt-Rite; Fit-Rite; PDQ.
For epoxy resin dies: Belle de St Claire; Tru-Fit.

Manipulation The resins are painted uniformly over the die avoiding puddles at any corners or line angles. The solvent evaporates leaving a film of polymer.

Properties According to brand and type, the film thickness varies between 10 and 20 μm per layer. The layers are additive and the pigments permit a check on coverage of successive layers.

Applications The uniform expansion of accurate dies to create space within or around a restoration to accommodate the luting cement.

6.5.2 Surface pore fillers

These are needed to block the porosity on the surface of gypsum models and dies to prevent fluid wax flowing into them, hardening and making the pattern impossible to remove. They are not required if die spacers are used.

Presentation Solutions of lubricants in appropriate solvents.

Common brands Hera IS99; Isolit; Microfilm; Ryco-Sep; Super-Sep.

Manipulation The solution is painted over the surface of the die and allowed to dry.

Properties The solutions enter the pores and leave a very thin film on the surface of the gypsum without changing the dimensions of the die.

Applications The sealing of gypsum surfaces (which are not to receive die-spacing solution) prior to the application of hot wax.

Further reading

Chong, Y.H., Soh, G., Setchell, D.J. and Wickens, J.L. (1990) The relationship between contact angles of die stone on elastomeric impression materials and voids in stone casts. *Dental Materials*, **6**, 162–166

Sarma, A.C. and Neiman, R. (1990) A study on the effect of disinfectant chemicals on physical properties of die stone. *Quintessence International*, **21**, 53–59

Torrance, A. and Darvell, B.W. (1990) Effect of humidity on calcium sulphate hemihydrate. *Australian Dental Journal*, **35**, 230–235

7 Waxes and thermoplastic baseplate materials

7.1 Waxes

Presentation Waxes are complex combinations of organic substances of fairly high molecular weight (15–20 carbon atoms). They are blended by the manufacturer to suit particular applications. *Basic constituents:*

1. *Animal sources:* beeswax from honeycombs; a brittle wax consisting of an amorphous mixture of hydrocarbons and esters. When mixed with paraffin wax it makes the paraffin less brittle at room temperature and reduces the flow at mouth temperature. Melting point about 75°C.
2. *Mineral sources:* paraffin wax from petroleum distillation; a polycrystalline wax made of straight-chain hydrocarbons. Brittle when solid. 'Needle' crystals which develop on cooling (45–80°C) change to 'plates' on cooling a further 10°C. Other mineral waxes: ceresin (higher melting point and greater hardness); microcrystalline (higher melting range, 70–100°C); ozokerite, montan and barnsdahl (earth waxes).
3. *Vegetable sources:* Carnauba from South American palm trees, a blend of straight-chain esters, melting point about 105°C, a hard, lustrous and tough wax, blends with paraffin to harden it and raise its solid–solid transition range (see Properties). Candelilla from plants; similar to carnauba, melting point about 70°C. Other vegetable waxes: Japan wax; ouricury; cocoa butter.
4. *Other additives.* Synthetic waxes. Gums and

resins, e.g. copal, dammer, mastic, sandarac and shellac.

Properties

1. *Solid–solid transition temperature:* on warming, waxes undergo a solid transition in which the stable, orthorhombic crystal lattice form starts to change to a hexagonal form just below the melting point. Because the change is progressive, waxes can be manipulated without flaking, tearing or becoming unduly stressed. Waxes which need to be rigid in the mouth (e.g. inlay waxes) must have a solid–solid transition temperature above 37°C.
2. *Coefficient of thermal expansion:* at $350 \times 10^{-6}/$°C, this is higher than that of any other dental material. On removal from the mouth a wax pattern could contract up to 0.6%. This is a potential source of error.
3. *Flow:* Waxes flow or deform when subjected to a load. The flow increases as the temperature is raised above the transition temperature. Inlay waxes for the direct technique have a large flow at about 40–45°C to give good detail, but negligible flow at 37°C.
4. *Internal stresses:* uniform heating is difficult because of their low thermal conductivity. Ensure that waxes are adequately heated before deforming them otherwise distortion will follow when the stresses are relieved on subsequent warming.

7.1.1 Modelling or baseplate wax

Uses Baseplate patterns; registration of jaw relationships; construction of trial dentures.

Special properties Easy to mould when softened; must not crack or tear; easy to carve; no changes when frequently melted and solidified; no residue after application of boiling water and detergent.

Alternatives to modelling wax For the creation of stable, thin, stress-resistant registrations it is possible to use an addition-cured silicone paste as an alternative to folded wax sheet.

Common brand Memosil C.D.

Manipulation The components are automatically mixed as they are extruded through the static mixing tip from the cartridge delivery presentation. The mixed material is applied directly to the lower teeth: the patient then gently closes together.

Special properties This material is transparent at all stages and this enables contacts to be checked *through* the registration. It is thixotropic and thus flows readily (but only under load), producing a thin layer. It has a setting time of 3 minutes, a high final hardness and good dimensional stability.

7.1.2 Inlay wax

Uses Preparation of inlay patterns either in the mouth (the direct technique) or on a model or die (the indirect technique).

Special properties Good flow above mouth temperature and rigid below; contrasting colour to tissues; low thermal contraction; easy to carve; no residue after burning out.

7.1.2.1 Alternatives to inlay wax
7.1.2.1.1 Aesthetic waxes: For the build-up of crowns, which it is intended should be tried in the mouth for the purposes of obtaining a perfect colour match with the adjacent teeth, waxes are available in colours which simulate those of the natural dentition. These are known as aesthetic or diagnostic waxes and are also used by ceramic technicians to visualize clinical crowns during their construction
Common brands: Chromowax; Yeti-Creation.
7.1.2.1.2 Acrylic resins: For the preparation of inlay, crown and bridge patterns in either the mouth or the laboratory, for making transfer copings or connections for metal copings, and for bite registration, an alternative to wax is self-curing acrylic.
Common brand: Duralay; Palavit GLC (light-cured); Pattern Resin.
Manipulation: The red- or blue-pigmented polymer powder and liquid monomer are mixed to a paste which is applied to either the tooth or a die coated with a separating medium. Alternatively a paint-on technique is used in which a fine brush is

dipped into the monomer and then into the polymer powder to create a bead. This is transferred to the tooth to die. The process is repeated until the pattern is complete. The advantage of building up the pattern from the fit surface is that the effects of polymerization shrinkage are largely overcome. Once set, it is invested and burns out like wax.
Special properties: High strength when set; this enables patterns to be removed and handled without damage or distortion, hence patterns made on dies can be tried in the mouth. No residue after burning out.

7.1.2.2 Wetting agents
Because waxes are hydrophobic and reject water and water-based materials such as investments, it is necessary to coat wax patterns with a wetting agent called a surfactant.

Presentation Solutions of bifunctional molecules with some groups which are attracted to the wax and others which are hydrophilic.

Common brands Debubblizer; Delar; Hera NE99; Lubrofilm; Pro-Wax; Vacufilm; Waxit; Wettax.

Manipulation Several coats are applied to the wax pattern with a brush, taking care not to trap air bubbles at re-entrant surface features.

Properties Wets the surface of the wax pattern and leaves a very thin layer of bifunctional molecules on the surface.

Applications The treatment of wax patterns prior to investment.

7.1.3 Sheet casting wax

Uses and presentation Supplied in sheets which have been rolled to a precise thickness. Used in the construction of metal denture bases. Preformed sections such as round, half-round and flat are also available.

Special Properties Adaptable (after being warmed) by using moist cotton wool. Burns out without leaving any residue.

7.1.4 Sticky wax (model–cement)

Uses   The temporary joining of articles such as fragments of a broken denture prior to repair

Special Properties   Brittle; adhesive; no flow at room temperature; easily removed by boiling water.

7.1.5 Carding and boxing-in wax

Uses   Mounting of teeth in sets; boxing-in of impressions prior to casting up in gypsum.

Special properties   Readily undergoes plastic deformation at room temperature; self adhesive.

7.2 Thermoplastic baseplate materials

Composition   One of the following:
1. Wax, similar to modelling wax.
2. Shellac (natural resin) plus inert ceramic or metallic fillers.
3. Polystyrene (synthetic polymer).

Special properties   Thermoplastic, such that they flow when warmed but are rigid at mouth temperature.

Further reading

Sykora, O. and Sutow, E.J. (1990) Comparison of the dimensional stability of two waxes and two acrylic resin processing techniques in the production of complete dentures. *Journal of Oral Rehabilitation*, **17**, 219–227

8 Investment materials

Investment materials are used to form rigid, heat-resistant moulds for the casting of inlays, crowns, bridges, splints and denture frameworks in corrosion-resistant alloys and for supporting components during soldering. The casting investment should expand to compensate for the shrinkage which occurs when the alloy solidifies and cools to room/mouth temperature.

Basic constituents.
Refractory: to expand and resist the heat and forces of casing.

Binder: to hold the refractory particles together and possibly to aid the expansion.

Presentation   A powder consisting of refractory and binder constituents, together with a reducing agent such as charcoal, and modifying elements such as boric acid and sodium chloride to restrain shrinkage due to dehydration. The powder is mixed with exactly the recommended quantity of water or liquid binding agent.
1. *Refractory constituents:* a particulate mixture of the allotropic forms of silica (SiO_2), such as cristobalite and quartz, each having a characteristic inversion temperature at which the silicon–oxygen bonds (which are oriented at about 90°C below the inversion temperature) rotate so that the silicon–oxygen bonds are then at 180°. This results in a greater expansion than would be expected from the usual linear relationship between dimensions and temperature.
2. *Binder constituents and types:* a material which mixes with water to form a pourable slurry with the refractory constituents, and which undergoes a setting reaction to produce a rigid mould. The types of binder commonly used are gypsum, phosphate and silica.

8.1 Gypsum-bonded investments

Gypsum here refers to the α-hemihydrate of calcium sulphate.

Common brands
Casting investments: Astracast; Beauty-Cast; Cristobalite Inlay; Dentacast; Goldstar; Hartex; Inlay-vest; Jeycast; Luster-Cast; Microvest; Shiny-Brite.
Soldering investments: Deguvest L; Hi Heat; Soldavest; Speed E.

Manipulation   Gypsum-bonded investments are vacuum-mixed with the correct amount of water and vibrated around the sprued pattern, held within a metal casting ring. At one time such rings were lined with asbestos tape, but to reduce the potential hazard to laboratory staff a ceramic fibre tape (e.g. Kaoliner or Kera-Vlies) is now used. When set, the investment is heated through 150–200°C to drive off the water and burn out the wax pattern. It is then heated to 700°C.

Properties Setting occurs when the α-hemi-hydrate hydrates to become the dihydrate (see 6.1)

$$CaSo_4 \cdot \frac{1}{2}H_2O + 1\frac{1}{2}H_2O \rightarrow CaSO_4 \cdot 2H_2O$$

As well as the thermal expansion (which occurs when the investment is heated to 700°C), additional expansion comes from:
1. Setting expansion when the dihydrate forms.
2. Hygroscopic expansion, obtained by immersing the setting investment in water.

Above 1200°C gypsum reacts with silica thus:

$$CaSO_4 + SiO_2 \rightarrow CaSiO_3 + SO_3$$
$$\text{gas}$$

SO_3 gas is corrosive; a source of porosity and a back-pressure product.

Gypsum-bonded investments are thus contra-indicated for high-fusing alloys, e.g. Co-Cr, Au-Pt.

Applications Investment of wax patterns for types I–IV dental gold alloys. Also used for silver and its alloys, and for stabilizing components during investment soldering

8.2 Phosphate-bonded investments

Magnesium oxide + ammonium phosphate.

Common brands Alpha-Cast MP; Argivest; Aurobond; Biosint-Supra; Calsite; Castorit-C, -Super; Cera-Fina; Combi-Vest; Croform Hi-Tech, W-B Precision; Cruta-Vest; Deguvest F, CF, HPG; Denti-Vest; Duceratin (for titanium alloys); DVP; Econo-Vest; Eurocast; Finavest; 'GC Vest; Hi Chrom 2; Hi-Temp; Jeyvest; Microtex 84; Nicrobond; Pallavest (for palladium alloys); Polycast; Rema Exakt; Rema Star; Widerit; Zeusvest.

Manipulation Phosphate-bonded investments are mixed with the correct amount of water and vibrated around the sprued pattern held within a plastic ring, which is removed from the set investment before the latter is heated, first through 150–200°C to drive off the water and burn out the wax pattern, and then to 1000–1100°C

Properties Setting occurs due to the reaction between the constituents in aqueous solution:

$$MgO + NH_4H_2PO_4 \rightarrow MgNH_4PO_4 + H_2O$$

The magnesium ammonium phosphate crystals grow and interlock to cause setting and this contributes to the overall expansion of the set investment.

Applications Investment of wax patterns for the high-fusing gold- and nickel-based alloys that are used in porcelain-fused-to-metal techniques. The investment of wax patterns for the cobalt–chromium alloys used in the construction of partial dentures.

8.3 Silica-bonded investments

Ethyl silicate.

Common brand Refractory S.

Manipulation A polymerized form of ethyl silicate is reacted with water to form a sol of poly(silicic acid) with the liberation of ethyl alcohol:

$$poly[Si(C_2H_5O)_4] + 4H_2O \rightarrow$$
$$poly[Si(CH)_4] + 4C_2H_5OH$$
$$sol$$

The sol is mixed with the refractory silica in the presence of magnesium oxide and a gel forms, causing the investment to set. The mould is then dried.

Properties During drying out, considerable shrinkage occurs due to loss of alcohol and water. The mould is then a solid mass of silica, which expands considerably when heated and compensates for both the setting shrinkage and the casting shrinkage of the alloy. The set investment has a very low porosity and vents are needed to permit the escape of air during casting.

Applications Formerly used for the investment of wax patterns for high-fusing dental alloys. Now superseded by phosphate-bonded investments.

Further reading

David, D.R. and Kennedy, M.P. (1990) Xeroradiographic determination of effective setting expansion of a cristobalite investment. *Dental Materials*, **6**, 29–34

9 Casting alloys

Any component made of a metal or alloy which is to be used in the mouth should be completely chemically inert. It should neither corrode (a chemical attack in which metal is actually lost from the component) or tarnish (a chemical attack in which a surface reaction discolours it).

9.1 Dental gold alloys (casting shrinkage: 1.25–1.50%)

There are now many dozens of dental casting alloys which contain one or all of the noble metals (gold, platinum and palladium) and the challenge is how to classify these alloys.

When gold was not as expensive as it is today, classification was easy as there were just four types of alloy. These are sometimes known as the specification alloys, as they comply with national and international standards, including BS 4425, which requires that they contain no less than 75% of the noble metals. The four types have characteristic mechanical properties which enable them to be classified as soft, medium, hard and extra-hard. Whilst these alloys are the most expensive, they are those which should be used whenever possible as they offer the greatest resistance to both tarnish and corrosion. Such alloys have densities in the range 15–19 g/cm^3. Although economic considerations now dictate that alloys containing far less gold than those of BS 4425 should be used, modern alloys can still be described in relation to the mechanical properties of the original four types.

To add to the confusion, the American Dental Association (ADA) now has an alternative classification for dental alloys, and this is intended to help dentists and technicians in selecting suitable materials. In this classification, those alloys which contain at least 60% of the noble metals and at least 40% of gold are called high noble. Those which contain at least 25% gold, platinum or palladium are

called noble, and those which contain less than 25% of these noble metals are classified as predominantly base.

9.1.1 The high-gold specification casting alloys (BS 4425: ADA high noble)

Presentation Stamped pieces of gold alloy. Density range 15–19 g/cm^3. Colour: red/yellow.

Type I (A or soft)	19–22 carat, 800–900 fine Au plus up to 10Ag-5Cu
Type II (B or medium)	18–19 carat, 750–780 fine Au plus up to 15Ag-10Cu-4Pd-1Pt-1Zn
Type III (C or hard)	15–19 carat, 620–750 fine Au plus up to 16Ag-11Cu-4Pd-3Pt-1Zn
Type IV (D or extra-hard)	14–17 carat, 600–700 fine Au plus up to 20Ag-16Cu-5Pd-4Pt-2Zn

Pure gold = 24 carat = 1000 fine. The compositions shown are maximum amounts. In these alloys the noble metal content is never less than 75%.

Common brands Users should refer to manufacturer's data sheets for details of types

Apollo 3, 4; Argenco 5, 10, 17; Chicago IV; Degulor A, B, C, i, M, MO, S; Dentalor; Duocast; Firmilay; Foundation; Harmony Line; JA; JB; JC; Kenbridge; Maingold G, SG; Mattibel G, R; Matticast R; Mattident G, R; Mattigold AE; Mattinax GA, R; Medinlay; Modulay; Neocast; Ney-Oro; Orplid; Platigo J; Pluto 2P; Protor; Trucast II, III; World 75.

Manipulation

	Melting range
Type I	900–1000°C
Type II	920–980°C
Type III	900–1000°C
Type IV	850–950°C

All types will melt in an air–gas flame and can be

cast into a mould made of gypsum-bonded investment, which has been heated to 700°C. Castings are allowed to cool to below red heat before being quenched. Ultrasonic cleaning and acid immersion are employed as part of the finishing techniques.

Castings in types I and II alloys are used as cast. Those in types III and IV alloys are soft when quenched and can be readily deformed. They can be heat-hardened as outlined below.

Typical heat treatments

Softening   Heat to red-heat (700°C) to produce a disordered solid solution and quench in water. The solid solution remains disordered and hence dislocations can move and alloy can be shaped by mechanical deformation.

Hardening   Heat to red-heat (700°C) to produce a disordered solid solution and then either slowly cool or hold at about 420°C for 10 minutes before bench-cooling. This allows the ordered solid solution to form a superlattice which can interfere with the movement of dislocations. The proportional limit and hardness are raised and the ductility and elongation are reduced.

Properties

	Proportional limit (MN/m^2)	Elongation to failure %	Brinell hardness BHN
Type I	85	25	75
Type II	60	24	100
Type III			
As cast	195	20	140
Hardened	290	10	180
Type IV			
As cast	360	15	150
Hardened	585	10	230

The *proportional limit* is an indication of the strength of the alloy and the support it will need. Type I alloys thus require plenty to prevent deformation in service, whereas type IV alloys will stand up to heavy loads without suffering permanent deformation.

The *elongation to failure* is an indication of how easy it is to burnish the alloy. Type I alloys are ductile and easy to burnish, whereas type IV alloys are more brittle and are not readily burnished.

Applications

Type I – Low stress inlays, e.g. for class III or V cavities.

Type II – Most types of inlays.

Type III – Crowns and bridges where no porcelain is required.

Type IV – Partial denture construction, particularly clasps.

Clasps can be bent into shape with the alloy in the heat-softened condition and then heat-hardened to raise the proportional limit.

9.1.1.1 High-gold content alloys for porcelain-fused-to-metal techniques (also known as metal–ceramic or bonding alloys)

Presentation   Stamped pieces of gold alloy (22–23 carat; 920–960 fine; density 17–19 g/cm^3; colour–straw) containing up to 6% platinum, 5% palladium, 1% silver and traces of indium, iron and tin to assist in forming a chemical bond with the porcelain. Copper, which turns the porcelain green, is absent.

Common brands   Albus 190; Armator; Argident yellow, 2A, 3; Bermudent; Ceramco; Classic III; Degudent G, H, N, U; Engelbond Elite; Esticor Ideal, Royal, Special, Swiss; Golden Multibond; Herador NH; Hi-T Multibond; Image; Jelenko O; JP 11, 80, 87, IV; Matticraft Alpha, E, G, JMP, S; Microbond Hi Life; Noble J; Orion; Orplid Keramik; Panabond Yellow; Porcast; Premium; RX Imperial 2; SMG; Szabo YPG; Will-Ceram P.

Manipulation   Melts between 1200 and 1250°C in a ceramic crucible by an oxy-gas flame and it is cast centrifugally, or in a platinum-wound electrical furnace under vacuum, in which case casting is assisted by compressed air (Heraeus). A carbon-free phosphate-bonded investment is used in either case and the casting should be slowly cooled for maximum hardness and strength.

Properties
Proportional limit   265 MN/m^2
Elongation to failure   3%
Hardness (maximum)   150 BHN

The trace elements indium, iron and tin diffuse to the surface of the alloy during the firing of the porcelain and add a chemical component to the porcelain–metal bond.

Applications   Porcelain-fused-to-metal-units, e.g. faced crowns and bridges.

The properties of these alloys are mimicked by all other types of dental casting alloys which contain noble metals. It is thus possible to have, for example, alloys with the same properties as the type III, high gold specification alloys which can be categorized as high-, medium- or low-gold. Although their mechanical properties will be similar to those listed above and their applications will be the same, the alloys with reduced noble metal contents tend to have inferior resistance to tarnish and corrosion

9.1.2 Medium-gold alloys

As the price of gold has increased, alloys which do not comply with BS 4425 have been introduced as alternatives for inlays, crowns and bridges, including those to which porcelain veneers are to be fired. In the latter case many new base metal alloys are being used, but for normal inlays and crowns alloys with a much reduced noble metal content are now available. Whilst their physical and mechanical properties are similar to those of the high-gold alloys, their resistance to tarnish and corrosion is distinctly inferior and it takes only a few repeated casts before the composition shifts, such that tarnish, at least, becomes inevitable once they are cemented in place.

In the UK the alloys recommended for use under the National Health Service are those which comply with BS 6042. This specification describes such alloys as semiprecious and requires that they contain not less than 30% of the noble metals gold, platinum and palladium and not more than 20% of base metals such as copper and zinc. The remainder is silver and in practice they are generally silver–palladium–gold–copper alloys. There are four types of casting alloys which have a similar

range of properties to the high-gold alloys, and there is also a range of copper-free, silver–palladium–gold alloys intended for use in restorations to which porcelain veneers are to be attached.

9.1.2.1 The medium-gold specification casting alloys (BS 6042)

Presentation   Stamped pieces of alloy containing various proportions of gold, platinum, palladium, copper, silver and zinc. If they comply with BS 6042 the noble metal content will be not less than 30% and the copper and zinc content will be not more than 20%. These alloys are yellow in colour and have densities in the range 13–15 g/cm^3.

Common brands   Argenco 4, 27, 75; Argicast B; Aurea; Baker Four; Cascowyte; Cehadentor; CJ 60; Duallor; Forticast; Galaxy; Hera GC; Improved 1 Star; JCB; Jel 2, 3, 4; Laboratory 22, 33, 44; Mattident 60; Maxigold; Medior; Midas; Midigold; Minerva 4; Mirafort 4; Modulor; Mowrey 20/46; Ney Cast III; Orocast; Panacast 60; Platigo G; Rajah; Saffron; Skillcast 60; Stabilor G, GL/NHS, NFIV; Sterngold 66; Sturdicast; Sunrise; World 50.

Manipulation   Melt between 850 and 950°C in an air–gas flame, but care should be taken not to overheat them. Cast into a mould made of gypsum-bonded investment. Allow to cool to below red-heat before being quenched. Used in the as-cast condition.

Properties   The mechanical properties (proportional limit, elongation to failure and hardness) are similar to those of the high-gold alloys of the same type. Variations in composition due to either poor batch control by the manufacturer or to poor quality control in the individual dental laboratory can lead to inferior tarnish resistance in service.

Applications   Each type should be used in the same stress situations as would the high-gold alloys.

9.1.2.2 Medium-gold content alloys for porcelain-fused-to-metal techniques

Presentation   Stamped pieces of white-coloured alloy containing 40–75% gold and a wide range of alloying additions, e.g. 20–45% palladium, 0–10% tin, 0–9% indium, 0–2% each of silver, cobalt and gallium. They have densities in the range 13–16 g/cm^3.

Common brands Argilite 2, 4; Argistar 45; Cameo; Cehadent Keramik; Ceramco White; Degubond 4; Degucast U; Dentabond; Deva M, 4; Doric Bonding Gold; Eclipse; Esticor Plus, Vnic; Engelbond PGX, 45; Galaxy; Herabond; Herador P; Improved Hi-T Multibond; JP I, IA, III; JPW; Matticraft M, Y, 45; M.P.V-Delta; NoSilver; Novabond; Olympia; Option; Orion Delphi; Panabond 45; PGX 45; Verinor; Vivostar.

Manipulation Melt between 1150 and 1300°C in a ceramic crucible either by an oxy-gas flame and centrifugally cast, or in a platinum-wound electrical furnace under vacuum and pressure cast. A carbon-free, phosphate-bonded investment is used. The casting should be slowly cooled for maximum hardness and strength.

Properties

Proportional limit	270–630 MN/m^2
Elongation	3–30%
Hardness	180–300 BHN

Silver-rich alloys can discolour the porcelain.

Applications. Substrates for porcelain-fused-to-metal crowns and bridges.

9.1.3 Low-gold alloys

These are either silver–palladium alloys or palladium-based alloys with a broad range of compositions. Those containing at least 25% of gold, platinum or palladium are considered noble under the ADA classification. The white golds in use in dentistry 25 years ago contained 30–45% silver, 20–25% palladium, 15–30% gold, 15–20% copper and 1% zinc.

9.1.3.1 Low-gold casting alloys (white gold, silver–palladium)

Presentation Stamped pieces of white alloy containing 40–70% silver, 20–35% palladium, 0–20% each gold and copper, 0–15% indium and small amounts of zinc and tin. Their density ranges from 10 to 12 g/cm^3.

Common brands Alba M; Albacast; Argenco 9, 18, 23, 26B; Cameolite; Castadur; Castell; Doric SP; Hera O; J-7; Jelcast; Maestro; Mattieco 25; Minigold; Palaural; Pallacast; Pallacon; Pallas 3, 4; Palliag M, MJ, W; Pallium 3; Pallorag; Palloro; Paloy; Panacast 5; Pangold; Pontallor 3, 4; Realor; Solarcast; Strator; Super Oralium; Tiffany; Topcast; Utiloy; Vista; White Economy; World 20.

Manipulation Melt between 875 and 1150°C in a ceramic crucible with an oxy-gas flame. Overheating, which results in gross porosity due to occluded gases, must be avoided. Cast into gypsum-bonded investment and quenched from red-heat to avoid overhardening.

Properties (as quenched)

Proportional limit	345 MN/m^2
Elongation to failure	9%
Hardness (maximum)	170 BHN
Casting shrinkage	1.15%

These alloys must not be slowly cooled, otherwise they will overharden and become brittle. They are also prone to rapid work hardening, which precludes excessive adjustment or burnishing. Tend to tarnish in the mouth.

Applications
1. Inlays, crowns.
2. Partial denture frameworks.

9.1.3.2 Palladium-based alloys for porcelain-fused-to-metal techniques

Presentation Stamped pieces of white metal with a density of about 11 g/cm^3. Two types are available:
1. *Palladium–silver alloys*, which contain 60–80% palladium, 30–35% silver, 2–9% tin and 2–7% indium. Their density ranges from 10–12 g/cm^3.
2. *Silver-free palladium alloys*, which contain 80% palladium, 4–8% gallium, 5–8% indium, 0–14% tin, 0–10% copper, 0–3% cobalt and 0–2% each of gold and ruthenium. Their density ranges from 11 to 12 g/cm^3.

Common brands

Palladium–silver alloys: Albabond; Alborium; Argicraft 1; Argilite 50; Esticor Economic; Integrity; Jelstar; JP 5, 92; Matticraft B; Microcast MC; Orion Argos; Pageant; Pangold Keramik; Pors-on 4; Protocol; Silver Pal-Bond; SP 70; SP 90; Will-Ceram W1; WLW.

Silver-free palladium alloys: Alabond E; Argipal; Argenco 34; Bond-on 4; Cast Well; Doric GII; Dynasty; Encore Plus; Esticor Opal; Legend; Matticraft C, H, 80; Naturelle Rx; Novabond 2; Orion Libra; Pal-Bond Extra, 3; Panabond 2; PG 2; Spirit; Topcraft.

Manipulation The alloys melt between 1200 and 1250°C and should be cast as soon as they are molten into carbon-free, phosphate-bonded investments, which have been heated to 850°C. Slow cooling is required prior to breaking out from the investment. Mild cleaning with ultrasonics and steam are recommended, and degassing under vacuum is advisable before oxidation at the same temperature. The framework should be ultrasonically cleaned prior to the application of the porcelain.

Properties

Proportional limit	650 MN/m^2
Elongation to failure	30%
Hardness	250 BHN

Applications Bridge frameworks of all sizes.

9.2 Chromium-containing alloys

Chromium confers a degree of stainlessness on alloys which contain at least 12% of the element. This chemical protection comes from a coherent passive film of chromium oxide on the surface which has the same volume as the metal it replaces.

9.2.1 Cobalt chromium (stellite)

Presentation Ingots or splash alloy (shot) containing up to 65% cobalt, 35% chromium and 7% molybdenum, with small quantities of carbon, tungsten, manganese, silicon and iron. In some alloys the cobalt is substituted by up to 30% nickel.

In one type of alloy the chromium is substituted by up to 10% titanium. The density of these white alloys ranges from 8 to 8.5 g/cm^3.

Common brands

For castings without porcelain facings
Biosil h, f; C&J 1, 2; Chromodur M; Croform Excel, Regular, Springhard; Crutanium (with titanium); Duraflex; Duralium; Hi Crome; JFB Alloy; Megallium; Micronium HS, N10; Niranium; Nobilium; Panachrome; Platinore; Remanium CC; Svedion; Victory; Virilium; Vitallium; Wironit; Wisil.

For porcelain-fused-to-metal substrates
Arcalloy; Arobond; Bio-Cast; Bondi-Loy; Ceramalloy; Dentitan; Dentobond; Discovery; Duceralloy U; Freebond; Maxibond; Medicast; Neobond II; Novarex; Remanium CD; Supranium; Vi-Comp.

Manipulation Melt 1250–1450°C by either an oxyacetylene flame or induction heating, often in an inert atmosphere (argon). The molten alloy is centrifugally cast into a mould made of phosphate- or silica-bonded investment which has been heated to between 1000 and 1100°C. Sand-blasting and electrolytic polishing are employed as part of the finishing techniques.

Properties

Proportional limit	550–650 MN/m^2
Elongation to failure	4%
Hardness (maximum)	370 BHN
Casting shrinkage	1.8–2.3%
Elastic modulus (E)	250 GN/m^2
(cf. type IV gold	100 GN/^{2})

Because the modulus of Co-Cr alloys is twice that of type IV dental gold, connectors in Co-Cr can be made only half as thick as those in gold and still be as rigid. The low elongation precludes substantial adjustment. The titanium-containing alloy, with an elongation of 10%, is more readily and safely adjusted if necessary. For all these alloys the high hardness enables a good polish to be produced with difficulty, but it lasts a long time.

Applications

1. Denture bases and connectors.
2. Sub-periosteal and endosseus implants.
3. Minimum-preparation bridges (Maryland).

9.2.2 Nickel–chromium

Presentation Ingots containing up to 80% nickel and 20% chromium. In some alloys the nickel is substituted by up to 10% cobalt, 5% molybdenum, 4% aluminium and 4% manganese. Traces of boron, carbon and iron are generally present and some alloys contain up to 2% beryllium. These require efficient extractors to reduce hazardous beryllium levels of the dust during finishing. The density of these white alloys is between 7.5 and 8.3 g/cm^3.

Common brands
With beryllium: Cristal B; DJ Metal; Duceranium U; Gemini; Litecast B; Multibond; Nobilium; NPX III; Resistal P; Rexillium III; Super-Cast; Talladium Premium; Talladium V; Thermabond; Ticon; Ticonium T3; Tristar; Ultratech; Unitbond; Verabond.
Beryllium-free: Doric Non-Precious; Electro-magma; Howmedica III; Jelbon; Jelspan; Microbond NP$_2$; NCM Alpha; Nirabond; Nobil-Ceram; Omega Alpha MS; Omega VK; Remanium CS; Roll-X; S-1; Talladium NoBel-T; Unibond; Wiron 88.

Manipulation Melt between 1150 and 1250°C by either an oxy-gas flame or induction heating. The molten alloy is cast into a mould made of phosphate-bonded investment which has been heated to between 900 and 1000°C. Sand-blasting and ultrasonic cleaning are employed as part of the finishing techniques.

Properties

Proportional limit	230 MN/m^2
Elongation to failure	4%
Hardness (maximum)	250 BHN
Casting shrinkage	1.4%

The proportional limit is much lower than that of cobalt–chromium alloys and much closer to that of a type III dental gold. However, their elastic modulus is 200 GN/m^2 (compared with 100 GN/m^2 for type III dental gold alloys), thus allowing rigid structures to be made with thin sections. This, combined with the ability of some of them to be etched to produce a microretentive surface and their affinity for porcelain, has made them popular for use in Maryland bridges and their variants.

Applications
1. Inlays, crowns and bridges.
2. Metal–ceramic units, e.g. crowns and bridges retained with a minimum of preparation of the adjacent teeth.

9.3 Silver alloys

Although it is electrochemically noble, silver tends to tarnish in the mouth and its alloys cannot be considered to be as corrosion resistant as those of gold.

9.3.1 Sterling silver

Presentation Stamped pieces of sterling silver containing up to 7.5% copper, the remainder being silver.

Common brand Ash casting silver.

Manipulation Melts between 900 and 920°C in an air–gas flame and is cast into a mould of Baker's sterling investment (gypsum-bonded) which has been heated to 700°C. Casting may be achieved by using the Solbrig system, in which the silver is melted in the hot investment cone. Once molten, a damp fibre sheet is placed firmly on top of the investment and above the silver. The steam pressure thus produced forces the silver into the mould.

Properties

Proportional limit	55 MN/m^2
Elongation to failure	22%
Hardness	25 BHN

The low proportional limit and hardness and the high ductility enable cemented silver splints to be readily removed without damaging the teeth or newly formed bone.

Applications Surgical cap splints used for fixation during the reossification of a fractured or surgically displaced mandible or maxilla. Cemented *in situ*, usually with black copper cement.

9.3.2 Silver–palladium alloys (gold-free)

Presentation   Stamped pieces of silver-coloured alloys containing:

1. Up to 25% palladium (these are classified as noble by the ADA system).
2. Less than 25% palladium (these are classified as predominantly base by the ADA system).
   The other elements are copper, indium and zinc.

Common brands

Noble: Ney (Ag-25Pd-14Cu-2Zn); W.L.W. (Ag-25Pd-14In). Predominantly base: Salivan (Ag-20In-5Pd).

Manipulation   Silver–palladium alloys have a low density and must be fully molten when cast: however, care must be taken not to overheat the alloys as they readily dissolve oxygen and this leads to porosity when they solidify. They should be rapidly cooled once cast to prevent overhardening.

Properties   The proportional limit and hardness are similar to those of high-gold alloys, but they are not as ductile. Silver alloys do not have the same tarnish resistance as those of gold.

Applications   Each type should be used in the same stress situations as would the corresponding gold alloys.

9.4 Dental solders

Solders are alloys with melting points lower than those of the components which they are being used to join together. The melting point of the solder is controlled by the composition which, although it differs from that of the components being joined, should contain as large a quantity of corrosion- and tarnish-resistant metal as possible. Dental solders are presented in the form of strip or wire.

9.4.1 Gold solders

These can be used to join the individual gold castings of multiunit restoration such as a bridge.

Solders for metal–ceramic restorations are copper-free and melt in the range 1050-1150°C. These alloys contain at least 80% gold, platinum and palladium with small amounts of silver, iron, tin and indium. Zinc is also present to lower the melting range.

Solders for cast components are gold–silver–copper alloys with small amounts of zinc and tin. They melt in the range of 750-850°C.

Common brands

For gold alloys: Argen; Auridium; Easy Flow; Engelbond Hi; Mattiflo; Nobil Solder; Solder Auro; Unilot; UniSolder.

For base metal alloys: Aucrom 1; Cromo Pal; DWL-Lot.

Manipulation   Can be used freehand or, for maximum accuracy, by aligning components in investment (gypsum-bonded for cast components and phosphate-bonded for metal–ceramic restorations). Components should be clean and smooth.

Antiflux, such as Contex, or a suspension of graphite, chalk or rouge, should be applied to the area where solder is not required. A small amount of flux, such as Anoxon, Uniflux or Veriflux, or a mixture of 45% sodium tetraborate (borax), 35% boric acid and 10% silica, should be applied to the area to be soldered. Investment is dried out prior to heating. Soldering takes place on a preheated block using a gas–air flame.

Applications

1. The joining of cast gold components of multiunit restorations.
2. The bonding of precision attachments to cast gold restorations.
3. The connection of wrought gold clasps to cobalt–chromium denture bases (requires a fluoride flux such as Oxynon).

9.4.2 Silver solders

These can be used to join stainless steel or cobalt–chromium components. When soldering stainless steel, as low a temperature as possible is desirable to prevent both the annealing of the work-hardened material and the formation of chromium carbide at the grain boundaries. This latter reduces the amount of chromium at the surface, with a corresponding loss of the protective passive oxide film of chromium oxide. Whilst outside dentistry a cadmium-containing alloy known as turbine solder (Ag-25Cu-15Cd-15Zn; melting range 580–660°C) is used for this purpose, cadmium is not acceptable as a component for *in vivo* use because of its toxic action and ready dissolution. Modern silver solders for dental use are thus silver–copper–zinc alloys, containing tin and indium to lower the melting range of normal silver solder (Ag-27Cu-10Zn), which has a melting range of 700–730°C.

Common brands Silver solders tend to be sold according to their melting range without a brand name.

Manipulation Can be used freehand or within gypsum-bonded investment, as described above. However, to break down the chromium oxide film on stainless alloys the flux must contain potassium fluoride. It must also contain a greater proportion of boric acid to allow it to fuse at a lower temperature.

Applications
1. The attachment of preformed orthodontic devices to removable appliances.
2. The bonding of wrought stainless steel or cobalt–chromium clasps to cobalt–chromium denture bases.

9.5 Cast titanium alloys

The casting of titanium (melting point 1668°C) and its alloys must be undertaken in vacuum arc furnaces, as the molten metal ignites spontaneously in air, and traces of oxygen, nitrogen or carbon in the metal make it brittle. The technology for its safe use in the dental laboratory is still under development, as are the investment materials needed to withstand such high temperatures. The most promising systems use magnesia as a refractory, melting under vacuum (air pressure < 10 Torr) and pressure casting with argon (> 50 Torr).

Potential applications for this light, corrosion-resistant metal and its alloys include denture bases and crowns. (see also 11.4.2).

Further reading

Biological effects

Dahl, B.L., Hensten-Pettersen, A. and Lyberg, T. (1990) Assessment of adverse reactions to prosthodontic materials. *Journal of Oral Rehabilitation*, **17**, 279–286

Namikoshi, T., Yoshimatsu, T., Suga K., Fujii, H. and Yasuda, K. (1990) The prevalence of sensitivity to constituents of dental alloys. *Journal of Oral Rehabilitation*, **17**, 377–381

Corrosion resistance

Cannay, S. and Öktemer, M. (1992) *In vitro* corrosion behaviour of 13 prosthodontic alloys. *Quintessence International*, **23**, 279–287

Muller, A.W.J., Maessen, F.J.M.J. and Davidson, C.L. (1990) Determination of the corrosion rates of six dental NiCrMo alloys in an artificial saliva by chemical analysis of the medium using ICP-AES. *Dental Materials*, **6**, 63–68

General properties

Brown, D. (1988) Oral golds. *Gold Bulletin*, **21**, 24–28

Brown, D. and Curtis, R.V. (1992) Alternatives to gold. *Dental Update*, **19**, 325–330

Chew, C.L., Norman, R.D. and Stewart, G.P. (1990) Mechanical properties of metal–ceramic alloys at high temperature. *Dental Materials*, **6**, 223–227

Soldering

Sobieralski, J.A., Schelb, E. and Prihoda, T.J. (1990) Torch versus oven preceramic soldering of a nickel–chromium alloy. *Quintessence International*, **21**, 753–757

Titanium casting

Blackman, R., Barghi, N. and Tran, C. (1991) Dimensional changes in casting titanium removable partial denture frameworks. *Journal of Prosthetic Dentistry*, **65**, 309–315

Hruska, A.R. (1990) A novel method for vacuum casting titanium. *International Journal of Prosthodontics*, **3**, 142–152

Takahashi, J., Kimura, H., Lautenschlager, E.P., Chern Lin, J. H., Moser, J.B. and Greener, E.H. (1990) Casting pure titanium into commercial phosphate-bonded SiO_2 investment moulds. *Journal of Dental Research*, **69**, 1800–1805

10 Principles of lost wax casting and casting faults

10.1 Principles of the lost wax casting process (Fig. 4)

Sprue

The diameter should be related to the size of the casting.

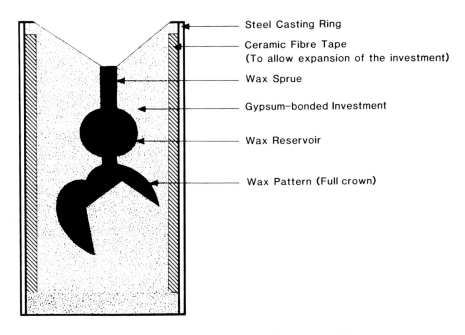

Figure 4 Cross-section of an invested pattern of a full crown prior to burning out of the wax.

Small inlays: sprue diameter 1.3 mm.
Most inlays: sprue diameter 2.0 mm.
Large inlays: sprue diameter 2.6 mm.
Large frameworks need multiple sprues.

Reservoir

This is attached to the sprue about 1 mm from the pattern. It helps avoid shrinkage porosity in the inlay by supplying molten alloy as the pattern solidifies.

10.1.1 Sequence of operations for the lost wax casting of an indirect inlay

1. Prepare tooth; take an impression; produce a die.
2. Prepare a wax pattern; attach sprue (and reservoir if required); mount on a crucible former.
3. Line the casting ring with damp ceramic fibre tape, e.g. Kaoliner or Kera-Vlies; fix casting ring and crucible former together; apply wetting agent to a pattern and sprue.

4. Mix investment with correct volume of water; vibrate it around pattern and sprue; allow to set.
5. Burn out wax; heat investment to cause expansion.
6. Heat alloy; apply flux; transfer investment; melt alloy; cast.
7. Allow to cool below red-heat; quench in water.
8. Remove casting from investment; clean it in an ultrasonic bath; acid-clean surface to remove oxides
9. Trim off sprue; adjust to fit; polish.
10. Lute on prepared tooth with a suitable cement, e.g. zinc phosphate, glass-ionomer, polycarboxy-late, zinc oxide–eugenol containing ethoxybenzoic acid or unfilled dimethacrylate.

10.2 Casting faults (and how to avoid them)

A casting may:
1. Be dimensionally inaccurate.
2. Have a rough surface and/or fins.
3. Be porous, contaminated or incomplete.

10.2.1 Dimensional errors (Fig. 5)

Problem	Likely cause	How to avoid fault
Too small	Too little mould expansion	Use correct temperature
Too large	Too much mould expansion	Use correct temperature and investment materials
Distorted	Stress relief of wax pattern	Warm wax thoroughly before creating pattern

10.2.2 Rough surfaces and fins

Problem	Likely cause	How to avoid fault
Rough surface	Breakdown of investment	Do not overheat mould or alloy
	Air bubbles on wax pattern	Use wetting agent and/or vacuum-investing technique
	Weak investment	Avoid using too much water when mixing investment or too much wetting agent on wax pattern
Fins	Cracking of investment	Avoid heating investment too rapidly

10.2.3 Porosity, contamination and incompleteness

Problem	Likely cause	How to avoid fault
Porosity		
Irregular voids	Casting shrinkage of alloy	Place sprues of correct diameter and reservoir at (or near) the bulkiest section of the pattern
	Turbulent flow of molten alloy Inclusion of particles of investment	Place sprues in correct position to prevent turbulence Heat mould upside down so that any loose particles fall out
Spherical voids	Gases dissolve in molten alloy and form bubbles when it cools	Do not overheat it for too long
Contamination		
Oxidation	Overheating in air	Do not use an oxidizing flame or heat for too long Use a flux to protect molten alloy
Sulphur	Breakdown of investment (particularly gypsum-bonded)	Do not overheat the investment
Incompleteness (Fig. 6)		
Rounded margins	Back-pressure of air due to low porosity of mould	Place pattern no more than 6–8 mm from the end of the casting ring. Use porous investments (or vents). Ensure there is no wax left and cast with sufficient force
Short castings	Alloy deficiency	Use enough alloy; make sure it is completely molten
	Mould too thin, too cold or had blocked sprues	Use correct diameter sprues and heat to correct temperature
	Insufficient casting force	Ensure casting machine is correctly balanced and accurately wound up

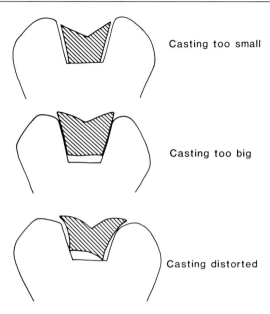

Figure 5 Possible dimensional deviations following casting.

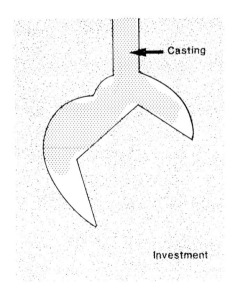

Figure 6 Rounded margins of an incomplete casting.

Further reading

Bertolotti, R.L. (1990) Casting metals. *Compendium of Continuing Education in Dentistry*, **11**, 300–308

Davis, D.R., Kawashima, S.S. and Nguyen, J.H. (1990) Effect of ring length and diameter on effective radial setting expansion. *Dental Materials*, **6**, 56–59

11 Wrought alloys

Metals and alloys which are formed *when they are solid*, by any process which involves their deformation by mechanical means into the desired shape, can be said to be *wrought*. Dental applications of wrought alloys are set out below.

11.1 Stainless steel

Steel is an alloy of iron and up to 2% carbon. Stainless steels contain at least 12% chromium to give them a passive (corrosion-resistant) oxide layer. Although stainless steel can be cast, its high ductility enables it to be mechanically shaped into useful artefacts.

Forms used in dentistry:

11.1.1 Sheet

Presentation Sheets of 18/8 austenitic stainless steel, some as thin as 0.1 mm. This alloy contains 18% chromium, 8% nickel, about 0.1% carbon and the balance is iron. Some alloys, known as 18/8/1 or stabilized austenitic stainless steels, in addition to the chromium and nickel, contain up to 1% titanium (or niobium) to prevent weld decay. The sheets are annealed (softened) by heating to 1050°C for 2 minutes and then quenched in order to relieve any work-hardening.

Manipulation The annealed steel sheet can be deformed by:

1. *Swaging:* hand beating with a soft mallet over a die. Intermediate annealling is necessary for maximum detail.
2. *Explosive forming:* a pressure wave is generated by detonating an explosive charge in a tank of water. The steel sheet, which is in contact with the die, is deformed as the pressure wave passes.
3. *Hydraulic forming:* a pressure of 70 MN/m^2 is produced by pumping oil into a pressure chamber, which contains the steel sheet held at the edges but in contact with the die.

In all cases the material work-hardens. After forming, the sheet is cut to size and tags or pieces of wire gauze (to regain the acrylic gum-work and teeth) are spot-welded into position. Polishing of the fitting surface follows.

Properties Very thin and light (0.1 mm as compared with 1.5 mm for an acrylic denture base). Highly resistant to fracture. High thermal conductivity (transmits heat rapidly to the palate).

Applications Fracture-resistant bases for upper dentures

11.1.2 Wire

Presentation Wires of austenitic stainless steel of various diameters and hardness values. During drawing down to size, wires undergo severe work-hardening. They are used in the extra-hard, hard and soft (annealed) condition. Annealing can be achieved by heating to 1050°C and quenching into water. Although the 18/8 stainless steels are not normally considered to be heat-hardenable, the transformation from austenite to ferrite can be induced by heating the wire at 450°C for 10 minutes. This raises the flexural rigidity but reduces the corrosion resistance. Such heat treatments also tend to change the colour of the wire by creating a thin oxide film on the surface.

For orthodontic use wires may be presented as coils or straight lengths of single-strand wire with a round cross-section, straight lengths of rectangular cross-section (more rigid), or as very flexible multistrand coils.

Manipulation Wires are bent to shape using the appropriate type of pliers.

Properties	Soft	Hard	Extra-hard
Proportional limit	280	1050	1450 MN/m^2
Elongation to failure	50	6	1%
Hardness	170	250	350 BHN
Modulus of elasticity	200	200	230 GN/m^2

Applications Components of orthodontic appliances. Rests and clasp arms for partial dentures. Lingual bars.

11.1.3 Preformed crowns

Presentation A range of bell-shaped molar crowns of various sizes made from work-hardened stainless steel.

Common brand Ion Ni-Chro.

Manipulation The tooth is prepared as for a full gold crown.

11.1.4 Other forms

Wrought stainless steel is also used for:
1. Dental instruments (see section 1.1).
2. Surgical implants: prosthetic devices such as joints; internal-fixation devices for immobilizing fractured bones.

    The alloy used is a surgical grade of stainless steel and contains up to 3% molybdenum to promote good resistance to chloride corrosion.
3. Tape: used for orthodontic bands (often spot welded).
4. Dentine pins and root posts (see section 4).

11.2 Gold alloys (wire)

Presentation and applications Gold alloy wires are either simple ternary alloys of gold, copper and silver, or platinized alloys containing 10–20% platinum and palladium. They can be used in the work-hardened condition for orthodontic appliances.

Common brands Baker Clasp wire; Pallacast Wire; 16/17 Platinized Wire.

Properties	Work-hardened
Proportional limit	550 MN/m^2
Elongation to failure	3%
Hardness	220 BHN
Modulus of elasticity	95 GN/m^2

(Note that this is less than half that of stainless steel.)

11.3 Chromium-containing alloys

11.3.1 Cobalt–chromium

Presentation and applications
1. Wires: These have a similar composition to casting alloys. They are used for components of partial dentures.
2. Wrought sections: Cobalt–chromium alloys are used for a wide range of surgical and dental implants. They have an excellent resistance to *in vivo* corrosion.

Properties	Work-hardened
Proportional limit	900 MN/m^2
Elongation to failure	1%
Hardness	225 BHN
Modulus of elasticity	210 GN/m^2

11.3.2 Cobalt–chromium–nickel

Several special alloy wires are available for specific uses, for example, Elgiloy (Co-20Cr-16Fe-15Ni-7Mo-2Mn), and Crozat. This alloy was originally developed for use in watch springs. It can be softened (annealed) by heating to 1230°C and then water-quenching. It can be hardened by heating in a dental furnace for 7 minutes at 482°C, or by passing an electric current through it until a paste such as Temper-Indicating-Paste is seen to flash. It is presented for orthodontic use in straight lengths of various hardness values. The softened material can be easily manipulated and then heat-treated. This raises the yield strength and lowers the ductility. The alloy is not easily soldered.

Wiptam (Co-30Cr-25Ni) is popular as an economical way of producing the root section of a post-crown. For this application the wire is sandblasted prior to having a gold core cast on to it. When cemented *in vivo* a galvanic couple such as this creates the ideal conditions for crevice corrosion.

11.4 Titanium alloys

11.4.1 Wires

Presentation Various titanium alloy wires are available including:
1. Commercially pure titanium, which always contains some oxygen in solution.
2. β-titanium: an alloy of titanium–11% molybdenum-6% zirconium–4% tin.
3. Titanium–5% aluminium–4% vanadium.
4. Titanium–aluminium (α-titanium) which is a nickel-free alloy capable of being welded. It hardens in the mouth over a period of 3–4 months due to the formation of titanium hydride.
5. Nickel–titanium alloys containing almost equal parts of the two major constituents plus small amounts of other constituents such as cobalt. Those which contain around 55 weight per cent nickel have a shape-retentive memory and a characteristic activation temperature. In simple binary alloys this is between −30°C and +100°C. By skilful alloying and processing this temperature can be made such that it is close to mouth temperature. Above this temperature, wires which have been lightly deformed will return to the shape which they were given at a much higher temperature (between 482 and

510°C). However, the shape-retentive memory effect, which is due to a transformation from a martensitic phase to one which is austenitic, is not generally used in dentistry. The low elastic modulus of these alloys gives them great pliability and they are useful additions to the range of archwires available to the orthodontist. Most are supplied as pre-formed arches of various designs; however, some are available as straight lengths and as tightly coiled springs.

Some of them show a property which has been called super-elasticity. This refers to their ability during deactivation to deliver a constant, light force as they spring back to between 8% and 2% of their zone of elastic deformation.

Common brands of nickel–titanium wires
Align; Chinese NiTi; Elastinol; Japanese NiTi; Marsenol; Ni-Tek; Ni-Ti; Nitanium; Nitinol; nt plus; Orthonol; Reflex; Rematitan; Sentalloy; Sentinol; Speed; Super Nitane; The Force; Titanal; Titanium Memory Wire; tp wire; Vitanol.

11.4.2 Wrought titanium and titanium–aluminium–vanadium

Titanium–aluminium–vanadium (Ti-5Al-4V) alloys are used in a wide range of surgical implants, including replacements for sections of incised mandible, endosseus blade and screw implants and denture studs.

Properties

Alloy	Yield strength MN/m²	Modulus of elasticity GN/m²
'Nitinol' (Ti-48Ni-2Co)	40	425
β-titanium (Ti-11Mo-6Zr-4Sn)	75	1100
Work-hardened titanium	100	500
Wrought Ti-5Al-4V	120	1100

11.4.3 Machined crowns

Presentation Blocks of commercially pure titanium.

Common brands Dux System; Procera.

Manipulation The model is scanned by a computerized digitizer and the information is used in the computer-aided design of the restoration. The fit surface is produced either by milling away the unwanted material or by eroding it away with an electric arc (spark machining). The outer surface is then prepared, and after hand-smoothing, porcelain with a low-fusing temperature is applied and fired.

Properties High strength, low density, good resistance to corrosion, radiolucent.

Applications The production of single crowns or multiple unit bridges.

11.5 Alternatives to orthodontic wires

11.5.1 Elastics (elastomerics)

Presentation Transparent or grey loops, chains or threads of natural polymers such as latex, or synthetic polymeric, preformed ligatures manufactured to close tolerances from natural or synthetic rubbers.

Common brands Alastics; Break-Away; Dentalastics; Dentaurum; E-Chain; Elasto-force; Energy Chain; Energy Ringlets; Memory Chain; Olympia; Ormco; Power Chain; Quick Ligs; Rocky Mountain.

Properties Ligatures of similar size have similar load/deflection characteristics; however, the force delivered decreases as they absorb water.

Applications Space closing, rotation of teeth and other tooth movements.

Further reading

Elastics

Huget, E.F., Patrick, K.S. and Nunez, L.J. (1990) Observations on the elastic behaviour of a synthetic orthodontic elastomer. *Journal of Dental Research,* **69,** 496–501

Wires

Kapila, S. and Sachdeva, R. (1989) Mechanical properties and clinical applications of orthodontic wires. *American Journal of Orthodontics and Dentofacial Orthopedics*, **96**, 100–109

Kusy, R.P. and Wilson T.W. (1990) Dynamic mechanical properties of straight titanium alloy archwires. *Dental Materials*, **6**, 228–236

Yoneyama, T., Doi, H., Hamanaka, H., Okomoto, Y., Mogi, M. and Miura, F. (1992) Super-elasticity and thermal behaviour of Ni-Ti alloy orthodontic arch wire. *Dental Material Journal*, **11**, 1–10

12 Polymeric denture base materials

Used for production of a base to provide support and retention for artificial teeth in the correct occlusal relationship for each individual patient.

12.1 Poly(methyl methacrylate): and other acrylic polymers

12.1.1 Heat-cured (heat-activated) poly(methyl methacrylate)

Applications
1. Denture bases (complete and partial).
2. Gumwork on metallic denture bases.
3. Manufacture of artificial teeth.

Presentation
1. *Powder:* clear or pigmented microspheres of poly(methyl methacrylate) polymer together with 0.5% by weight of initiator, usually dibenzoyl peroxide. The size of the powder particles can influence the doughing time and improved mechanical properties are obtained by the use of co-polymers and methyl methacrylate with vinyl chloride and vinyl acetate. The impact resistance can be improved by using a polymer bead made by co-polymerizing methyl methacrylate and butadiene styrene in an emulsion and coating the beads with a layer of methyl methacrylate. These are called microdispersed rubber phase polymers. Poly(HEMA), which is a hydrophilic polymer, is added to some to improve the wettability and aid retention.
2. *Liquid:* clear volatile methyl methacrylate monomer, boiling point 100.3°C, containing 0.01% of hydroquinone as a stabilizer. Some

materials contain up to 6% of cross-linking agents such as ethylene glycol dimethacrylate (EGDMA). One material contains 4-META, which forms a chemical bond between the acrylic and basemetal denture alloys, thus reducing the interfacial stresses between the two components and so reducing the cracking of the acrylic.
3. Occasionally presented as a premixed gel formed from polymer and monomer. These gels are press-packed and heat-cured.

Common brands Acron Rapid; Acron Standard; Betacryl II; Croform Exten; Doric; Hydrocryl (with poly(HEMA)); LP-22; Luxon; MDA; Meadway; Meliodent; Metrocryl Universal; Microlon; Minacryl Universal; Paladon 65; Plastex; Redilon; SR Ivocap; Stellon; Super-Cure; Trevalon; WHW.

High-impact, micro-dispersed rubber-phase polymers: Acron Hi; Acrygel (premixed gel); Hircoe; Lucitone 199; Macromer; Optilon 399; Trevalon Hi.

Manipulation
Mixing: The polymer is thoroughly mixed with the liquid monomer at a ratio of 3–3.5 : 1 by volume, such that there is always enough monomer present to wet all the polymer. It is allowed to stand in a closed pot until the 'dough' stage, when it is then packed in a stone or plaster mould or flask.

Changes on mixing.

Stage 1: Sandy; the polymer and monomer form a wet, sand-like mixture.

Stage 2: Tacky: the surface of the polymer dissolves in the monomer and the mixture sticks to the pot.

Stage 3: Doughy: more polymer dissolves and the mixture becomes smooth and dough-like; it breaks when pulled with a slight snap. *The mould is packed at this stage*.

Stage 4: Rubbery: further dissolution, but too stiff to mould.

Note: All the above stages are physical processes and no polymerization occurs until activated.

Packing: Avoid contamination of dough with dirt, plaster or perspiration. Ensure there is an adequate quantity of dough and use enough packing pressure.

Curing: The addition polymerization reaction is exothermic and care must be taken to prevent the internal temperature of the dough from reaching 100.3°C, otherwise gaseous porosity will result.

Curing cycles (water baths)

1. Long low temperature: 72°C for 16 hours followed by a *slow* cool to avoid high residual stresses generated by the thermal expansion differences between the plaster mould and the denture base
2. Short low temperature: 72°C for 2 hours plus short high temperature (100°C for 2 hours) followed by *slow* cool. After careful separation of the denture from the mould, the acrylic flash is removed and the denture is polished using pumice suspended in water. Care must be taken not to overheat the denture at this stage.

Properties

Tensile strength	70 MN/m^2
Elongation to fracture	2% (brittle)
Impact strength	Low
Modulus of elasticity	3.5 GN/m^2

(*Note*: the modulus of elasticity of cobalt–chromium casting alloy is 250 GN/m^2 and that of type IV dental casting gold is 100 GN/m^2)

Water absorption	2% (at saturation)

Excellent aesthetics; translucent; easily pigmented. Easy to process and repair.

12.1.2 Self-cured (cold-cured, autopolymerized) poly(methyl methacrylate)

Applications

1. 'Pour-and-cure' denture bases (using agar-agar moulds).
2. Denture repairs and relines.
3. Removable orthodontic appliances.
4. Special trays (material contains an inert filler such as chalk or slate).
5. Post-dam on upper dentures.
6. Direct filling resins and dies.

Presentation

1. *Powder:* clear or pigmented microspheres of poly(methyl methacrylate) polymer (generally finer than that used in heat-cured acrylic), together with 0.5% by weight of dibenzoyl peroxide as an initiator. Several materials incorporate 4-META as an agent to promote bonding to the metallic components of dental appliances, especially those made of stainless steel, cobalt–chromium, nickel–chromium or silver alloys.

   Orthodontic base polymers generally contain 5–20% poly(ethyl or butyl methacrylate) or some contain either polystyrene or poly(2-ethyl-hexyl-methacrylate). These polymers are added to improve the anti-slump properties of these materials during manipulation.
2. *Liquid:* clear, volatile methyl methacrylate monomer containing 0.01% hydroquinone as stabilizer and up to 2% of a chemical activator such as the tertiary amines dimethyl-*p*-toluidine or dihydroxy-*p*-toluidine. Sulphinic acid derivatives can also be used as activators.

Common brands

Denture bases, reline and repair: Acron Self Cure; Austenal Chairside Reline; Casco; Croform Repair; Degupress; De Trey RR; Kerr's Fast-Cure; Meta-Dent and Meta Fast (with 4-META); META FAST; NHP; Palapress vario; Perm; Pour-N-Cure; QC 20; Rebaron; Redilon DB; Redifast; Reprodent Hard; Simplex Rapid; Stabilo Temp; Vertex Regular; Vertex SC; Vita K + B.

Orthodontic appliances: De Trey Orthoresin; Forestacryl; Orthocryl; Ultracryl; Unicryl; Vertex Orthoplast.

Special tray: Formatray; Ostron 100; Palavit L; Reditray; Vertex Trayplast.

Manipulation In general, the powder and liquid are mixed to a fluid consistency, since doughing and polymerization occur concurrently. No external heat is required to activate the initiator.

Denture bases are moulded by the pour-and-cure technique in which the fluid powder–liquid mixture is allowed to flow into an agar-agar mould containing the artificial teeth.

Orthodontic appliances are formed on a plaster model which has been saturated with water and then coated with a layer of sodium alginate-separating medium, by building up a powder–liquid mix around the wire components. This is done by adding loose powder to monomer painted over the model, and then alternately infiltrating the polymer powder with monomer liquid and vice versa until the appliance has the required thickness. Polymerization is allowed to occur in warm water contained in a pressurized hydroflask, or polyclave. A hydroflask is also used to prevent porosity and promote polymerization of self-curing acrylic used in the repair of denture bases.

Special tray acrylic is moulded over a wax and/or ceramic tape-covered stone model.

Alternatives to acrylic for special trays Polymers which can be softened in hot water into a pliable dough and then formed over the model are available as multicoloured pellets. These become translucent when heated and regain their colours when cooled. (See also 13.8.5.)

Common brands HydroMold; TrayDough.

Direct filling acrylic, which has been superseded by composite resin, used to be inserted into the prepared and lined cavity as soon as it was mixed and held in position under pressure with a mylar matrix strip.

All forms of self-cured acrylic can and should be finished to produce smooth surfaces using a range of abrasives. Overheating must be avoided.

Properties Compared with heat-cured acrylic, self-cured materials are generally more porous; only 80% as strong; of greater initial dimensional accuracy (this can change when they absorb water); higher in residual monomer content (may be up to 5% at first compared with 0.5% for heat-cured acrylic); softer and less abrasion-resistant.

12.1.2.1 Self-cured higher acrylics For relining dentures at the chairside, alternatives to methyl methacrylate are available. These are higher acrylics which undergo addition polymerization reactions that are less exothermic than that of methyl methacrylate. As a result they are less traumatic to the mucosa.

Presentation
1. Powder: poly(ethyl methacrylate) together with dibenzoyl peroxide as *initiator.* Supplied with:
2. Liquid: *n*-butyl methacrylate monomer together

with a tertiary amine as *activator.*

Common brands Colacryl Chairside Reline; Dura-Liner II; Kooliner.

12.1.3 Alternative methods of producing denture bases

12.1.3.1 Microwave curing

Presentation Poly(methyl methacrylate) powder with dibenzoyl peroxide initiator; stabilized methyl methacrylate monomer with reduced amounts of tertiary amine activator.

Common brand Acron MC.

Manipulation The wax pattern is invested in a special, fibre-reinforced, polymeric flask using a modified dental plaster (Advastone). Curing of the acrylic dough takes 3 minutes in a microwave oven.

Properties Apart from the faster processing, the resultant denture base contains less residual monomer than the traditional heat-cured base, and it is free from porosity. The curing process results in only a small amount of shrinkage and a dense polymer with minimal water absorption. These latter two properties result in improved stability and fit.

Applications The production of dentures which have *no* metallic components.

12.1.3.2 Injection moulding

Presentation Cartridges of pink or clear thermoplastic methacrylate co-polymer, or acetal homo- and co-polymer.

Common brands Methacrylate co-polymer: Luxene Astron Vinyl; Flexiplast; Polyan Acetal polymer: Dental D.

Manipulation The cartridges are either heated to make the acrylic co-polymer into a plastic mass, which is injected via a Polypress into the flask. The process uses carbon dioxide at a pressure of 10 atmospheres and takes less than a second. The pressure is maintained until the co-polymer has cooled and become rigid, or they are cold-injected and heat-cured. The acetal polymers are injected via an MG Newpress.

Properties High strength and fracture resistance are attributed to the homogeneity of these materials and their high density. No monomer is used and hence none remains after processing. The co-polymers show minimal water absorption and long-term dimensional stability. The acrylic co-polymers can be relined and repaired when necessary.

Applications The production of complete denture bases or the addition of polymer to metal partial dentures. The acetal polymers are also suitable for use in the construction of permanent and removable posterior bridges and orthodontic appliances. Soft versions of both types of material are available and are suitable for making bite-guards.

12.2 Polycarbonate

Presentation

1. Denture base polymer: vacuum-packed pellets of pigmented polycarbonate (-O-R-O-CO-O-R-O-CO-), which is a thermoplastic resin.
2. Temporary crowns: glass-fibre-reinforced, pre-formed, polycarbonate crowns (for anterior and premolar teeth).

Common brands Denture bases: Bayer's Andoran. Crowns: Directa; Ion polycarbonate crowns.

Manipulation *Denture bases:* The polymer is injection-moulded at about 355°C under a pressure of 410 kN/m^2. Methylene dichloride is employed in the solvent polishing of polycarbonate.

Temporary crowns are trimmed, ground, crimped and shaped without risk of fracture.

Properties

Tensile strength	65 MN/m^2
Elongation to fracture	60% (ductile)
Impact strength	High (nine times that of acrylic)

Water absorption   0.4% (at saturation)
Good aesthetics: translucent
Complex processing technique (dentures)

Applications Temporary crowns and rarely as high-impact-resistant denture bases.

12.3 Vulcanite

Presentation Sheets of pure rubber (the *cis*-isomer of polyisoprene) containing 32% sulphur and suitable metal-oxide pigments.

Manipulation The sheets of rubber are adapted on to a denture model and the flask is closed. Curing of the rubber takes place in an autoclave at 168°C under a steam pressure of 620 kN/m^2. Under these conditions the rubber is cross-linked by the sulphur (vulcanization) and becomes a tough, rigid solid.

Applications Formerly used for denture bases but now completely superseded by acrylic, which has better aesthetics and is easier to process.

Further reading

Denture base materials

Eichold, W.A. and Woelfel, J.B. (1990) Denture base acrylic resins: friend or foe. *Compendium of Continuing Education in Dentistry*, **11**, 720–725

Frangou, M., Huggett, R. and Stafford, G.D. (1990) Evaluation of the properties of a new pour denture base material utilizing a modified technique and initiator system. *Journal of Oral Rehabilitation*, **17**, 67–77

Jagger, R.G. and Huggett, R. (1990) The effect of cross-linking on sorption properties of a denture-base material. *Dental Materials*, **6**, 276–278

Ladizesky, N.H., Chow, T.W. and Ward, I.M. (1990) The effect of highly drawn polyethylene fibres on the mechanical properties of denture base resins. *Clinical Materials*, **6**, 209–225

Rawls, H.R., Starr, J., Kasten, F.H. *et al.* (1990) Radiopaque acrylic resins containing miscible heavy-metal compounds. *Dental Materials*, **6**, 250–255

Rodford, R.A. (1990) Further development and evaluation of high impact strength denture base materials. *Journal of Dentistry*, **18**, 151–157

13 Concomitant denture materials and laboratory polymers

13.1 Artificial teeth

Presentation Sets of teeth in various mould shapes, made of injection-moulded acrylic, or porcelain. The acrylic is usually cross-linked (typically with ethylene glycol dimethacrylate) to make it resistant to the action of monomer (which can cause surface crazing). A recent development uses high molecular weight dimethacrylate resins instead of acrylic.

Common brands The brand names of teeth appear to change frequently. There are many different brands and as many qualities. Isosit SR and Orthosit are the brand names of the dimethacrylate teeth.

Manipulation Acrylic teeth bond readily to poly(methyl methacrylate) denture base material but porcelain teeth do not and require mechanical anchorage by either pins or diatoric (undercut) holes.

Properties Both types have excellent aesthetics.
Abrasion resistance: Porcelain best
Anelastic dampin: Acrylic best (less click on contact)
Thermal expansion: Acrylic is the same as denture base, porcelain much lower, can lead to stresses at interface
Adjustment: Porcelain difficult to grind and polish; acrylic easy
Cost: porcelain about 5 times the cost of acrylic teeth

13.2 Permanent soft (resilient) linings

A permanent dental material is one whose need for replacement is dictated by clinical rather than material changes. Soft linings are more compliant than conventional poly(methyl methacrylate) ones. There are three types:

1. Plasticized acrylic.

2. Siloxane polymers.
3. Polyphosphazene elastomers.

13.2.1 Plasticized acrylic

Presentation Sheets of either poly(ethyl methacrylate) and poly(ethyl acetate), poly(vinyl acetate) and poly(vinyl chloride), or organo-fluorine elastomer. Or as powder–liquid systems in which the powder is either poly(ethyl methacrylate) or poly(methyl methacrylate) and the liquid some type of alkyl methacrylate monomer, e.g. methylethyl- or n-butyl methacrylate, sometimes with the addition of ethyl acetate. The liquid also contains 25–55% of a plasticizer such as di-n butyl phthalate, butyl phthalyl butyl glycolate or 2-ethyl hexyl diphenyl phosphate. The powder also contains a small amount of dibenzoyl peroxide as an initiator for the polymerization of the monomer

Common brands
Flexible sheets: Ardee; Nous; VinaSoft.
Heat cured systems: Coe Super-Soft; Neotone; Palasiv 62; Reprodent Soft; Softic 49; Total; Vertex Soft.

Manipulation The flexible sheet is bonded to the denture base with an acrylic solvent. The powder and liquid of the heat-cured systems are mixed to form a dough and either adapted to a clean denture base, or processed against the acrylic dough. Heat-curing at 72°C for 16 hours or 72°C for 2 hours plus 100°C for 2 hours then follows.

Properties The plasticizer lowers the glass transition temperature (Tg) of the normally hard and brittle acrylic and makes it rubbery and soft. Note that poly(ethyl methacrylate) has a Tg of 65°C whereas poly(methyl methacrylate) has a Tg of 105°C. The latter will require more plasticizer to reduce its Tg and make it soft. The softness decreases as the plasticizer leaches out into the oral fluids. There is a good adhesive bond between this type of lining and denture base acrylic.

13.2.2 Siloxane polymers

Presentation Supplied as a base paste which contains α-Ω-dihydroxy end-blocked poly(dimethyl siloxane) and 15–40% of inert filler. There are two variants, namely heat- and self-cured materials. Each employs a cross-linking agent. The heat-cured materials use acryloxyalkyl silane and dibenzoyl peroxide is used to initiate the cross-linking reaction which is activated by heat. The heat-cured lining of this type is supplied with a silane bonding agent to attach it to the acrylic denture base, (silane is γ-methacryloxypropyltrimethoxysilane). The self-curing materials use such cross-linking agents as triethoxy-silananol, ethyl polysilicate, tetraethoxy-silane and methyl triacetoxysilane. This latter agent is catalysed by water and acetic acid is produced as the byproduct of the cross-linking reaction. The other agents are catalysed by either dibutyl tin dilaurate or stannous octoate and alcohol is the byproduct of the cross-linking reaction. The self-cured materials are supplied with a bonding agent consisting of silicone polymer in a solvent.

Common brands
Heat-cured: Mollopast-b; Permaflex; Polyliner 40.
Self-cured: Cardex-Stabon; Flexibase; Mollosil; Per-Fit; Simpa; Ufi Gel P.

Manipulation Applied to either a clean, adhesive-coated denture base, or processed against adhesive-coated acrylic dough. They cure either by heating or autopolymerization.

Properties These polymers have an inherently low glass transition temperature which makes them soft and resilient at mouth temperature. Their resilience is unaffected by oral fluids. They are not naturally adhesive to acrylic and this can cause problems. Growth of *Candida albicans* is more prevalent under silicone materials than under acrylic soft linings.

Soft lining materials generally have a low modulus of elasticity and absorb a lot of energy when they are stressed by undergoing elastic deformation. By absorbing this energy during mastication, the mucosa is afforded some protection. Care is needed in keeping them clean; hypochlorite cleansers tend to cause bleaching and hardening; oxygenating cleansers may cause surface bubbling to occur in some materials.

13.2.3 *Polyphosphazene polymers*

Presentation Supplied as sheets of a fluoro-alkoxy-substituted polyphosphazene elastomer containing acrylic cross-linkers, poly(methyl-methacrylate) beads, barium sulphate, peroxide initiators and pigment. The acrylic cross-linkers penetrate the elastomer and enable it to be bonded to acrylic denture bases and cured to provide a resilient lining.

Common brand Novus.

Manipulation Strips of the elastomer are placed on a stone model and covered with a sheet of polythene during a trial packing under pressure against the denture. After removal of excess material the model is again put under pressure to allow the elastomer to adapt to its new shape. The denture base is then painted with monomer and curing is achieved by curing the denture and liner under pressure at 74°C for 8 hours. Finishing can be accomplished using sharp, fine carbide burs or sandpaper followed by smoothing with wet pumice.

Properties Absorbs more water than either plasticized acrylic or siloxane polymer, but does not support the growth of fungus. The hydration acts to improve its energy absorption and it maintains its resilience over many years. Forms a permanent bond to acrylic denture bases without the need for special bonding agents.

13.3 Tissue conditioners (functional impression materials)

Presentation
1. *Powder:* acrylic polymers or co-polymers, e.g. poly(ethyl methacrylate). Supplied with:
2. *Liquid:* a mixture of an aromatic ester, e.g. butyl phthalyl butyl glycolate, or di-*n* butyl phthalate plus benzyl salicylate together with ethyl alcohol. The ester behaves as a *plasticizer* and the alcohol is a *penetrant*, which speeds up the process.

Common brands Coe Comfort; Colacrl Soft Reline; Dura Conditioner; GC Soft-Liner; Kerr's

FITT; Lynal; Recon; Soft Oryl; Tempo; Viscogel.

Manipulation   The powder and liquid are mixed in the recommended ratio to produce a fluid paste. This is applied to the mucosal surfaces of a clean denture which is then seated in the mouth. The tissue conditioner forms a physical gel and stiffens up in 5–10 minutes to form an elastic, resilient layer.

Properties   A viscoelastic medium which flows under a steady load but is highly elastic and resilient under sudden loads. The plasticizer and alcohol are leached out by the oral fluids (generally within a week or two) and the conditioner hardens. It is only intended for temporary use. They should be cleaned only with soap and water.

Resilience is defined as the capacity for storing and returning energy in a rapid deformation.

13.4 Peripheral seal

Presentation
1. *Powder:* poly(ethyl methacrylate) together with dibenzoyl peroxide as *initiator.* Supplied with:
2. *Liquid:* n-butyl methacrylate monomer together with a tertiary amine as *activator.*

Common brand   Peripheral Seal; Reprodent.

Manipulation   The powder and liquid are mixed to form a stiff paste and this is applied to the borders of the fitting surface of the denture, which is replaced in the mouth, where a peripheral seal is formed as the material polymerizes.

Properties   The higher methacrylates are less irritant to the mucosa than methyl methacrylate and their polymerization exotherm is much less. Both properties enable this material to be used with safety in the mouth.

Note: The glass transition temperatures of the methacrylate polymers are as follows; methyl 105°C; ethyl 65°C; n-butyl 20°C; 2-ethoxy ethyl 15°C.

13.5 Denture cleansers

The purpose of denture cleansers is to remove organic deposits such as food debris and plaque and the inorganic components of calculus, without harming the denture in any way, or the patient whilst using it or afterwards in the mouth. There are several types:

1. Soap and water.
2. Alkaline peroxides.
3. Hypochlorite solutions.
4. Dilute acids.
5. Abrasive powders and pastes.

13.5.1 Soap and water

Presentation   Block or bars of stearate derivatives.

Common brands   Any common toilet soap free from phenolic (carbolic) compounds.

Manipulation   The soap is applied to the denture using a soft, damp brush and all surfaces and crevices are cleaned. This should ideally occur after every meal.

Indications   Useful for the conscientious denture wearer. Safe on all types of denture base and concomitant materials, including soft linings and tissue conditioners.

Limitations   Will not remove stubborn deposits, stains and hardened calculus.

13.5.2 Alkaline peroxides

Presentation   Tablets or powder containing soluble percarbonates and/or peroxides, which dissolve in warm water to produce an alkaline solution of hydrogen peroxide. They also contain sodium carbonate and citric acid to make then effervesce when they first dissolve and an indicator to colour the water!

Common brands   Boots; Efferdent; Steradent.

Manipulation   Dentures are soaked overnight in a

freshly made up solution. Organic debris creates oxygen bubbles from the solution and these carry the debris to the surface, where the bubbles burst and the debris falls to the bottom of the vessel in which they are soaking. Dentures should be brushed with a soft brush after an overnight soak. They should be rinsed well before being replaced in the mouth.

Indications   Remove most organic deposits. Safe to use on all components made from acrylic, metal or porcelain, but note the limitations below.

Limitations   Limited effect on hardened deposits. Can cause surface and sub-surface bubbling in tissue conditioners.

13.5.3 Hypochlorite solutions

Presentation   Dilute solution of sodium hypochlorite ready for use. Usually contains a corrosion inhibitor.

Common brand   Dentural.

Manipulation   As for the alkaline peroxide cleansers, that is soak, brush, rinse. The hypochlorite makes hard deposits brittle so that they can be more easily brushed away.

Indications   Removes soft and hard deposits, *but:*

Limitations   Can cause bleaching of acrylic. Can corrode cobalt–chromium and stainless steel. Tends to leave an odour of bleach.

13.5.4 Dilute acids

Presentation   Two types:
1. *Type A:* liquid: consisting of a 5–10% solution of either hydrochloric or phosphoric acid, suitably coloured.
2. *Type B:.* Tablet: containing an acid salt such as sodium bisulphite and compounds which dissolve in water to produce a low-pH, oxygen-releasing solution. The tablet also contains a carbonate or bicarbonate which generates carbon

dioxide when first placed in water. This helps the tablet to disintegrate. Also contains detergent, peppermint flavouring and a suitable colouring.

Common brands
Type A: Denclen.
Type B: Deep Clean.

Manipulation
1. *Type A:* This applies locally to hard deposits using a brush or cotton wool. The calculus dissolves and can be brushed away. The denture is well-rinsed before being replaced in the mouth.
2. *Type B:* The tablet is dissolved in warm water and the dentures are soaked overnight. After soaking they should be brushed and thoroughly rinsed. Plaque tends to turn brown in this solution and can be removed by brushing with a normal dentifrice.

Indications   Very effective on stubborn inorganic deposits.

Limitations   Caution is needed when using these acid cleansers over long periods on all base metal alloys, as corrosion is possible.

13.5.5 Abrasive powders and pastes

Presentation   Mixtures of abrasives or abrasives in an inert fluid carrier.

Common brands   Dentu-Creme; Smoker's toothpaste.

Manipulation   Applied as a slurry or paste with a brush to all parts of the denture.

Indications   Probably the least satisfactory type of denture cleanser. Soft deposits can be removed but hard, inorganic deposits remain. They can only be removed at the unacceptable expense of wearing away the denture acrylic.

Limitations   Severe abrasion of polymeric denture base materials and teeth is possible. Paste can be difficult to remove completely after use.

13.6 Denture adhesives (fixatives)

Presentation Powders, ointments, liquid preparations and shaped sheets. The powders are various mixtures of natural gums such as karaya, tragacanth, gelatin and pectin, and synthetic materials such as sodium carboxymethylcellulose and poly(ethylene oxide). When moistened, the gums soften and swell to form a gel which is thickened by cellulose present as an additive. Other additives include antibacterial and wetting agents, inert fillers and flavourings.

The ointments and liquid preparations are water-based formulations containing sodium carboxymethylcellulose and poly(ethylene oxide). The sheets consist of flexible layers of mixtures of natural and synthetic gums, which have been rolled into sheets and cut into the approximate shapes of upper and lower dentures.

Common brands Cushion grip (sheet); Dentu-Hold; Firmdent; Fittydent; Kolynos; Poli-Grip; Seabond; Snug; Super Sterafix; Super Poli-Grip; Super-Wernet's.

Manipulation The powders are sprinkled on to the wet fitting surface of the denture, whereas the ointments and liquid preparations are applied to a dry denture. The powders form viscous gels which, like the ointments and liquids, displace air from between the denture and the mucosa, aiding retention.

Indications Useful as an aid to retain dentures either during their construction phases or where these are physical limitations to any other sort of effective retention. Sometimes used as a vehicle to apply drugs to the oral mucosa.

Limitations Indiscriminate use without clinical supervision is not advisable. The misuse of such retentive aids can lead to premature bone resorption and loss of positive sources of retention.

13.6.1 Magnetic retention

Magnetic forces have been used in dentistry for many years. In the early days the magnets, which were made from Al-Ni-Co or Pt-Co alloys, were bulky and of low magnetic energy. The ferrites, which followed them, were an improvement. The dental magnets of the 1990s contain elements described as rare earths. The most common are those based on samarium with cobalt ($SmCo_5$) or neodymium with iron and boron ($Nd_2Fe_{14}B$).

Presentation Magnets for dental use are generally of the closed-field type and are supplied with either pre-formed ferromagnetic keepers in various shapes or ferromagnetic alloys, which can be cast to fit, for example, a root canal. Some are supplied as closed units, which possess a protective coating to separate the magnet from oral fluids.

Common brands Dyna DE; Innovadent; Jackson SSI; Magnadent; Parkell.

Properties Rare earth magnets create forces about 30 times as strong as those produced by conventional ferromagnetic materials. They are biologically compatible even though they may corrode slightly. Corrosion is preventable by encapsulation at the expense of some force loss. They possess high peak energy product values, which create strong attractive or repulsive forces, and high coercive forces, which provide resistance to demagnetization.

Applications Magnets have been used successfully to retain overdentures (in which the keeper is cemented into a decoronated tooth). They can also be used for the retention of maxillo-facial prostheses. There is growing interest in using them in orthodontics, particularly for moving maxillary molars via the repulsive force of the magnets. Cemented ferromagnetic keepers should be checked for secureness before a patient is subjected to magnetic resonance imaging.

13.7 Fit-checking materials

A wide range of materials has been used for this purpose, including pastes and wax films. Theoretically, any material which can be applied as a thin film and then preferentially displaced into regions of poor fit or from regions of tight fit can be used. At least one manufacturer markets a siloxane-based material for this purpose.

Common brand Fit-Checker.

Presentation A tube of white base paste and a small tube of transparent catalyst paste. A liquid retarder is also provided for use when the room temperature is high. The chemistry of the setting reaction is based on that of the silicone impression materials, although whether this is a condensation or addition-curing material is not clear.

Manipulation Equal lengths of base and catalyst paste are mixed for 20 seconds to produce a homogeneous mix, which is added to the fitting surface of the prosthesis and placed in the patient's mouth. After 3 minutes the prosthesis can be removed and the regularity of silicone layer assessed.

Properties Flow to produce a thin film under load-bearing areas. Sets within 3 minutes. Easy to remove cleanly from the denture after use.

Applications The assessment of the fit of the mucosal surfaces of denture bases or the inner surfaces of crowns.

Note: Whilst this particular material is packed and marketed for this purpose, more commonly the indicator materials described in section 4.5.2 are used to assess the fit of dentures.

13.8 Light-cured laboratory materials

The use of light-activated polymers has been extended to laboratory materials and several presentations are available. All contain diacrylate resin monomers, suitable pigments and agents which, under the influence of light of the appropriate wavelength, produce the free radicals needed to promote addition polymerization.

13.8.1 Composite inlays and onlays

The use of composites as fillings in large cavities in posterior teeth has not proved to be satisfactory. Access is not easy and this makes adaptation of the composite and the creation of good contact points difficult. Because of their bulk there are curing problems, and their polymerization shrinkage when bonded to a tooth can distort it and create

discomfort for the patient. As well as these problems, or possibly because of them, their in-service performance is unpredictable.

To overcome many of these problems systems have been developed in which the composite is formed as an inlay or onlay on a model and is cured outside the mouth. The restoration is then cemented into a cavity, which has been prepared to accept it, using a dual-cure, dimethacrylate resin cement.

All systems seek to do this but the technology varies.

Common brands

1. *Brilliant Dentin (Coltène): Presentation:* An indirect system, which provides four shades of Brilliant Dentin composite containing 0.5 μm, radiopaque, barium glass filler, and a pre-programmed, heat/light-curing unit, the DI-500.

   Manipulation: An impression is taken and a stone model is produced. This is coated with Lab Separator. The inlay is built up sequentially and each increment is exposed for 40–60 seconds to a normal blue-light source. The inlay can be characterized with Paint On Colors before it is placed in the DI-500 tempering unit, where it is exposed to blue light at a temperature of 120°C for a preset time.

   On removal, the fitting surface is roughened using carbide burs before it is cemented into place. Duo-Cement and Duo-Bond are recommended for this, the latter being used to coat both the inlay and the cavity. The cavity may be lined with a glass-ionomer cement, its dentine may be coated with a dentine-bonding agent, and its enamel should be etched. Best results are obtained if cementation is carried out under rubber dam.

2. *E.O.S. (Vivadent): Presentation:* A semidirect system which provides two shades of radiopaque, microfine Heliomolar as its composite, and two silicone pastes – viscous Redphase P for taking an impression and rigid Bluephase P for producing a model.

   Manipulation: An impression is taken using Redphase P in a polyamide quadrant tray. The set impression is coated with Nobond separating medium and a die is created at the chairside using Bluephase P. This is coated with Dentin Protector and composite is added to build up the inlay without distorting the silicone die. After each increment is added it is exposed to a normal blue-light source. On completion, the inlay is given a further exposure from each aspect for 1 minute. It is separated from the die and its fitting surface is light-cured for 1 minute. This surface is then relieved by burs and the outer surface is polished prior to being cemented in place with a dual-cure cement. Dual-Cement and Special Bond II are recommended, the latter being used to coat both the inlay and the cavity.

3. *Kulzer Inlay System (superseded by Charisma Inlay): Presentation:* An indirect system which provides three shades of Estilux Posterior CVS or Charisma composite for occlusal surfaces and a radiopaque base composite BXR or Colorfluid. Tempering can be brought about in a Dentacolour XS laboratory unit or in a Translux Lightbox, which is attached to the output of a Translux blue-light surgery curing unit.

Manipulation: An impression is taken and a stone model is produced. This is coated with Insulating Gel, a separating medium. The radiopaque base composite is applied and cured in either the unit or the light-box for 90–120 seconds. The occlusal composite is added (ideally in a single layer) and similarly exposed. The cured inlay is finished with fine carbide burs, and this is followed by a further period in the unit or light-box for 2–3 minutes. The fitting surface is roughened using a 40 μm diamond finishing bur and the occlusal surface is polished prior to cementation. Kulzer Adhesive and Kulzer Adhesive Bond or Twinlook (dual-cure cement) are the recommended materials for this.

4. *SR-Isosit Inlay/Onlay System (Vivadent): Presentation:* This is an indirect system which uses seven shades of a microfine composite, which also contains a radiopacifying agent. Its hardware consists of an Ivomat, which is a pressure chamber capable of applying 6 atmospheres of steam at a temperature of 120°C

Manipulation: An impression is taken and *two* stone models (the master and the working) are produced. The working model is coated with SR-Separating Fluid and activated SR-Isosit-N Fluid. The inlay is built up on this model and then placed in the Ivomat heat/pressure unit, where it is cured in steam at 120°C and 6 bar for 10 minutes. The fitting surface of the inlay is ground to fit the master model and sand-blasted using alumina powder at low pressure. The borders are roughened and the non-fitting surface is polished prior to cementation. Dual Cure cement and Special Bond II are the materials recommended for this procedure.

Other brands Clearfil CR Inlay; Concept; Conquest; Herculite XRV-Lab; TrueVitality.

Properties of composite inlays

Considerable aesthetic appeal and early evidence suggest they have both good inherent resistance to wear and they appear to cause a minimum of wear on opposing teeth. Wear grooves which develop as the resin-based cement wears away can be cleaned out and repointed with fresh cement.

Applications The production of inlays and onlays for posterior teeth and veneers for anterior teeth.

13.8.2 Denture base material

Common brands De Trey Triad Denture System; Extoral VLC Reline; LiteLine; WIL-O-dont (gel).

Presentation Pigmented and filled resin in sheet, rope form, or as a gel. Once manipulated the resin is activated in a visible light-curing unit which utilizes several collimated light sources.

Manipulation Sheet material is adapted to the model and light-cured for 2 minutes. Acrylic teeth are then attached to this base with light-cured resin and gingival contouring follows, prior to a final light-curing cycle of about 10 minutes. The gel is adapted around orthodontic wires, given a primary cure under an ultraviolet lamp and then exposed to intense blue light to complete the cure.

Advantages For dentures no investing or packing is required (hence no separation from a mould). Teeth are set in resin which is then rapidly cured.

Orthodontic appliances do not require curing in a hydroflask.

Properties Claimed to be both colour stable and dimensionally stable. However, laboratory tests suggest a higher shrinkage than conventional poly(methyl methacrylate) denture base resin and an inferior impact strength.

Applications
1. Full and partial denture bases.
2. Denture relines and repairs.
3. Base plates for wax rims.
4. Orthodontic appliances.
5. Obturators.

13.8.3 Surface treatment agents

Common brands GC Permacure System; Extoral VLC Glaze.

Manipulation Denture bases or acrylic veneers are roughened and cleaned before a thin layer (10 μm) of resin is painted over the surface. Curing takes place in a light unit (such as the Permacure UC-1 or the Prolite II or 3) for 20 minutes.

Advantages Produces a smooth, hard and abrasion-resistant layer. No polishing is required.

Properties Claimed to be twice as hard as poly(methyl methacrylate). This gives improved resistance to wear and a surface lustre. Does not adhere to metal or porcelain.

Applications
1. Surface treatment of denture bases, veneer crowns and orthodontic treatment.
2. Fixing of resin stain of acrylic crowns and veneers.

13.8.4 Light-cured resin veneers

The use of light-activated polymers has been extended to materials processed in the laboratory as alternatives to porcelain for use in aesthetic veneers on either precious or base metal alloy substrates.

Common brands Compatit R; Elcebond; Visio-Gem.

Presentation A range of cervical, dentine, enamel, opaque and intensive shades of diacrylate resins presented in tubes from which they can be extruded by a turning movement of thumb and forefinger. Each resin incorporates visible light-activated compounds, which produce the free radicals needed for polymerization when exposed to visible light with a wavelength in the range of 460 nm. Two light sources, the Visio Alfa and the Visio Beta, are used for the preliminary and final curing of Visio-Gem respectively.

Manipulation The veneer is built up in stages using the various shades on a metal substrate, which must have good mechanical retention aids designed into it. Each stage receives a short exposure to the Visio Alfa light (wavelength 406 nm), which increases its viscosity. Once the veneer is complete it is permanently cured under vacuum for 15 minutes in the Visio Beta unit (wavelength 300–1600 nm). During this intense exposure any internal yellowing which can develop on curing is bleached out. The vacuum eliminates the effects of air-inhibition of the polymerizing resin.

Advantages The production of customized aesthetic effects using a minimum amount of time and material.

Properties Harder and four times as abrasion-resistant as poly(methyl methacrylate). Resists surface staining. Colour-stable once cured. Retention is by mechanical means only.

Applications Aesthetic, durable veneers on precious and base metal alloy substrates.

13.8.5. Miscellaneous light-cured laboratory materials

Light-curing polymers are now available as replacements for traditional materials in the following applications:

Custom trays – Citotray; Convertray; Individo Lux; Paladisc LC; Palatray; T-Lux.

Model blocking out – Blocset.

Modelling resin for casting – Palavit G LC.

They are cured in units such as the Individo Light Box or a Traylight unit.

Further reading

Composite resin inlays/onlays

Asmussen, E. and Peutzfeldt, A. (1990) Mechanical properties of heat treated restorative resins for use in the inlay/onlay technique. *Scandinavian Journal of Dental Research*, **98**, 564–567

De Gee, A.J., Pallav, P., Werner A. and Davidson C.L. (1990) Annealing as a mechanism of increasing the wear resistance of composites. *Dental Materials*, **6**, 266–270

Jackson, R.D. and Ferguson, R.W. (1990) An esthetic, bonded inlay/onlay technique for posterior teeth. *Quintessence International*, **27**, 7–12

Peutzfeldt, A. and Asmussen, E. (1990) A comparison of accuracy in seating and gap formation for three inlay/onlay techniques. *Operative Dentistry*, **15**, 129–135

Scherer, W., Caliskan, F., Kaim, J., Moss, S. and Vijayaraghavan, T. (1990) Comparison of microleakage between direct placement composites and direct composite inlays. *General Dentistry*, **38**, 209–211

Wendt, S.L. and Leinfelder, K.F. (1990) The clinical evaluation of heat-treated composite resin inlays. *Journal of the American Dental Association*, **120**, 177–181

Denture adhesives

Chew, C.L. (1990) Retention of denture adhesives–an *in vitro* study. *Journal of Oral Rehabilitation*, **17**, 425–434

Karlsson, S. and Swartz, B. (1990) Effect of denture adhesive on mandibular denture dislodgement. *Quintessence International*, **21**, 625–627

Light cured laboratory resins

Benington, I.C. and Cunningham, J.L. (1991) Sorption determination of hollow VLC resin obturators. *Journal of Dentistry*, **19**, 124–126

Clancy, J.M.S., Hawkins, L.F., Keller, J.C. and Boyer, D.B. (1991) Bond strength and failure analysis of light-cured denture resins bonded to denture teeth. *Journal of Prosthetic Dentistry*, **65**, 315–324

Passon, C. and Goldfogel, M. (1990) A direct technique for the fabrication of a visible light-curing resin provisional restoration. *Quintessence International*, **21**, 699–703

Magnetics

Bondemark, L. and Kurol, J. (1992) Force–distance relation and properties of repelling SmCo$_5$ magnets in orthodontic clinical use: an experimental model. *Scandinavian Journal of Dental Research*, **100**, 228–231

Gillings, B.R. and Samant, A. (1990) Overdentures with magnetic attachments. *Dental Clinics of North America*, **34**, 683–709

Resilient denture liners

Graham, B.S., Jones, D.W., Thomson, P.J. and Johnson, J.A. (1990) Clinical compliance of two resilient denture liners. *Journal of Oral Rehabilitation*, **17**, 157–163

Tissue conditioners

Murata, H., Shigeto, N. and Hamada, T. (1990) Viscoelastic properties of tissue conditioners – stress relaxation test using Maxwell model analogy. *Journal of Oral Rehabilitation*, **17**, 365–375

14 Dental porcelain

Dental porcelain can be described as a translucent, composite material, in which crystals of ceramics such as alumina (Al_2O_3) and quartz (SiO_2) are suspended in a non-crystalline (amorphous) glassy matrix, which contains pigments to provide colour.

Its natural translucency and its ability to be made to mimic the shades and characteristics of natural teeth make it useful as an aesthetic restorative material. However, its inherent brittleness (which is due to the presence of microcracks, and their ability to grow rapidly from either the internal or external surfaces of stressed restorations) is a major failing, and can lead to catastrophic disintegration. Prevention of such failures is aided by bonding the porcelain to strong and rigid metal substrates (sections 9.1.1.1, 9.1.2.2, 9.1.3.2, 9.2.1, 9.2.2), or by adding crystals of ceramics, which interfere with the movement and growth of microcracks and thus reinforce the porcelain.

General applications

Dental porcelains were used in the 18th and 19th centuries to produce artificial teeth, an application for which they are still used (section 13.1). In the first half of the 20th century, feldspathic porcelains (containing only small amounts of quartz in a matrix made up of feldspars) were developed for jacket and post crowns. Because of their low strength, catastrophic failures were frequent.

The 1960s saw the invention of the aluminous porcelains, in which crystals of alumina (Al_2O_3) were added to reinforce the glassy matrix.

Simultaneously, alloys and porcelains evolved which could be combined to utilize the strength of the metal and the aesthetics of the porcelain. Developments of materials, handling techniques, equipment and cementing procedures during the 1980s now enable porcelain to be used as laminate veneers, inlays, onlays, crowns and even as all-porcelain bridges.

14.1 Feldspathic and aluminous porcelains

14.1.1 Jacket and post-crown applications

Presentation A white powder, consisting of the quenched and ground produce of the pyrochemical reaction between feldspar, quartz and kaolin, mixed together in the approximate ratio $80:15:5$. The powder also contains metal oxide pigments which are stable when heated, and organic pigments which disintegrate on firing. These latter are used to identify dentinal and incisal edge porcelains during the preparation of crowns and facings. Aluminous porcelains, especially those used for the cores of jacket crowns, contain up to 40% of alumina (Al_2O_3) as a reinforcing agent (crack stopper). However, alumina is opaque and this limits its usefulness when translucency is required.

Common brands Carrara; Ceramco; Doric; Flexo-Cram; Vita.

Manipulation The powder is made into a paste with an aqueous medium and is applied to the platinum foil crown matrix closely adapted to a die, or to a cast metal substrate. The particles are brought into intimate contact by spatulation, vibration, brushing and absorption of water with a tissue. After drying at the mouth of the furnace, firing takes place at a temperature recommended by the manufacturer. During firing the porcelain particles fuse together and air from the spaces between them diffuses to the surface. Sometimes vacuum firing is recommended to encourage this. Slow cooling follows and, after characterization with appropriate features and pigments, a glaze is produced by a longer firing.

Properties

Tensile strength
(not reinforced with alumina)   70 MN/m^2
Tensile strength
(reinforced with alumina)   50 MN/m^2
Firing shrinkage   30–40%

Porcelain is chemically inert. Its glossy surface deters the retention of plaque and it has excellent aesthetics.

Applications
1. Jacket crowns.
2. Post-crowns.
3. Artificial teeth for dentures.

14.1.2 Laminate veneers, inlays and onlays

Presentation White powder with a composition similar to that shown above, usually containing calcined alumina. In at least one brand this has been precoated with glassy matrix material to improve wetting.

Common brands Cerinate Porcelain Laminate; Chameleon; Cosmotech Porcelain; Ducera-Lay; Indirect Porcelain System; IPS Corum; Microbond Porcelain Facings; Mirage; Vitadur N.

Manipulation Whilst these materials can be built up on platinum foil-covered stone dies, they are usually produced on refractory ceramic dies, which can be introduced into the furnace to support the porcelain during firing (section 6.4). The fitting surfaces of veneers are roughened to promote bonding using either alumina powder under low pressure or a buffered gel based on hydrofluoric acid, such as ammonium bifluoride. Similar surface treatments can be given to the fitting surfaces of porcelain inlays and onlays prior to their cementation with resin-based cements (sections 2.1.12 and 2.1.13).

Properties Similar to those shown above. More abrasion resistant, aesthetic, colour stable and retentive than polymeric veneers and inlays.

Applications
1. Laminate veneers.
2. Inlays.
3. Onlays.

14.1.3 Porcelain for veneers bonded to metal (porcelain-fused-to-metal, metal–ceramic restorations)

Presentation   A white powder with a similar basic composition to that shown above. However, additional alkali oxides are present and these encourage the growth of leucite (K_2O, Al_2O_3, $4SiO_2$).

This raises the coefficient of thermal expansion of the porcelain such that it almost matches that of the metal substrate. This prevents the creation of high interfacial stresses, which could lead to delamination during service.

Common brands   Biopaque; Ceramco II; Cosmo-tech; Creation; Doric M-K; Duceram; Duceratin (for titanium frameworks); Matchmaker; Surprise; Ultra-Pake; Vintage Opal; Vita-Omega; Vita Spray-On; Vita-VMK 68N.

Manipulation   The metal substrate is covered with a layer of opaque porcelain and fired prior to the build-up of layers of pigmented and translucent porcelains to produce the required contour and appearance.

Properties   When porcelain is fused to a metal substrate, bonding occurs via several mechanisms:
1. The physical action of surface wetting (van der Waals force).
2. Mechanical retention in surface irregularities on cooling.
3. Chemical attraction from the dissolution and diffusion into porcelain of oxides of such metals as tin, indium and iron (in gold–platinum metal–ceramic alloys), aluminium and chromium (in nickel–chromium and cobalt–chromium metal–ceramic alloys).
4. Compression bonding as a result of a slight mismatch in the thermal expansion coefficients of the metal and the porcelain, such that the porcelain contracts and lightly compresses the metal substructure.

Applications
1. Jacket crowns.
2. Maryland bridges.
3. Multiunit bridges.

14.1.4 Porcelain bonded to metal foils

14.1.4.1 The twin-foil technique (as developed by McLean and Sced)   The purpose of this technique is the reinforcement of porcelain jacket crowns by bonding the porcelain to platinum foil, thus preventing the opening of microcracks and their propagation through the porcelain leading to catastrophic failure.

Presentation   Platinum foil, 0.05 mm thick for posterior teeth or 0.025 mm thick for anterior teeth, together with a porcelain formulated for bonding to metals, e.g. Vita-VMK.

Manipulation   An inner platinum foil, 0.025 mm thick, is adapted to the die with a tinner's joint and a 1 mm skirt around the margin. A second foil is then adapted over the first (0.025 mm thick for anterior teeth) and this is removed and degreased before receiving a 0.5 μm layer of tin by electroplating. After washing, it is fired in vacuum to $1000°C$, at which temperature the tin forms a metallurgical bond with the platinum. Air is admitted to the furnace and the tin coating oxidizes. After cooling, a porcelain crown is built up on the oxidized, tin-plated platinum foil. This is fired in the usual way. The inner platinum foil is removed and the crown is ready for cementing in position.

Properties   Bond strength 55 MN/m^2 (cf. bond strength of VMK 68 to Degudent: 28 MN/m^2).

The improved resistance to failure by the catastrophic propagation of cracks is a great advantage. It is much cheaper than a cast noble metal unit, despite the cost of the platinum.

Application   Reinforced porcelain jacket crowns for anterior and posterior teeth.

14.1.4.2 Aesthetic foils

Presentation   Foils, 50–60 μm thick, of noble

metals whose porcelain contact surface area is good. Strength and economy are achieved by combining gold with platinum and palladium in a complex sandwich.

Common brands   Ceplatec; Renaissance.

Manipulation   Foils are adapted to dies using one of several techniques and feldspathic porcelains are built up on the surface.

Properties   The foil acts as a reinforcing layer to prevent the propagation of cracks. The gold in contact with the porcelain provides enriched aesthetics.

Applications   Porcelain jacket crowns.

14.2   Reinforced porcelains

Several techniques have evolved to increase the strength of porcelain without resorting to a metal substrate.

14.2.1 High-ceramic cores

Presentation   These utilize alumina (Al_2O_3) or leucite as reinforcing agents within core materials.

Common brands   Optec HSP; Vita Hi-Ceram; Vita In-Ceram.

Manipulation   Special techniques are needed to produce the optimum results. For example, Vita In-Ceram requires the production of an alumina substructure. This is formed on a special plaster die and is sintered at 1120°C for 2 hours to fuse partially the alumina particles to one another. The porous substructure which results is coated with glass powder. During a further firing at 1100°C for 4 hours this infiltrates the pores and eliminates them as a source of weakness. Filling the pores also improves the translucency of the core on to which the required anatomical crown can then be built.

Properties   The strength of these reinforced cores is superior to all other ceramics.

Applications
1. Cores for anterior or posterior porcelain crowns.
2. All-porcelain anterior bridges of up to 3 units.

14.2.2 Ion exchange reinforcement

Presentation   A fluid containing low-fusing potassium salts.

Common brands   Ceramicoat.

Manipulation   The fluid is painted on to the surface of the porcelain, dried at 150°C for 20 minutes and then at 450°C for 30 minutes. The salt is rinsed off with water when the ceramic has cooled.

Properties   At high temperature potassium ions from the applied salt are exchanged for sodium ions from within the glassy matrix of the porcelain. On cooling, the potassium ions (which are bigger than the sodium ions) remain within the surface, producing low-temperature ionic crowding. This creates a compressive stress that has to be overcome before a surface crack can propagate and cause failure. Reinforcement is the result. No deleterious effects on aesthetics or fit.

Applications   The reinforcement of any type of ceramic restoration.

14.3   Ceramic crowns

4.3.1 Castable ceramic crowns

Glass–ceramics, which can be cast using the lost wax process rather like dental alloys, can be used as an alternative to cast metal and metal–ceramic restorations. They are semicrystalline glasses in which the crystals help to deflect and divert microscopic cracks thus giving the crown the strength needed for both laboratory finishing and *in vivo* service.

Common brands   Ceramapearl; Dicor.
1. *Ceramapearl – Presentation:* Ingots of castable apatite ceramic in a disposable crucible.

Manipulation: The glass is melted at 1520°C and cast centrifugally into a mould made from a special phosphate-bonded investment. It is heated at 750°C for 10 minutes to anneal the glass and allow the release of residual stress. After removal and cleaning, it is re-embedded in investment and heated to 855°C for an hour. The resulting restoration is a glass–ceramic apatite with high strength but no inherent colour. Pigments are fired on to the restoration by heating it in air at 820°C.

2. *Dicor – Presentation:* Small ingots of glass made from SiO_2-K_2O-MgO-MgF_2 and containing minor amounts of Al_2O_3, ZrO_2 and fluorescing agents. These ingots are supplied in a disposable crucible.

Manipulation: A wax pattern of a full crown is invested in phosphate-bonded investment which, when set, is heated to 900°C for 30 minutes. The glass ingot is melted by heating to 1370°C in an electric furnace for 6 minutes. Centrifugal casting in a motor-driven machine then follows. After bench-cooling to room temperature, the amorphous and transparent glass casting is removed and inspected for defects. It is then reinvested and placed in a ceraming oven where it is heated through a specific time/temperature cycle. During this 'ceraming' process the fluoride acts as a nucleating agent and crystals of tetrasilic fluormica develop throughout the casting. These crystals make the casting translucent and give it enough strength to be ground to produce any necessary contacts and to make occlusal adjustments. Colouring can be added by using a thin layer of porcelain glaze and shades. These are fired as often as necessary in an ordinary porcelain furnace.

Properties: Non-toxic and non-irritant. Inert in the oral environment. In Dicor the interlocking of the mica crystals gives the material a transverse strength which is twice that of porcelain. Hardness and elastic modulus similar to enamel. Radiographically similar to enamel. Can be fired repeatedly without degradation during the colouring and glazing stages, although some shrinkage occurs on casting.

Applications
1. Laminate veneers.
2. Inlays and onlays.

3. Crowns for anterior or posterior teeth.

14.3.2 Hot transfer-moulded glass–ceramics

These use leucite-reinforced ceramics, which are formed by the lost-wax principle by a high-temperature pressing procedure.

Presentation Cylinders of leucite-reinforced ceramic and a press ceramic furnace, EP 500.

Common brand IPS Empress.

Manipulation Crowns are modelled in wax on a light-curing die material, which reproduces the shade of the remaining part of the tooth. The pattern is invested in a special fluid investment. The leucite-reinforced ceramic is plasticized at 1100°C in the EP 500 furnace and then injected at a pressure of 3.5 bar into the investment. Pressure is maintained and the ceramic is forced into the fine detail of the investment. On cooling, the ceramic core can be ground to produce a core which represents the dentine and to this the appropriate incisal material is added. The restoration can be characterized, stained and glazed.

Properties No shrinkage after the pressing procedure. No ceraming process is required. The pressed shape remains stable during multiple firings. The material has a high flexural strength. Radiopacity similar to enamel.

Applications
1. Aesthetic crowns for anterior or posterior teeth.
2. Inlays and onlays.
3. Laminate veneers.

14.4 Computer-aided design/manufacture (CAD/CAM) ceramic inlays (also known as computer integrated manufacturing systems)

Presentation Pre-fired blocks of feldspathic porcelain or glass–ceramic.

Common brands Bioram-M; Cerec Dicor MGC;

Macor-M; Mark II; Vita-Cerec.

Manipulation An optical impression of an inlay cavity is produced with an intraoral television camera using the principles of triangulation. Its internal dimensions are computed, and the pre-formed block is machined at the chairside, silane-coated and cemented in place using a dual-cure, resin-based composite luting cement.

Properties The machining tends to crack the ceramic, and such cracks are a source of weakness. The marginal gap is considerable.

Applications Inlays for posterior teeth.

14.5 Porcelain repair materials

Presentation Pigmented powders and unfilled dimethacrylate resin together with a silane bonding agent.

Common brands Aristoprime; C & B-Metabond; Cerinate Prime; Fusion; Mirage ABC; Monobond S; Prisma Ceraprime; Porcelite Primer; Scotchprime; Silibond; Silistor; Ultra-Bond.

Manipulation The damaged porcelain is roughened with a diamond bur and, where possible, undercuts are created. The surface may be treated with hydrofluoric acid to aid retention. This is available either as a 4% solution or as a gel containing 8–10% hydrofluoric acid, e.g. Ceram-etch; PorceLock; Stripit; Ultradent Porcelain Etch. If one of these is used in the mouth, *extreme* care is necessary and the use of rubber dam is absolutely essential along with copious washing and aspiration if damage to any other tissues is to be avoided. Alternatively, the surface may be cleaned with an oil-free prophylaxis paste, washed and dried before the silane bonding agent is applied. One material uses a hydrolysed bond enhancer (Silicer) to stabilize microcracks in the ceramic surface prior to the application of the silane bonding agent. With some materials the resin and powder are mixed and the repair is built up; with others a light-curing composite is used. Once set, it is contoured and smoothed.

Properties Whilst silane promotes bonding between the porcelain and the dimethacrylate, the bond is enhanced by mechanical retention or chemical etching.

Applications The repair and restoration of chipped porcelain veneers on multiple unit bridges.

Further reading

General reviews

Futterknecht, N. and Jinoian, V. (1992) A renaissance of ceramic prosthetics? *Quintessence of Dental Technology*, **15**, 65–78
Piddock, V. and Qualtrough, A.J.E. (1990) Dental ceramics – an update. *Journal of Dentistry*, **18**, 227–235
Qualtrough, A.J.E., Wilson, N.H.F. and Smith, G.A. (1990) The porcelain inlay: a historical review. *Operative Dentistry*, **15**, 61–70

CAD/CAM systems

Mormann, W.H., Brandestini, M., Lutz, F., Barbakow, F. and Gotsch, T. (1990) CAD-CAM ceramic inlays and onlays: a case report after 3 years in place. *Journal of the American Dental Association*, **120**, 517–552
Taira, M., Wakasa, K., Yamaki, M. and Matsui, A. (1990) Dental cutting behaviour of mica-based and apatite-based machinable glass ceramics. *Journal of Oral Rehabilitation*, **17**, 461–472

Castable ceramics

Rappold, A.P. and Ireland, E.J. (1990) Fabrication of a crown to fit an existing partial denture using castable glass. *Operative Dentistry*, **15**, 224–227

Porcelain fused to metal

Adachi, M., Mackert, J.R., Parry, E.E. and Fairhurst, C.W. (1990) Oxide adherence and porcelain bonding to titanium and Ti-6Al-4V alloy. *Journal of Dental Research*, **69**, 1230–1235
McLean, J.W., Kedge, M.I. and Hubbard, J.R. (1976) The bonded alumina crown. 2. Construction using the twin foil technique. *Australian Dental Journal*, **21**, 262–268
McLean, J.W. and Sced, I.R. (1976) The bonded alumina crown. 1. The bonding of platinum to aluminous dental porcelain using tin oxide coatings. *Australian Dental Journal*, **21**, 119–127
Murakami, I., Vaidyanathan, J., Vaidyanathan, T. K. and Schulman, A. (1990) Interactive effects of etching and pre-oxidation on porcelain adherence to non-precious alloys: a guided planar shear test study. *Dental Materials*, **6**, 217–222

Reinforced ceramics

Dietschi, D., Maeder, M., Meyer, J-M. and Holz, J. (1990) *In vitro* resistance to fracture of porcelain inlays bonded to tooth. *Quintessence International*, **21**, 823–831

Hondrum, S.O. and O'Brien, W.J. (1988) The strength of alumina and magnesia core crowns. *International Journal of Prosthodontics*, **1**, 67–72

Kon, M., Ishikawa, K. and Kuwayama, N. (1990) Effects of zirconia addition on fracture toughness and bending strength of dental porcelains. *Dental Material Journal*, **9**, 181–192

Reghi, R.R., Daher, T. and Caputo, A. (1990) Relative flexural strength of dental restorative ceramics. *Dental Materials*, **6**, 181–184

Taira, M., Namura, Y., Wakasa, K., Yamaki, M. and Matsui, A. (1990) Studies on fracture toughness of dental ceramics. *Journal of Oral Rehabilitation*, **17**, 551–563

Repairs to porcelain

Bertolotti, R.L. and Paganetti, C. (1990) Adhesion monomers utilised for fixed partial denture (porcelain/metal) repair. *Quintessence International*, **21**, 579–582

Gregory, W.A. and Moss, S.M. (1990) Effects of heterogeneous layers of composite and time on composite repair of porcelain. *Operative Dentistry*, **15**, 18–22

Sidhu, S.K. and Capp, N.J. (1990) A comparative study of porcelain repair materials. *Clinical Materials*, **5**, 29–42

15 Preventive materials

15.1 Cleansing aids

15.1.1 Toothbrushes

Presentation Toothbrushes are presented in many different shapes and sizes. However, despite the morphological variations, most consist of flexible nylon monofilaments, assembled in groups and mounted in a matrix of holes drilled in moulded polystyrene or polypropylene handles. The tips of the groups of filaments (tufts) are trimmed by the manufacturer to suit the current style. A few models utilize natural bristles or combinations of nylon filaments and natural bristles. Both bristles and filaments absorb water over a period of time; this makes them soft and ductile and they eventually distort and lose their efficacy as plaque removers.

Common brands Addis-Wisdom Quest; Aquafresh Flex; Braun (electrical); Butler G.U.M.; Colgate Double Action; Gibbs Mentadent P; J & J Reach; Kent OK, Nova, Visa, KB425; Kitty Dentafit (electrical); McLeans; Oral-B 10, 20, 30, 32, 35, 40, Indicator, Plus, Right Angle; Proxabrush; Sensodyne Search; Tau-Marin.

15.1.2 Dentifrices

Presentation Powders, pastes or gels consisting of mixtures of mild abrasives, such as calcium phosphates and pyrophosphates (hydrated and anhydrous), calcium carbonate, alumina and aluminium hydroxide and aluminium trihydrate, silica gels and even acrylic microspheres. The silica gels consist of abrasive xerogels and aerogels whose role is as a thickener. These forms of silica have a refractive index that can be matched to that of water, thus making them transparent.

The pastes are made up with water and contain a humectant to stop them drying out, such as glycerol (which is sweet and warming) or sorbitol (which is sweet and cooling). They may contain additives such as alginates, antibiotics, astringent salts, chloroform, enzymes, fats and oils. Most contain sweeteners such as sodium saccharinate, flavourings such as peppermint, many are coloured, and most contain surfactants to make them foam and to disperse the flavouring. They also contain foam controllers, such as sodium dodecyl sulphate and sodium dodecyl benzene sulphonate.

Many contain therapeutic agents including up to 0.8% of fluoride, either as sodium monofluorophosphate, sodium fluoride or stannous fluoride. One brand (Corsodyl) contains 1% of chlorhexidine gluconate for the treatment and prevention of gingivitis, and several contain agents such as formalin, potassium chloride, potassium nitrate, sodium citrate, strontium acetate hemihydrate or strontium chloride hexahydrate, all of which appear to desensitize exposed dentine and cementum by mechanisms such as the partial occlusion of dentinal tubules or the reduction of intradental nerve activity following normally painful stimuli.

One brand (Zendium) contains the enzymes amylglucosidase and glucose oxidase which produce hydrogen peroxide. This reacts with another constituent (potassium thiocyanate) to form hypothiocyanate — a bacterial inhibitor. Others employ an antibacterial agent called triclosan (2,4-dichloro phenoxy)phenol, which is active against a wide spectrum of Gram-positive bacteria, Gram-negative bacteria, fungi and yeasts, all of which are present in dental plaque. This appears to be most effective when it is held on a co-polymer such as methoxylene and maleic acid. Zinc citrate has also been used as an antimicrobial agent to inhibit the growth of plaque and to reduce the deposition of calcium, which produces calculus.

An additive found in many dentifrices of the 1990s is 5% pyrophosphate (P_2O_7) whose role is to control the deposition of calculus and make any that is laid down weaker and easier to remove.

Common brands Aim; Aquafresh; Clinomyn; Colgate; Close-up; Corsodyl; Crest; Denivit; Emoform; Eucryl; Euthymol; Elgydium; Gibbs SR; Kingfisher; Macleans; Mentadent P; Pearl Drops; Phillips; Protect; Sensitive; Sensodyne; Signa; Topol; Wisdom Dental Gel; Zendium, etc.

Manipulation About 1 cm of paste or gel should be applied to the dentition via a moist brush (which is well designed and not too worn) using one of the currently approved techniques.

Properties The major benefit from using a dentifrice comes from the actual use of the brush to displace plaque. The abrasive is only of secondary importance. The therapeutic agents are beneficial and the desensitizing additives can be useful in certain cases. The flavourings and astringent salts are psychologically important.

15.1.3 Prophylaxis paste

Presentation Mild abrasives such as pumice, zirconium silicate and kieselguhr in non-reactive, water-soluble bases often based on glycerine. Some contain fluoride and flavouring oils, and others are free from these constituents.

Common brands Nupro; Orapol; Oraproph; Zircate and many others, often just called prophy-paste.

Manipulation Applied to the surfaces to be cleaned with either a rotating brush or rubber cup.

Properties When used occasionally by the dentist no excessive wear occurs. If the enamel is to be acid-etched, a paste which is free from both fluoride and oil should be used. In the absence of information about the fluoride and oil content, a

slurry of pumice powder in water is a safer alternative.

Applications
1. Removal of food and tobacco stains from enamel.
2. Primary polishing of restorations.
3. The removal of acquired pellicle prior to the acid-etching of enamel.

15.1.4 Disclosing agents

Presentation Tablets or solutions of harmless organic dyes such as erythrosin or basic fuchsin.

Common brands Dis-Plaque; Plaque Check; Toothguard and many others, often without a specific brand name.

Manipulation The tablets are dissolved in the mouth and the solutions are added to water. The resulting solution in each case is swirled around the teeth and gums and then spat out.

Properties The red, blue or green vegetable dyes diffuse preferentially into the dental plaque.

Applications The disclosing of plaque on teeth and dentures, thus indicating the efficiency of cleansing procedures.

15.2 Fluoride agents

15.2.1 Fluoride mouthwashes

Presentation Flavoured solutions containing either 0.05% or 0.2% sodium fluoride along with anti-plaque agents of varying degrees of efficacy.

Common brands A.C.T.; Eludril; En-De-Kay Fluorinse; Fluoriguard; Mouthguard; Point Two; Reach Anti-Plaque.

Uses and properties The undiluted rinse is swirled around the mouth either daily (0.05%) or weekly (0.2%) and then spat out. The topical fluoride converts some of the surface hydroxy-apatite into acid-resistant fluorapatite.

15.2.2 Fluoride tablets

Presentation   Flavoured tablets containing either 0.5 mg or 1.0 mg of sodium fluoride.

Common brands   Fluotabs; Luride 0.5/1.0.

Uses and properties   The tablets are dissolved in the mouth and the solution swallowed each day in those regions where the normal water supply contains less than 0.3 p.p.m. of fluoride. The fluoride becomes systemic and enters the developing enamel or unerupted teeth.

15.2.3 Fluoride drops

Presentation   Flavoured and sweetened solutions of sodium fluoride.

Common brands   Fluodrops; Luride drops.

Uses and properties   The drops are added to the food or drink of the very young in those areas where the water contains less than 0.3 p.p.m. of fluoride. The fluoride becomes systemic and enters the developing enamel of unerupted teeth, forming acid-resistant fluorapatite.

15.2.4 Fluoride gels

Presentation   Gels of various viscosities, created by adding hydroxyalkyl cellulose thickening agents to flavoured solutions of acidulated phosphate fluoride (APF) or 0.4% stannous fluoride.

Common brands   Alpha-Gel; En-De-Kay; Hifluor-Gel; Luride; Omnigel; Protect; Rafluor New Age.

Manipulation   The gel is applied to the entire dentition at one time by using two flexible trays which contain close-fitting paper of foam absorbent liners soaked in the gel. Exposure time is 4–5 minutes, followed by a period when rinsing should be discouraged. The stannous fluoride gel is for use at home, and should be applied with a dry toothbrush over the surfaces of the teeth. Rinsing should be avoided for 30 minutes.

Properties   Some gels are very fluid and others are more jelly-like. All show pseudoplastic behaviour, that is, they appear less viscous when stressed. This means that they flow readily around the tissues when removed. The presence of phosphate ions in a solution of pH 4 prevents the dissolution of phosphate from the enamel and controls the amount of fluoride entering the enamel to form calcium fluorapatite, which itself makes the superficial enamel more resistant to caries.

15.2.5 Fluoride varnishes

Presentation   Tubes or cartridges of an alcoholic solution of natural resins containing 50 ng of sodium fluoride per millilitre.

Common brand   Duraphat.

Manipulation   The varnish can be applied via a cotton swab or from the cartridge via a blunt needle to caries-exposed sites and the hypersensitive necks of teeth. Two to three applications per year are recommended.

Properties   Covers the teeth for several hours and provides a topical caries prophylaxis along with a temporary treatment of the sensitive necks of teeth.

15.3 Fissure sealants

Used for the protection of the deep and narrow fissures of posterior teeth from accumulating food debris and plaque by filling them with a durable material, which is retained without the need for any mechanical preparation of the tooth.

In the past both methyl-2-cyanoacrylate with a silicate filler and polyurethane-containing sodium monofluorophosphate have been tried as fissure sealants, but they have proved to lack the necessary durability. Occasionally these materials are used as a means of retaining topical fluoride in position for longer than possible with gels and mouthwashes.

Acrylic resin containing amine fluoride has also been used for this purpose.

Fissure sealants in current use are described below:

15.3.1 Bowen's resin

Presentation

1. *Type A:* Chemically activated: two low-viscosity components, one of which is a dimethacrylate resin which may contain a small amount of inert filler or up to 1% titanium dioxide (this is an opacifier to assist detection *in vivo*). One component contains dibenzoyl peroxide as an initiator, and the other an activator such as a tertiary amine or sulphinic acid. Several contain small amounts of fluoride.
2. *Type B:* Blue-light-activated: a single low-viscosity resin which contains similar light-sensitive initiators to those used in other light-curing systems, such as composite filling materials and cements.

Common brands

1. *Type A:* Chemically activated: Concise White Sealant System; Delton; Oralin (pink or clear); UltraSeal XT.
2. *Type B:* Blue-light-activated: Alpha-seal; Delton Light-Curing; Estiseal; Den-Mat Resto-Seal; Helioseal; Luma-Seal; Oralin Light-Curing; Prisma-shield; Sealite; Ultra-Seal; Visar Seal; Visio-Seal.

Manipulation Either type has to be bonded to enamel by the mechanical retention brought about by cleaning, acid-etching (40–50% phosphoric acid, 1–2 minutes), washing and drying. The resin must be applied to the etched surface before the patient licks it and thus contaminates it with salivary proteins. The components of type A are mixed together prior to being applied to the etched surface. Type B systems require a source of visible blue light which is applied for an adequate period (usually 30–60 seconds).

Properties These materials show good retention when correctly handled and are about 60% effective over 2 years.

15.3.2 Glass-ionomer cements

Presentation, brands etc. See section 2.1.10.

Manipulation Teeth are not acid-etched but are cleaned with prophylaxis paste and washed, and the debris is removed with citric acid or poly(acrylic acid) solution. The thickly mixed cement is applied and allowed to set without disturbance. Any excess is then removed with sharp instruments and the surface varnished to prevent premature dissolution.

Properties Somewhat soluble, but fluoride ions leach out from the cement to form fluorapatite in the adjacent enamel.

15.4 Mouthguards (mouth protectors, dental guards, gum shields)

The purpose of these devices is to give protection to those indulging in contact sports, who are likely to be subjected to blows to the mouth, and in particular to the mandible. They are made from resilient polymers and the best ones are constructed to fit a model produced from impressions of the particular patient's dentition. In service they are intended to absorb energy by elastic deformation, thus protecting anterior teeth from a direct blow, and posterior teeth and restorations from cusp damage when the mandible is subjected to high forces. During impact the energy absorbed by the mouthguard also reduces that transmitted to the mandibular condyle, capsule and disc and helps prevent damage to these organs. They may also prevent serious intercranial damage such as subdural haemorrhage, as when the condyle is forced upwards and backwards into the base of the skull by a direct blow to the chin.

These are three presentations of these materials:

15.4.1 Standard sizes from stock

These are rather like soft impression trays. Whilst they have arch form, they have a flat occlusal fitting surface and no retentive possibilities. They are bulky and difficult to manage and also impair speech.

15.4.2 Mouth-formed guards

Presentation   Two formats are available:

(a) Vinyl blanks, which are softened by immersing them in very hot water for 30 seconds and then shaping them in the mouth by the occlusal forces and the fingers as they cool and their plasticity disappears.

(b) Self-polymerizing powder/liquid systems in which the mixed constituents are poured into a moulding shell and seated in the mouth for 5 minutes to allow the soft polymer to form.

Common brands   Type a: Redigard; Type b: Dental Guards.

Properties   Whilst they have reasonable adaptation to the teeth and gums, they are rather bulky.

15.4.3 Custom-made mouthguards

These are the most satisfactory type of guard available at present.

Materials   They are made either from plasticized vinyl polymers or polymers with inherently low glass transition temperatures. These latter include a co-polymer of poly(vinyl acetate) and polyethylene, and acetal co-polymers. Polyurethane and rubber latex have also been used. Transparent sheet (1–3 mm thick) made of thermoplastic polymers such as poly(butadiene-styrene), which is rigid at mouth temperatures, is available for the production of splints.

Common brands   *Soft polymers:* Bioplast; Copyplast; Drufosoft; Flexital; Luxene; Protexoflex; Vanguard.

   Rigid polymers: Biocryl; Drufolon E; Erkoflex; Imprelon.

Manipulation   Sheets (3 mm thick) of the thermoplastic co-polymer are placed over a model of the dentition produced from an impression of the patient's maxillary arch. The model should be coated with cold-mould seal to prevent water uptake during the moulding process, during which they are softened by radiant heat and vacuum formed on a machine such as the Biostar or Vacuformat-U. On cooling, their peripheries are trimmed to extend within 2 mm of the mucolabial folds, so that the mouthguard covers all the teeth and vertical portions of the hard palate. The acetal co-polymers are injection moulded via a Piston Jet manual injection machine.

Properties   Close adaptation makes them comfortable to wear: speech is not seriously impaired. Said to last a season – but clearly this depends on the sport, the wearer and the length of the season.

Applications

1. Mouthguards for contact sports; night guards for bruxists.
2. Thermoplastic sheet of this type can also be used when duplicates of study models are required.
3. Diagnostic occlusal appliances (used to hold occlusal registration material).
4. Splints.

15.5 Tooth-bleaching materials

Uses   Employed to improve the appearance of teeth which have become stained either due to ageing, or to chemical changes associated with the incorporation of therapeutic agents such as tetracycline or fluoride.

Presentation

1. Bleaches for use in the dental surgery containing 30–35% hydrogen peroxide, sometimes mixed with silica to form a gel, or with salts containing calcium, phosphate and fluoride ions to encourage remineralization. Others consist of a low concentration of hydrochloric acid and a fine abrasive contained within a water-miscible paste.
2. Bleaches for use by the patient containing either 10% carbamine peroxide or between 1.5 and 6% hydrogen peroxide. They are slightly acidic.

Common brands

For surgery use: *Acid + pumice flour* – Prema.
For home use: *Carbamine Peroxide-based* – DentaLite; Dentlbright; Just White; Nu-Smile; Opalescence; Proxigel; Rembrandt Lighten; White & Brite.

Hydrogen peroxide-based – Natural White; Peroxyl.

Manipulation Surgery bleaching utilizes heat, light, acid gels or abrasives, or combinations of these. The heat and light come from a powerful bleaching light, and the acid gels are applied for 30 minutes. All systems require several applications.

Home bleaching requires the removal of plaque followed by the wearing of a soft tray containing gel for up to four hours. The tray is similar to a custom-made mouthguard.

Properties The agents do not have any adverse effects on gold, amalgam, porcelain or microfilled composites, although some hybrid composites can be roughened by the gels. The bleaches should not be allowed to come into contact with dentine.

Tooth hypersensitivity is possible after treatment, as are soft tissue lesions

Ageing stains respond best to these agents. If no major improvement occurs after several applications, veneering of the teeth should be considered.

Further reading

Bleaching

Darnell, D.H. and Moore, W.C. (1990) Vital tooth bleaching: the 'white and brite' technique. *Compendium of Continuing Education in Dentistry*, **11**, 86–94
Haywood, V.B., Leech, T., Heymanh, H.O., Crumpler, D. and Bruggers, K. (1990) Nightguard vital bleaching: effects on enamel surface texture and diffusion. *Quintessence International*, **21**, 801–804

Dentifrices

Mann, P.H., Harper, D.S. and Regnier, S. (1990) Reduction of calculus accumulation in domestic ferrets with two dentifrices containing pyrophosphate. *Journal of Dental Research*, **69**, 496–501

Fissure sealants

Conry, J.P., Pintado, M.R. and Douglas, W.H. (1990) Measurement of fissure sealant surface area by computer. *Quintessence International*, **21**, 27–33
Rock, W.P., Weatherill, S. and Anderson, R.J. (1990) Retention of three fissure sealants resins. The effects of etching agent and curing method. Results over 3 years. *British Dental Journal*, **168**, 323–325

Fluorides

Arends, J., Ruben, J. and Dijkman, A.G. (1990) The effect of fluoride release from a fluoride-containing composite resin on secondary caries: an *in vitro* study. *Quintessence International*, **21**, 671–674
Nystrom, G.P., Holtan, J.R. and Douglas, W.H. (1990) Effects of fluoride pretreatment on bond strengths of a resin bonding agent. *Quintessence International*, **21**, 495–499

Mouthguards

McCarthy, M.F. (1990) Sports and mouth protection. *General Dentistry*, **38**, 343–346

16 Periodontal and surgical packs

16.1 Dressings/packs

These are used to keep wounds clean and separated from food, saliva and bacteria whilst healing proceeds. If they have analgesic, antihaemorrhagic and bacteriostatic effects and they adhere to the soft tissues as well, this is an advantage. All sorts of setting pastes and viscoelastic gels have been used and even cyanoacrylate adhesives have been tried. Several commercial products are available:

16.1.1 Two-paste systems

16.1.1.1 Eugenol-containing dressings

Common brand Wards Wondrpak.

Presentation Two pastes, one containing eugenol and an inert filler, such as talc, the other containing zinc oxide in a mixture of natural resins and oils and isopropyl alcohol.

Manipulation The pastes are mixed to produce a homogeneous consistency in 30 seconds. This is applied to the tissues and allowed to set.

Properties Sets slowly to produce a semirigid dressing. Eugenol, despite its bactericidal properties, can sometimes cause an allergic reaction.

16.1.1.2 Eugenol-free dressings

Common brands Coe-Pack; Periodontal Pack; Zone.

Presentation Two pastes, one containing zinc oxide in a non-reactive oily base. The other contains a long-chain fatty acid in an inert base such as talc. Two per cent of chlorhexidine is incorporated as an antibacterial agent.

Manipulation The pastes are mixed to produce a homogeneous consistency in 30 seconds and then applied to the tissues.

Properties Sets with an exothermic reaction to form a rigid dressing in 3-7 minutes. The absence of eugenol prevents the allergic reactions sometimes seen.

16.1.2 Single-paste systems

These consist of a mixture of inorganic compounds held in a volatile solvent.

Common brand Peripac.

Presentation A single, viscous paste containing calcium phosphate and zinc oxide and the volatile solvent tetraethyl glycol dimethyl ether.

Manipulation The paste is applied to the tissues and the solvent evaporates, leaving the inorganic constituents held in close contact with themselves and the soft tissues.

Properties The loss of solvent is a fairly slow process, especially from thick sections, but as it evaporates the dressing shrinks.

16.1.3 Powder–liquid systems

The components of these materials are similar to those found in tissue conditioners and they behave in a similar manner.

Common brand Peripac Improved.

Presentation A powder which is composed of poly(ethyl methacrylate) and zinc oxide and a liquid which contains *n*-butyl phthalate (as a plasticizer), alcohol (to assist the plasticizer in its penetration of the polymer particles), and poly(acrylic acid) to give the material some degree of adhesion to the soft tissues. By weight, 2% of the powder is chlorhexidine acetate, which is included to give the dressing antibacterial properties.

Manipulation Measured quantities of the powder and liquid are mixed together in 15 seconds to produce a pliant gel which can be syringed around the tissues.

Properties Sets in about 10 minutes to a rubber-like consistency. May be left *in situ* for 7–10 days. The chlorhexidine acetate is said to reduce postoperative pain and inhibit plaque formation in the area. The plasticizer may produce superficial damage to composites and (to a lesser extent) to glass-ionomer fillings, but any damage can be eliminated by prophylaxis after the dressing has been removed.

16.1.4 Light-curing systems

Presentation Light-proof tube of pink, translucent, urethane methacrylate monomers, which can be light-cured.

Common Brand Barricaid.

Manipulation Can be dispensed either directly on to dried tissues or from a mixing pad. The material can be moulded; however, rubber gloves require lubricating with water or saliva to prevent adhesion of the uncured resin. Buccal and lingual sites are exposed in turn to blue light for 40 seconds each. Contouring is possible once it has cured, using finishing burs in a low-speed handpiece.

Properties Strongest of the periodontal dressings and least prone to absorb water and become unhygienic. Translucent and flexible.

Applications Periodontal wound dressings.

16.1.5 Mucous membrane dressings

Presentation Either a powder consisting of pectin, gelatin and carboxymethylcellulose, or the same constituents in a liquid paraffin–polyethylene base as an ointment. Sometimes contain medicaments.

Common brands
Powder: Orahesive.
Ointment: Orabase.

Applications The dressing is applied to the mucosa to protect lesions from the oral environment. Moisture causes the natural and synthetic gums to swell and form a viscous, protective gel which is gradually eroded by saliva.

16.2 Suture materials

Both absorbable (A) and non-absorbable (NA) types are available:

Presentation Monofilament; multifilament.

Composition
Natural: Catgut (A)
                            Cotton (NA)
                            Silk (NA)

Synthetic: *Polymers*
                            Nylon (A)
                            Polyacrylonitrile (NA)
                            Polydioxanone (A)
                            Polyester (NA)
                            Poly(glycolic acid) (A)
                            Polypropylene (NA)
                            Metals
                            Stainless steel (NA)
                            Tantalum (NA)

Handling As there is no measurable difference in the rate of wound healing whether the suture is tied loosely or tightly, loose suturing, which lessens the pain and reduces cutting of the soft tissues, is recommended.

16.3 Implantable Biomaterials

Ceramics, metals and composite materials are all in use as various forms of implant; some are preformed and others are used in bulk.

16.3.1 Metals and alloys

Inert metals such as commercially pure titanium or Ti-6Al-4V alloys (section 11.4) are used for the basis of wrought, endosseous implants, and cobalt–chromium alloys (section 11.3) can be cast to produce periosteal implants.

16.3.1.1 Endosseus implants

Presentation Many different formats, including blades and multi-component units, the lower sections may be made from titanium or titanium–aluminium–vanadium alloy, which may or may not be either plasma-sprayed or coated with hydroxyapatite. These are screwed into a hole which has been tapped carefully into the bone of either the maxilla or mandible.

Common brands A.M.S.; Astra; Bonefit; Calcitek; Core-Vent; Discimplant; IMZ; Innovative Dental Products; Intoss; ITI-Straumann; Nobelpharma (Brånemark System); Osseodent; Steri-Oss.

Manipulation and properties The bone is prepared so as to cause minimal trauma and the titanium fixtures are inserted and left *in situ* without load for 3–6 months to allow healing and initial osseointegration. Abutments, which pass through the gum, are then added and the appropriate prostheses are fitted. Titanium and the molecular layer of oxide which forms on its surface are biocompatible and bone grows into intimate contact with it thus providing retention.

Applications The retention of fixed or removable prostheses in upper and lower jaws.

16.3.2 Ceramics

Presentation and applications Various forms are available including:
1. Natural hydroxyapatite granules (from coral) for

augmentation of the alveolar ridge.

2. Synthetic, densely sintered hydroxyapatite in blocks and shaped components for correcting alveolar ridge discrepancies in the anterior maxilla, and preformed plastic surgery components such as orbital floor implants.

3. Porous, rounded, non-resorbable hydroxyapatite granules (0.8 to 1.8 mm diameter) for alveolar ridge augmentation and filling periodontal defects. These granules may be mixed with particles of cancellous bone.

4. Resorbable tricalcium phosphate granules in various sizes, for encouraging growth where active bone metabolism is present.

5. Single crystal alumina rods for use as transdental implants via the roots of teeth.

6. Polycrystalline alumina rods and shaped root implants and blocks for transdental fixation, orthograde and retrograde fillings.

7. Polycrystalline alumina which is laser-machined to produce a screw thread for use as artificial roots.

8. A mixture of hydroxyapatite and calcium sulphate hemihydrate for filling periodontal defects and extraction sockets.

Common brands

1. Interpore 2000.
2. Alveorestor; Osprovit.
3. Alveograf; Calcitite; Ostrix-NR; Periograf.
4. Osticon; Ostilit; Ostrix-B, -C, -PM.
5. Saphilox.
6. Alveoform; Biolox; Diakor 8-18.
7. C.B.S.
8. Hapset.

Manipulation Granules are deposited from a syringe into sub-periosteal pockets. Preformed shapes and blocks are trimmed prior to sterilization. They are anchored with sutures until collagen starts to invaginate their structure. The plaster and hydroxyapatite are mixed with water to form a setting paste.

Properties These materials are inert and well-tolerated by the hard and soft tissues. Loss of retention after insertion can result in loss of the implant. If bony ingrowth can be achieved, considerable stabilization is possible. In the mixture

the set plaster is slowly absorbed leaving the hydroxyapatite behind.

16.3.3 Ceramic–polymer composites

Presentation Sheets, block or preformed shapes of porous poly(tetra-fluoro-ethylene)(PTFE)-vitreous carbon fibre composites.

Common brands Proplast.

Manipulation The preformed shapes and blocks are trimmed prior to sterilization. They are anchored with sutures until collagen starts to invaginate their structure.

Properties Inert, non-resorbable and well-tolerated by the hard and soft tissues. Bony ingrowth occurs into the porous structures, providing considerable stabilization.

Applications

1. Augmentation of the alveolar ridge.
2 Recontouring of temporomandibular joint condyles.

16.4 Augmentation material

Presentation Expanded PTFE or nylon web coated with hydrophobic co-polymer of poly(vinyl chloride)/polyacrylonitrile (PVC/PAN), or hydrophobic silicone rubber.

Common brands Gore-Tex (GTAM) – PTFE-based; Versapor – nylon-based.

Manipulation and properties The inert biomaterial is applied so as to provide cover for three-dimensional spaces and to preserve any blood clots. Can be left in place for up to 9 months for bone to form via guided tissue regeneration. The open microstructure of the material allows for tissue integration.

Applications

1. Ridge augmentation.

2. Repair of osseous defects.
3. Closure of extraction sockets.

16.5 Soft maxillofacial polymers

Over the centuries many materials have been tried as replacements for tissues of the face which have been lost either by disease or traumatic mutilation. During the 20th century, polymers such as polyurethane and poly(vinyl chloride) have been tried. However, in the 1990s the polymers of choice for replacing soft tissues are the silicones.

Presentation Silicone polymers for maxillofacial and other prosthetic applications are presented either as single component (high temperature vulcanizing – HTV) or two-component (room temperature vulcanizing – RTV) systems.

Common brands Cosmesil SM4; Dow Corning MDX 4/4516; Silskin II.

Manipulation The RTV silicones are mixed, packed into foil-covered gypsum moulds, and cured at room temperature for 24 hours. The HTV materials are cured either by immersing the packed mould in boiling water for an hour, or by a two-stage procedure. This latter is required for the form of HTV silicone which has to be shredded, rolled and packed before being put through a first set cure of 120°C for 4 hours. This is followed by a final cure at 204°C for 3 hours. Microwave curing can also be used. Bonding to tissue is achieved using silane-based adhesive agents, which eventually hydrolyse to produce acetic acid.

Properties Soft-tissue prostheses have to withstand the onslaughts of a wide range of environmental conditions without becoming unhygienic, hardening, tearing, becoming detached or changing colour. The silicones achieve many of these requirements, with the HTV materials possessing the best mechanical properties. Both types age. The RTV materials are the easiest to mould.

Applications Soft tissue prostheses of all types.

Further reading

Augmentation materials

Cortellini, P., Pini Prato G., Baldi, C. and Clauser, C. (1990) Guided tissue regeneration with different materials. *International Journal of Periodontics and Restorative Dentistry*, **10**, 137–151

Dental implants

English, C. (1990) An overview of implant hardware. *Journal of American Dental Association*, **121**, 360–368

Ichikawa, Y., Akagawa, Y., Hirosama, U. and Tsuru, H. (1992) Tissue compatibility and stability of a new zirconia ceramic *in vivo*. *Journal of Prosthetic Dentistry*, **68**, 322–326

Kent, J.N., Block, M.S., Finger, I.M., Guerra, L., Larsen, H. and MISIEK, D.J. (1990) Biointegrated hydroxyapatite-coated dental implants: 5 year clinical observations. *Journal of the American Dental Association*, **121**, 138–144

Lemmons, J.E. (1990) Dental implant biomaterials. *Journal of the American Dental Association*, **121**, 716–719

Szmulker-Moncler, S. and Subruille, J.H. (1990) Is osseointegration a requirement for success in implant dentistry? *Clinical Materials*, **5**, 201–208

Traisel, M., Le Maguer, D., Hildebrand, H.F. and Iost, A. (1990) Corrosion of surgical implants. *Clinical Materials*, **5**, 309–318

Periodontal dressings

Von Fraunhofer, J.A. and Argyropoulos, D.C. (1990) Properties of periodontal dressings. *Dental Materials*, **6**, 51–55

Soft maxillofacial polymers

Conroy, B. (1985) Maxillofacial prosthetics and technology. In (eds N.L. and Williams J.Ll.) *Maxillofacial Injuries*, vol 2, Edinburgh, Churchill Livingstone, pp. 869–998

Polyzois, G.L., Frangou, M.J. and Andreopoulos, A.G. (1991) The effects of bonding agents on the bond strengths of facial silicone elastomers to a visible-light activated resin. *International Journal of Prosthodontics*, **4**, 440–444

Wolfaardt, J.F., Cleaton-Jones, P., Lownie, J. and Ackermann, G. (1992) Biocompatibility testing of a silicone maxillofacial prosthetic elastomer: soft tissue study in primates. *Journal of Prosthetic Dentistry*, **68**, 331–338

17 Orthodontic materials

The construction of orthodontic appliances, both fixed and removable, requires the use of a wide range of dental materials. Most of these have been described in detail in the following sections:

Wires

Gold alloys 11.2
Nickel–titanium alloys 11.4
Stainless steel 11.1.2
Titanium alloys 11.4

Elastics 11.5.1

Acrylic base resins 12.1.2

Cements
Acrylic 2.1.12
Dimethacrylate 2.1.13
Glass-ionomer 2.1.10
Zinc phosphate 2.1.6
Zinc polycarboxylate 2.1.9

Special orthodontic materials include:-

17.1 Orthodontic brackets

These are bonded to teeth using one of the following mechanisms:

1. An adhesive cement, such as polycarboxylate or glass-ionomer, both of which form chemical bonds to enamel and many metals, including stainless steel.
2. Mechanical bonding in which fluid resins flow into the asperities of acid-etched enamel and the structured surfaces of the bracket.
3. A combination of the two mechanisms, with mechanical bonding to the enamel and chemical bonding to the bracket. This latter requires the fitting surface of the bracket to be primed in some way to encourage resin-based cements to form adhesive bonds.

Presentation

1. *18/8 Stainless steel:* (with molybdenum to increase their resistance to corrosion): these may be cast or wrought. The cast brackets incorporate a built-in structure of slots, whereas the wrought brackets generally have a retentive mesh welded to their fitting surface.
2. *Polymeric brackets:* Polycarbonate was tried but found to suffer from excessive wear. They have been superseded by reinforced polymers, which contain ceramic filler particles to improve their wear resistance, or they have built-in metal slots to accommodate the wire.
3. *Ceramic brackets:* Manufactured either by machining single crystals of alumina (these are

transparent) or by injection moulding and firing of alumina or zirconia (these are polycrystalline and thus translucent).

Common brands
Stainless Steel: Microlok; Ormesh.
Polymeric: Igloo; Mirage.
Ceramic: Single crystal – E.F.G.; Gem; Starfire
Polycrystalline – Allure III; Fascination; Harmony; Illusion; Intrigue; Quasar; Transcend.

Manipulation and properties

1. Stainless steel brackets may be retained with either an adhesive cement such as polycarboxylate or glass-ionomer, or any of the resin-based cements. They need only be clean and dry prior to use, and re-cycling is possible after any residual cement has been completely removed.
2. Polymeric brackets require their fitting surface to be primed with a monomer before they are bonded. Resin-based cements are the only ones suitable for this.
3. Ceramic brackets are continuously evolving. When first presented it was recommended that their smooth fitting surface should be coated with a silane primer to enhance the bond between the bracket and resin-based cement. However, on debonding of these brackets the weakest link was frequently found to be the enamel itself, and this has led to the creation during manufacture of a grooved fitting surface, and advice against the use of silane primers. Ceramic brackets are the least visible.

17.2 Orthodontic bonding adhesives

17.2.1 Adhesive cements

For details of polycarboxylate and glass-ionomer cements, several of the latter of which are designated 'type V – for orthodontic use', see sections 2.1.9 and 2.1.10. The advantage of these cements is the continuous loss of fluoride from their structure whilst they are in place. The fluoride is beneficial to those parts of the teeth which are likely to be denied access to saliva during the course of the orthodontic treatment.

17.2.2 Orthodontic bonding resins

Presentation   These are based either on acrylic or diacrylate resins. The acrylic is usually methyl methacrylate monomer and poly(methyl methacrylate) polymer powder. The diacrylate is generally the bis-GMA resin used by many of the manufacturers of composites. The resins are supplied both in filled and unfilled forms. The unfilled resins are intended for use on structural surfaces (such as acid-etched enamel) in the hope that their slightly inferior strength will be advantageous when the bracket is debonded. Some systems contain as little as 1% of filler.

The resins are made to set as the result of activating a chemical initiator which starts the polymerization. Activation may be either by another chemical or visible, blue light.

The so-called no-mix systems require the initiator (which is contained in a fluid carrier) to be painted on to both the etched enamel and the bracket. A layer of resin (which contains the chemical activator) is then sandwiched between the two coated surfaces. This system relies on the use of a very thin layer of resin to produce bonding. If the resin layer is too thick it will only polymerize at the edges, the middle will remain soggy and thus weak.

Common brands
Chemically-cured: Challenge; Classic-2; Concise System; Direct On II; Excel; Extend-A-Bond; Maxibond; Maximal; Phase II.
Light-cured: FluorEver; Insta-Bond VL; Light-Bond; Transbond; Translux; UltraLight.
No-Mix Systems: Advantage; Direct; Mono-Lok; Quasar; Rely-a-bond; Superbond; Ultratrim.

Manipulation and Properties   Filled and unfilled resins are applied according to preference and either chemically cured or light-cured according to type. Light-curing systems require 30 seconds under metal brackets and 10 seconds under ceramic brackets. The lightly filled resins are easier to debond and are recommended for use under non-yielding ceramic brackets. Remnants which remain attached to the tooth are said to be easier to remove than filled resins.

Applications   The temporary attachment of me-tallic, polymeric and ceramic orthodontic brackets to acid-etched enamel.

Further reading

Orthodontic brackets

Smith, N.R. and Reynolds, I.R. (1991) A comparison of three bracket bases. An *in vitro* study. *British Journal of Orthodontics*, **18**, 15–20

Orthodontic bonding

Chan, D.C.N., Swift, E.J. and Bishara, S.E. (1990) *In vitro* evaluation of a fluoride-releasing orthodontic resin. *Journal of Dental Research*, **69**, 1576–1579
Howell, S. and Weekes, W.T. (1990) An electron microscopic evaluation of the enamel surface subsequent to various debonding procedures. *Australian Dental Journal*, **35**, 245–252
Sadowsky, P.L., Retief, D.H., Cox P.R. *et al.* (1990) Effect of etchant concentration on the retention of orthodontic brackets: an *in vivo* study. *American Journal of Orthodontics and Dentofacial Orthopedics*, **98**, 417–421

18   Radiographic materials

Presentation   Pieces of X-ray film of various sizes packed between sheets of black paper to prevent exposure to light. A thin lead sheet is positioned on the side away from the X-ray tube to prevent fogging of the film due to the scattering of X-rays. The film consists of a base covered with a radiation-sensitive emulsion.

The base: A thin sheet of clear plastic, such as polyester, coated with an adhesive and emulsion on both sides. The emulsion is coated with a protective layer to prevent abrasion during handling and storage.

The emulsion: Constituents are:
1. *Silver halides:* usually silver bromide with a little silver iodide to increase the sensitivity. The overall sensitivity of the film depends on the grain size of the halide particles. The exposure latitude depends on the ranges of grain sizes present.
2. *Gelatine:* added to aid manufacture. It is transparent and swells when wet. It can thus absorb developing and fixing chemicals. It also holds the reacted and non-reacted species apart.

3. *Additives:* added to improve performance. These include sensitizing dyes, bacteriostatic agents, humectants and wetting agents.

Manipulation   The sequence of necessary operations is: exposure, develop, rinse, fix, wash, dry.

1. *Exposure:* On exposure to electromagnetic radiation such as X-rays or visible light, the silver halides dissociate and become active silver and halogen radicals. The halogen radicals are absorbed by the emulsion and the silver forms a latent image. The amount of silver produced is proportional to the exposure received.

2. *Developing:* When immersed in a reducing agent, the silver halides become silver. Those grains which contain active silver radicals are reduced preferentially. A negative image is thus produced. Developers are generally hydroquinone in alkaline solution. Additives include sodium sulphate to retard oxidation of the developer, and potassium bromide to restrain any unexposed silver bromide from being reduced and thus rinsing/fogging the film. The developing time is affected by the temperature of the solution and its age. The colder and older the developer, the slower the development will be.

3. *Fixing:* After a brief rinse, the unexposed silver bromide is removed by fixing the film in a solution of sodium or ammonium thiosulphate.

4. *Washing/drying:* The film must then be thoroughly washed to remove all developing and fixing chemicals. It must then be dried before it can be handled.

Faults

1. Film too dark suggests:
   (a) Fogging prior to development: keep unexposed films well away from the X-ray machine.
   (b) Overexposure to X-rays.
   (c) Overdevelopment: too long in fresh developer at too high a temperature.
2. Film too light suggests:
   (a) Underexposure to X-rays.
   (b) Underdevelopment.

Warning: Chronic exposure to X-rays can cause burns, carcinomas, necrosis of the tissues, leukaemias and sterility. *Thus:*

1. Avoid unnecessary exposures.
2. Allow patients to hold their films *in situ* during the production of a radiograph.
3. Protect the patient with a lead-lined apron.
4. Protect yourself by keeping your distance from the source of X-rays, ideally behind a radiation shield.

Further reading

Kaplan, I. and Dickens, R.L. (1990) Lightening of dark radiographs with a superproportional reducing agent. *Quintessence International*, **21**, 737–740

Appendix

Major suppliers of dental materials in the UK

Advanced Healthcare Ltd (Shofu), Tonbridge, Kent, 0892-870500

Amalreco Ltd, Leigh, Lancs, 0942-671491

Ash, Claudius, Sons & Co Ltd, Potters Bar, Herts, 0707-46433

Associated Dental Products Ltd, Swindon, Wilts, 0793-770256

Attenborough, C. & L.E. Ltd, Nottingham, 0602-473562

Austenal Ltd, Harrow, Middx, 081-863-9044

Bayer plc, Newbury, Berks, 0635-39000 ext. 3536

Billericay Dental, Witham, Essex, 0376-500222

Bracon Ltd, Hurst Green, Sussex, 058-086631

British Gypsum Ltd, Newark, Notts, 0474-4251

Cardozo, F.E., Ltd, Pinner, Middx, 081-866-3081

Ceramco Europe, Weybridge, Surrey, 0932-856240

Chaperlin & Jacobs Ltd, Sutton, Surrey, 081-641-6996

Clark Dental, Wickford, Essex, 0268-733146

Colgate Palmolive Ltd, Guildford, Surrey, 0483-302222

Coltène (UK) Ltd, Burgess Hill, West Sussex, 0444-235486

Cooper Health Products Ltd, Aylesbury, Bucks. 0296-32601

Core-Vent UK, London W13, 081-998-0879

Cottrell & Co Ltd, London W1, 071-580-5500

Courtin Ltd, Capel, Surrey, 0306-711278

CR Dental, Southall, Middx, 081-571-3954

Crest Professional Services Ltd, Egham, Surrey, 0784-474003

C.T.S. Dental Supplies, Reigate, Surrey, 0737-240948

Davis, J. & S. Ltd, Potters Bar, Herts, 0707-46330

Degussa Ltd, Wilmslow, Cheshire, 061-486 6211

Den-Mat, London E3, 0800-581303

Dental Express (Supplies) Ltd, Orpington, Kent, 0689-891451

Den-Tal-Ez Products (GB) Ltd, Hemel Hempstead, Herts, 0442-69301

Dent-O-Care, London NW10, 081-459-7550

Dentomax Ltd, Bradford, W. Yorks, 0274-308044

Dentoral Ltd, Smethwick, W. Midlands, 021-558-6041

Deproco UK Ltd, London EC4, 071-583-1570

De Trey Division, Dentsply Ltd, Weybridge, Surrey, 0932-853422

Downs Surgical Ltd, London W1, 071-486-3611

E.B. Dental Supplies Ltd, Doncaster, S. Yorks, 0302-368264

Ellman International (UK) Ltd, Northampton, 0604-37870

Engelhard Sales Ltd, Chessington, Surrey, 081-397-5292

Evacryl Dental Supply Co, London NW2, 0800-282545

Evident Dental Co Ltd, London NW1, 071-722-0072

Fairfax Dental Ltd, London SW15, 081-780-1360

Firmadent European, Sudbury, Suffolk, 0787-79947

Forestadent Ltd, Milton Keynes, Bucks, 0908-568922

Gibbs Oral Hygiene Service, London W1, 071-409-6272

Girrbach Dental Products Ltd, Wellingborough, Northants, 0933-400770

Glover Dental Supplies Ltd, Shrewsbury, Shropshire, 0743-241291

Harald Nordin (UK) Ltd, Worthing, W. Sussex, 0903-204427

Hawley Russell & Baker Ltd, Potters Bar, Herts, 0707-55579

Healthco (UK) Ltd, Enfield, Middx, 081-366-4412

Hoben Davis Ltd, Newcastle-under-Lyme, Staffs, 0782-622285

Howmedica International Ltd, London N16, 081-800-7444

Hudson Ltd, Sheffield, S. Yorks, 0742-683175

Intoss UK Ltd, London N7, 071-700-1440

Ivoclar-Vivadent Ltd, Leicester, Leics, 0533-364055

Jeydent, London E17, 081-527-1218

Johnson & Johnson Ltd, Maidenhead, Berks, 0628-822222

Johnson Matthey Dental Products, Birmingham, W. Midlands, 021-200-2120

Kent Dental/Hejco, Gillingham, Kent, 0634-364411

Kerr (UK) Ltd, Peterborough, Cambs, 0733-260998

Mason Dental Ltd, Bradford, W. Yorks, 0274-306683

Meadway, Old Woking, Surrey, 0483-77328

Metrodent Ltd, Huddersfield, W. Yorks, 0484-544444

Minerva (Cardiff) Ltd, Cardiff, S. Glam, 0222-490504

3M Health Care Ltd, Loughborough, Leics, 0509-613121

Nobelpharma UK Ltd, Harrow, Middx, 081-863-9044

Optident Ltd, Bingley, W. Yorks, 0274-551154

Oradent Ltd, Windsor, Berks, 0753-857714

Oral B Laboratories, Aylesbury, Bucks, 0245-442492

Oral Plastics Ltd, Lytham St Annes, Lancs, 0253-723181

Ortho-Care UK Ltd, Bradford, W. Yorks, 0274-392017

Orthologic Ltd, Potters Bar, Herts, 0707-46434

Orthomax Dental Ltd, Bradford, W. Yorks, 0274-733842

Panadent Ltd, London SE1, 071-403-1808

Precision Orthodontics Ltd, Esher, Surrey, 0372-65273

Precious Metal Techniques Ltd, London W1, 071-486-3881

Prestige Dental Products Ltd, Bradford, W. Yorks, 0274-721567

ProCare Dental, Bradford, W. Yorks, 0274-734321

P.S.P. Dental Manufacturing Co Ltd, Belvedere, Kent, 081-311-7337

Quality Endodontic Distributors Ltd, Peterborough, Cambs, 0733-371565

Quayle Dental Manufacturing Co Ltd, Worthing, W. Sussex, 0903-204427

Schein Rexodent, Southall, Middx, 081-574-0335

Schottlander Ltd, Letchworth, Herts, 0462-480848

Scientific Metal Co Ltd, London EC1, 071-831-1956

Selbe Trading Ltd, London NW4, 081-203-3859

Shofu Dental Products Ltd, Tonbridge, Kent, 0892-870800

Skillbond plc, High Wycombe, Bucks, 0494-448474

SmithKline Beecham Dental Services, Brentford, Middx, 081-975-4344

Spendental Manufacturing & Design, Ryde, Isle of Wight, 0983-66159

Stafford-Miller Ltd, Welwyn Garden City, Herts, 0707-331001

Staident International, Staines, Middx, 0784-455454

Talladium UK, Gerrards Cross, Bucks, 0753-889569

Terec Dental Group, Sunbury-on-Thames, Middx, 0932-786296

Ventura Oral Systems, Halifax, W. Yorks. 0422-381003

Warner-Lambert Health Care, London WC1, 071-242-4444

White, S.S. Manufacturing Ltd, Gloucester, Glos, 0452-307171

W.H.W. Plastics, Hull, Humberside, 0482-29154

Wright Health Group Ltd, Dundee, Tayside, 0382-833866

Part Four

Alphabetical list of commercial dental materials

Trade name	Type of material
A	
A.C.T.	fluoride mouthwash
A.M.S.	endosseous implant
A.R.T. Bond	multipurpose adhesive
ABC	self-cured resin cement
ABC Dual	dual-cured resin cement
Absolute	impression elastomer
Acculoid	impression agar
Achatit-Biochromatic	silicate cement
Acron Hi	high-impact denture acrylic
Acron MC	microwave curing acrylic
Acron Rapid, Standard	heat-cure denture acrylics
Acron Self-Cure	self-cure acrylic
Acupren	impression elastomer
Acusil	impression elastomer
Acrygel	high-impact denture acrylic
Adapt-Rite	die-spacing resin
Adaptic	early conventional self-cured composite
Adaptic LCM	light-cured microfine composite
Adaptic Universal	self-cured hybrid composite
Adaptic II	light-cured hybrid composite
Addis-Wisdom Quest	toothbrush
Adherence M5	dual-cured resin cement
Advantage	orthodontic bonding resin
Advastone	die stone
Agarloid	impression agar
AH26	endodontic sealant
Airblock	oxygen inhibition gel
Alabond E	silver-free Pd bonding alloy
Alastics	orthodontic elastomer
Alba M	low-gold casting alloy
Albabond	palladium–silver bonding alloy
Albacast	low-gold casting alloy
Alborium	low-gold casting alloy
Albus 190	high-gold bonding alloy
Alginoplast	impression alginate
Align	nickel–titanium wire
Alike	temporary crown and bridge (C & B) resin
Alka-Liner	calcium hydroxide cement
All-Bond	dentine/metal bonding agent
All-Bond 2	multipurpose adhesive
Alpha Titanium	titanium–aluminium alloy
Alpha-Bond	glass-ionomer cement
Alpha-Cast MP	phosphate-bonded investment
Alpha-Core	composite core paste
Alpha-Gel	fluoride gel
Alpha-Seal	light-curing fissure sealant
Alphadur 700	die stone
Alure III	ceramic bracket
Alveoform	ceramic implant
Alveograf	ceramic implant
Alveorestor	ceramic implant
Amalcap Plus	amalgam alloy

Amalgambond	adhesive resin cement
Amalgam Liner	light-cured cavity liner
Ames Copper	black copper cement
ANA 2000	amalgam alloy
Anchorex	preformed endodontic post
Anchorextra	preformed endodontic post
Andoran	polycarbonate denture base
Anoxon	soldering flux
Apollo 3, 4	high-gold casting alloys
Aqua Ionofil	glass-ionomer filling cement
Aqua Ionobond	glass-ionomer lining cement
Aqua Meron	glass-ionomer luting cement
Aqua-Fil	glass-ionomer filling cement
AquaBoxyl	zinc polycarboxylate cement
Aquacem	glass-ionomer cement
Aquafresh	dentifrice
Aquafresh Flex	toothbrush
Aqualox	zinc polycarboxylate cement
Arcalloy	cobalt–chromium bonding alloy
Ardee	plasticized acrylic liner
Argen	gold solder
Argenco 4, 27, 75	medium-gold casting alloys
Argenco 5, 10, 17	high-gold casting alloys
Argenco 9, 18, 23, 26B	low-gold casting alloys
Argenco 34	silver-free, Pd bonding alloy
Argicast B	medium-gold casting alloy
Argicraft 1	palladium–silver bonding alloy
Argident Yellow, 2A, 3	high-gold bonding alloys
Argilite 2, 4	medium-gold bonding alloys
Argilite 50	palladium–silver bonding alloy
Argipal	silver-free Pd bonding alloy
Argistar 45	medium-gold bonding alloy
Argivest	phosphate-bonded investment
Aristaloy	amalgam alloy
Aristaloy 21	amalgam alloy
Aristocore	composite core paste
Aristofil DP	light-cured microfine composite
Aristolux	light-cured microfine composite
Aristonol	zinc oxide–eugenol cement
Aristoprime	porcelain repair system
Arjalloy	amalgam alloy
Armator	high-gold bonding alloy
Arobond	nickel-chromium bonding alloy
Aroma Fine	impression alginate
Artalloy	amalgam alloy

Ash Casting Silver	sterling silver casting alloy
Astra	endosseus implant
Astracast	gypsum-bonded investment
Aucrom 1°	gold solder
Aurafil	light-cured hybrid composite
Aurea	medium-gold casting alloy
Auridium	gold solder
Aurobond	phosphate-bonded investment
Austenal Chairside	self-cure acrylic
Azure	hard die stone

B

Baker Four	medium-gold casting alloy
Baker Clasp Wire	wrought gold alloy wire
Barricaid	periodontal dressing
Barrier	dentine isolation material
BaseLine	glass-ionomer cement
BaseLine VLC	glass-ionomer cement
Basic	light-cured cavity liner
Bayer Cement	zinc polycarboxylate cement
Baysilex	impression elastomer
Beauty-Cast	gypsum-bonded investment
Belle de St Claire	die spacing resin
Bermudent	high-gold bonding alloy
Beta-Dur 700	die stone
Beta-Quartz	glass–ceramic insert
Betacryl II	heat-cure denture acrylic
Bifix	dual-cure cement
Bifluorid 12	varnish
Bio-Cast	cobalt–chromium bonding alloy
Biocryl	thermoplastic polymer sheet
Biolox	ceramic implant
Biomer	self-cured resin cement
Biopaque	metal–ceramic porcelain
Bioplast	thermoplastic sheet
Bioram-M	CAD/CAM inlay ceramic
Biosil h, f	cobalt–chromium casting alloys
Biosint-Supra	phosphate-bonded investment
Biostar	vacuum-forming unit
Biotrey	silicate cement
Bis-Fil-I	light-cured hybrid composite
Bis-Fil-M	light-cured microfine composite
Bite Registration Paste	registration paste
Bitestone	occlusal registration stone
blend-a-gum	impression elastomer
blend-a-print	impression alginate

blend-a-scon — impression elastomer
Blendant — early conventional self-cured composite
Blocset — light-cured model block out
Blu-Mousse — impression elastomer
Blue Core Build-up — composite core paste
Bluejey — die stone
Bluephase P — silicone die elastomer
Blueprint Asept — impression alginate
Blueprint Cremix — impression alginate
Bond-on 4 — silver-free Pd bonding alloy
Bondalcap — polycarboxylate cement
Bondi-Loy — cobalt–chromium bonding alloy
Bondlite — dentine bonding agent
Bonefit — endosseus implant
Boots — denture cleanser
Brånemark System — endosseous implant
Braun — electrical toothbrush
Break-Away — elastomeric ligature
Brilliant — light-cured hybrid composite
Brilliant Dentin — inlay composite
Butler G.U.M. — toothbrush
BXR — inlay composite

C
C.B.S. — ceramic implant
C&B Metabond — self-cure resin cement
C&J 1, 2 — cobalt–chromium casting alloy
CA 37 — impression alginate
CA Agent — dentine conditioner
Calcimol — calcium hydroxide cement
Calcitek — endosseus implant
Calcitite — ceramic implant
Calsite — phosphate-bonded investment
Calspar — impression plaster
Calxyl — calcium hydroxide paste
Cameo — medium-gold bonding alloy
Cameolite — low-gold casting alloy
Carboco — zinc polycarboxylate cement
Cardex-Stabon — self-curing silicone liner
Care — calcium hydroxide cement
Carrara — jacket crown porcelain
Casco — self-cure acrylic
Casowyte — medium-gold casting alloy

Cast Well — silver-free, Pd bonding alloy
Castadur — low-gold casting alloy
Castell — low-gold casting alloy
Castorit-C, -Super — phosphate-bonded investments
Cavalite — light-cured cavity liner
Cavex Clearfil — self-cured hybrid composite
Cavinol — zinc oxide–eugenol cement
Cavisol II — varnish
Cavit, Cavit-G, Cavit-W — temporary filling
Cavitemp — temporary filling
Cehadent Keramik — medium-gold bonding alloy
Cehadentor — medium-gold casting alloy
Cemper — self-cure resin cement
Ceplatec — aesthetic foil for porcelain
Cera-Fina — phosphate-bonded investment
Ceram-Core — glass-ionomer cement
Ceram-Etch — ceramic etchant
Ceram-Fil B — glass-ionomer filling cement
Ceramalloy — cobalt–chromium bonding alloy
Ceramapearl — castable glass–ceramic
Ceramcem — glass-ionomer cement
Ceramco — jacket crown porcelain
Ceramco — high-gold bonding alloy
Ceramco II — metal-ceramic porcelain
Ceramco White — medium-gold bonding alloy
Ceramicoat — ceramic ion exchange medium
Ceramicor — dentine pin
Ceramite H, V — die ceramics
Ceramlin — glass-ionomer cement
Ceramlite — glass-ionomer cement
CeramSave — glass-ionomer cement
Cerec Dicor MGC — machinable glass–ceramic
Cerinate Prime — porcelain silane bonding agent
Cerinate Porcelain — inlay/onlay, veneer porcelain
Ceri-Temp — temporary crown & bridge resin
Certain — light-cured hybrid composite
Cervident — early dentine bonding agent
Challenge — orthodontic bonding resin
Chameleon — laminate veneer porcelain
Charisma — light-cured hybrid composite
Charisma Inlay — inlay composite
Chelon-Fil — glass-ionomer filling cement
Chelon-Silver — glass-ionomer/cermet cement
ChemFil Superior — glass-ionomer filling cement
Chicago IV — high-gold casting alloy
Chinese NiTi — nickel–titanium wire

Chloropercha	endodontic sealant
Chromowax	diagnostic wax
Chromodur M	cobalt–chromium casting alloy
Cidex	cold disinfectant solution
Cimpat	temporary filling
Citotray	light cured tray resin
Citricon	impression elastomer
CJ 60	medium-gold casting alloy
Classic III	high-gold bonding alloy
Classic-2	orthodontic bonding resin
Clearfil Bond	dentine bonding agent
Clearfil Core	composite core paste
Clearfil CR Inlay	composite inlay system
Clearfil New Bond	dentine bonding agent
Clearfil Photo Bond	adhesive resin cement
Clearfil Ray-Posterior	light-cured hybrid composite
Clinomyn	dentifrice
Clip	temporary filling
Close-up	dentifrice
Coe Super-Soft	plasticized acrylic liner
Coe Alginate	impression alginate
Coe Comfort	tissue conditioner
Coe-Flo	impression paste
Coe-Pack	periodontal dressing
Cohere	impression hydrocolloid
Colacryl Chairside	self-cure higher acrylic liner
Colacryl Soft Reline	tissue conditioner
Colgate Double Action	toothbrush
Colgate	dentifrice
Coltex	impression elastomer
Coltoflax	impression elastomer
Coltosol	temporary filling
Combi-Vest	phosphate-bonded investment
Command Ultrafine	light-cured hybrid composite
Command Ultra-fine Color	light-cured colouring composite
CompaAdhesiv	dual-cure resin cement
CompaColor	light-cured colouring composite
CompaFill MH	light-cured microfine composite
Compafin	abrasive paste
CompaLay	composite inlay system
CompaMolar	light-cured hybrid composite
Compatit R	light-cured laboratory resin
Compolite	self-cured hybrid composite
Compolite II	light-cured hybrid composite
Composipost	preformed endodontic post
Comspan	self-cured resin cement
Concept	composite inlay system
Concise	self-cured hybrid composite
Concise Crown Build-up	composite core paste
Concise System	orthodontic bonding resin
Concise White Sealant	self-cure fissure sealant
Conquest	composite inlay system
Contex	antiflux
Contour	amalgam alloy
Convertray	light-cured tray resin
Copalite	varnish
Copyplast	thermoplastic polymer sheet
Coradent	composite core paste
Core-Shade	glass-ionomer cement
Core-Vent	endosseous implant
Coreform	composite core paste
Corelite	composite core paste
Corex	impression elastomer
Corsodyl	dentifrice
Cosmesil SM4	soft maxillofacial polymer
Cosmic	early conventional self-cured composite
Cosmotech Vest	die ceramic
Cosmotech Porcelain	laminate veneer porcelain
Cosmotech	metal–ceramic porcelain
Cover-Up II	adhesive resin cement
Creation Bond	dentine bonding agent
Creation	metal–ceramic porcelain
Creation 3 in One	dentine bonding primer
Crest	dentifrice
Cristal B	nickel–chromium bonding alloy
Cristobalite Inlay	gypsum-bonded investment
Crobrit	temporary C & B resin
Croform	cobalt–chromium casting alloy
Croform Excel, Regular	cobalt–chromium casting alloys
Croform Exten	heat-cure denture acrylic
Croform Hi-Tech	phosphate-bonded investment
Croform Repair	self-cure acrylic
Croform Springhard	cobalt–chromium casting alloy

CromoPal	gold solder
Crozat	wrought Co-Cr-Ni-Fe wire
Cruta-Gel	laboratory hydrocolloid
Cruta-Vest	phosphate-bonded investment
Crutanium	cobalt–chromium casting alloy
Crystacal R, D	die stones
Crystal Bond	retentive surface
Cupraloy	amalgam alloy
CuRay-Dual	
Match	dual-cure cement
Cushion Grip	denture fixative
Cytco	preformed endodontic post

D

D.I. 500	composite inlay curing oven
D.S.A.	impression alginate
D&Z	diamond bur
De Trey	
Orthoresin	self-cure acrylic
De Trey RR	self-cure acrylic
De Trey Triad	
System	light-cured denture resin
De Trey's Zinc	zinc phosphate cement
Debubblizer	surfactant
Deep Clean	denture cleanser
Degubond 4	medium-gold bonding alloy
Degucast U	medium-gold bonding alloy
Degudent G,	
H, N, U	high-gold bonding alloys
Degufill-H	light-cured hybrid composite
Degufill-M	light-cured microfine composite
Deguform	laboratory elastomer
Degulor A, B,	
C, i	high-gold casting alloys
Degupress	laboratory elastomer
Degupress	self-cure acrylic
Deguvest F,	
CF, HFG	phosphate-bonded investments
Deguvest L	soldering investment
Delar	surfactant
Delphic	self-cured hybrid composite
Delton	
Light-Curing	light-cure fissure sealant
Delton	self-cure fissure sealant
Den-Mat	
Core Paste	composite core paste
Den-Mat	
Crown Reline	self-cured resin cement
Den-Mat	

Rembrandt	light-cured colouring composite
Den-Mat	
Resto-Seal	light-cure fissure sealant
Denclen	denture cleanser
Denivit	dentifrice
Denlok	dentine pin
Denstone	die stone
Dentabond	medium-gold bonding alloy
Dentacast	gypsum-bonded investment
Dentacolour XS	laboratory light box
Dental D	injection mouldable polymer
Dental Guards	mouthguard resin
Dentalastics	elastomeric ligature
Denta-Lite	tooth-bleaching agent
Dentalor	high-gold casting alloy
Dentatus	dentine pin
Dentaurum	orthodontic elastomer
Denthesive	dentine bonding agent
Denti-Vest	phosphate-bonded investment
Dentin	
Protector	dentine isolation material
Dentin	
Bonding Agent	dentine bonding agent
Dentitan	cobalt–chromium bonding alloy
Dentlbright	tooth-bleaching agent
Dentobond	cobalt–chromium bonding alloy
Dentomat,2,3	automatic amalgamators
Dentu-Creme	denture cleanser
Dentu-Hold	denture fixative
Dentural	denture cleanser
Denturama	crown post
Detail	bite registration elastomer
Detascal E	impression elastomer
DeTrey	
Gutta-percha	temporary filling
Deva M, 4	medium-gold bonding alloys
DI-500	composite inlay tempering unit
Diaket	endodontic sealant
Diakor 8-18	ceramic implant
Dicor	castable glass–ceramic
Dicor MGC	dual-cured resin cement
Die-Keen	die stone
Diemet	model resin
Direct	orthodontic bonding resin
Direct-On II	orthodontic bonding resin
Directa	polycarbonate crown
Dis-Plaque	disclosing agent
Discimplant	endosseous implant
Disclosing Wax	occlusion/fit indicator

Discovery	cobalt–chromium bonding alloy	Durafill Bond	light-cured resin cement
Discovery	glass-ionomer filling cement	Duraflex	cobalt–chromium casting alloy
Dispersalloy	amalgam alloy	Duralay	self-cure wax alternative
DJ Metal	nickel–chromium bonding alloy	Duralingual	retentive mesh
Doric Acrylic	heat-cure denture acrylic	Duralit	model stone
Doric Bonding		Duralit S	hard die stone
Gold	high-gold bonding alloy	Duralium	cobalt–chromium casting alloy
Doric Dy-Rok	hard die stone	Duralloy	amalgam alloy
Doric GII	silver-free, Pd bonding alloy	Duraphat	fluoride varnish
Doric HTZ	die ceramic	Durelon	zinc polycarboxylate cement
Doric MDS	laboratory elastomer	Dux System	wrought titanium crown
Doric M-K	metal–ceramic porcelain	DVP	phosphate-bonded investment
Doric Non-		DVP Investment	die ceramic
Precious	Be-free, Ni-Cr bonding alloy	DWL-Lot	gold solder
Doric Porcelain	jacket crown porcelain	Dycal	calcium hydroxide cement
Doric Silicone	impression elastomer	Dycron	die stone
Doric SP	low-gold casting alloy	Dynasty	silver-free Pd bonding alloy
Dow Corning			
MDX 4/4516	soft maxillofacial polymer	**E**	
Dropsin	zinc phosphate cement	E.O.S.	composite inlay system
Drufolon E	thermoplastic polymer sheet	E-Chain	orthodontic elastomer
Drufosoft	thermoplastic sheet	Easy Flow	gold solder
DSD Fine Grain	low-copper amalgam alloy	Eclipse	medium-gold bonding alloy
DSD Autofine	low-copper amalgam alloy	Econo-Gel	laboratory hydrocolloid
Dual Cement	dual-cure resin cement	Econo-Vest	phosphate-bonded investment
Dual Cure	dual-cure resin cement	E.F.G.	ceramic bracket
Duallor	medium-gold casting alloy	Efferdent	denture cleanser
Dublikat	laboratory hydrocolloid	Elastigel	impression alginate
Dublisil	laboratory elastomer	Elastinol	nickel–titanium wire
Ducera-Lay	die ceramic	Elasto-force	orthodontic elastic
Ducera-Lay	laminate veneer porcelain	Elcebond	light-cured laboratory resin
Duceralloy U	cobalt–chromium bonding alloy	Electro-Magma	Be-free, Ni-Cr bonding alloy
Duceram	metal–ceramic porcelain	Elgiloy	wrought Co-Cr-Fe-Ni wire
Duceranium U	nickel–chromium bonding alloy	Elgydium	dentifrice
Duceratin		Elite	impression elastomer
Investment	phosphate-bonded investment	Elite Cement	zinc phosphate cement
Duceratin		Eludril	fluoride mouthwash
Porcelain	metal-ceramic porcelain	Emoform	dentifrice
Dugulor M,		Empress	impression alginate
MO, S	high-gold casting alloys	En-De-Kay Gel	fluoride gel
Duo-Bond	dual-cure resin	En-De-Kay	
Duo-Cement	dual-cure resin cement	Fluorinse	fluoride mouthwash
Duocast	high-gold casting alloy	Encore Plus	silver-free Pd bonding alloy
Duoloid	impression hydrocolloid	Endomethazone	endodontic sealant
Duomat	automatic amalgamator	Energy Chain	orthodontic elastomer
Dupliplast	laboratory hydrocolloid	Energy	
Dura Conditioner	tissue conditioner	Ringlets	orthodontic ligature
Dura-Liner II	self-cure higher acrylic liner	Engelbond Elite	high-gold bonding alloy
Durafill	light-cured microfine composite	Engelbond Hi	gold solder

Engelbond	
PGX, 45	medium-gold bonding alloys
Enhance	flexible abrasive disc/strip
EP 500	press ceramic furnace
Erkoflex	thermoplastic polymer sheet
Esticor Economic	palladium–silver bonding alloy
Esticor	
Ideal, Royal	high-gold bonding alloys
Esticor Opal	silver-free Pd bonding alloy
Esticor Plus,	
Vnic	medium-gold bonding alloys
Esticor	
Special, Swiss	high-gold bonding alloys
Estilux	light-cured microfine composite
Estilux Color	light-cured composite laminate
Estilux	
Posterior CVS	inlay composite
Estiseal	light-cured fissure sealant
Eucryl	dentifrice
Eurocast	phosphate-bonded investment
Euthymol	dentifrice
Exact	impression alginate
Exact	impression compound
Exaflex	impression elastomer
Exatec	preformed endodontic post
Excel	orthodontic bonding resin
Express	impression elastomer
Extend-A-Bond	orthodontic bonding resin
Extoral VLC	
Glaze	light-cured surface treatment
Extoral VLC	
Reline	light-cured denture resin
Extrude Extra	impression elastomer
Extrude	impression elastomer

F

F 21	polyester cement
Fascination	ceramic bracket
Fermit	temporary filling
Fidelity	impression alginate
Filpin Nova	dentine pin
Filpost	preformed endodontic post
Finavest	phosphate-bonded investment
Finesse	self-cured hybrid composite
Firmdent	denture fixative
Firmilay	high-gold casting alloy
Fit Checker	fit-checking elastomer
Fit-Rite	die-spacing resin
fittydent	denture fixative

Fix	impression tray adhesive
Flask-Stone	model stone
Flexi-Anterior	preformed endodontic post
Flexi-Cast	preformed crown post
Flexi-Flow	titanium-reinforced composite
Flexi-Post	preformed endodontic post
Flexibase	self-curing silicone liner
Flexiplast	injection-moulding acrylic
Flexistone	laboratory elastomer
Flexital	injection-mouldable polymer
Flexo-Ceram	jacket crown porcelain
Flint Edge	amalgam alloy
Fluodrops	fluoride drops
FluorEver	orthodontic bonding resin
Fluoriguard	fluoride mouthwash
Fluoroseal	light-cured cavity liner
Fluorothin	zinc silicophosphate cement
Fluotabs	fluoride tablets
FO-Pin	dentine pin
Forestacryl	self-cure acrylic
Formasil	laboratory elastomer
Formatray	self-cure tray acrylic
Forticast	medium-gold casting alloy
Foundation	high-gold casting alloy
Freebond	cobalt–chromium bonding alloy
Fuji Ionomer	
I/III	glass-ionomer cements
Fuji Lining	
LC	glass-ionomer cement
Fuji II LC	light-cured glass-ionomer filling cement
FujiCap II	glass-ionomer filling cement
Fujirock	die stone
Ful-Fil	light-cured hybrid composite
Fusion	porcelain repair system
Fynal	ethoxybenzoic acid (EBA) cement

G

Galaxy	medium-gold casting alloy
GC Caviton	temporary filling
GC Dentin	
Cement	glass-ionomer cement
GC Permacure	
System	light-cured surface treatment
GC Soft-Liner	tissue conditioner
GC Smooth Cut	diamond bur
GC Vest	phosphate-bonded investment
Geloform	laboratory hydrocolloid

Gem	ceramic bracket	Herador NH	high-gold bonding alloy
Gem-Base	glass-ionomer cement	Herculite	light-cured hybrid composite
Gem-Bond	dual-cured resin cement	Herculite	die stone
Gem-CC1	self-cured hybrid composite	Herculite	
Gem-Cem	glass-ionomer cement	XRV-Lab	composite inlay system
Gem-Core	glass-ionomer/cermet cement	Hermetic	endodontic sealant
Gem-Fil	glass-ionomer filling cement	Hi Crome	cobalt–chromium casting alloy
Gem-Lite 1	light-cured hybrid composite	Hi Heat	soldering investment
Gem-Ortho	glass-ionomer cement	Hi Chrom 2	phosphate-bonded investment
Gem-Seal	glass-ionomer cement	Hi-Dense	glass-ionomer/cermet cement
Gemini	nickel–chromium bonding alloy	Hi-Fi	glass-ionomer cement
Genesis	light-cured impression elastomer	Hi-T Multi-	
Geristore	dual-cure hybrid composite	bond	high-gold bonding alloy
Gi-Mask	laboratory elastomer	Hi-Temp	phosphate-bonded investment
Gibbs Menta-		HiDi	diamond bur
dent P	toothbrush	Hifluor-Gel	fluoride gel
Gibbs SR	dentifrice	Hinriplast	hard die stone
Glasionomer II	glass-ionomer filling cement	Hircoe	high-impact denture acrylic
Gluma, 2000	dentine bonding agents	HL72	early conventional self-cured
Golden Multi-			composite
bond	high-gold bonding alloy	Hold	impression tray adhesive
Goldex	model resin	Howmedica III	Be-free, Ni-Cr bonding alloy
GoldLink, 2	resin/metal bonding agents	Hydent	occlusion/denture fit indicator
Goldstar	gypsum-bonded investment	Hydrocal	model stone
Gore-Tex		Hydrocryl	denture acrylic
(GTAM)	augmentation polymer sheet	Hydrogum	impression alginate
Green-Mousse	impression elastomer	HydroMold	thermoplastic resin
GT Root-Post	preformed endodontic post	Hydrosil	impression elastomer
Guardian	blue-light protective glasses	Hydrosystem	wetting agent
Gypsogum	impression plaster	Hydroxyline	varnish

H		**I**	
Hapset	ceramic implant	ID210, ID220	cold disinfectant solutions
Harmony Line	high-gold casting alloy	Identoflex	flexible abrasive
Harmony	ceramic bracket	Igloo	polymeric bracket
Hartex	gypsum-bonded investment	Illusion	ceramic bracket
Harvard Cement	zinc phosphate cement	Image	high-gold bonding alloy
Healthco	blue-light protective glasses	Imperva	Bond dentine bonding agent
Heliocolour	light-cured paste laminate	Impredur	model resin
Heliolink	light-cured resin cement	Impregum F	impression elastomer
Heliomolar	light-cured microfine composite	Imprelon	thermoplastic polymer sheet
HelioProgress	light-cured microfine composite	Imprex	impression elastomer
Helioseal	light-cure fissure sealant	Imprint	impression elastomer
Hera GC	medium-gold casting alloy	Improved 1 Star	medium-gold casting alloy
Hera IS99	gypsum pore-filler	Improved Hi-T	
Hera NE 99	surfactant	Multibond	medium-gold bonding alloy
Hera O	low-gold casting alloy	IMZ	endosseus implant
Herabond	medium-gold bonding alloy	Indiloy	amalgam alloy
Herador P	medium-gold bonding alloy	Indirect Porcelain	veneer and bonding system

Individo Lux	light-cured tray resin/light box
Infinity	dual-cure cement
Inlayvest	gypsum-bonded investment
Innovative Dent. Prod.	endosseus implant
Insta-Bond VL	orthodontic bonding resin
Insulating Gel	separating medium
Intact	glass-ionomer cement
Integrity	palladium–silver bonding alloy
Interface	light-cured cavity liner
Interpore 2000	ceramic implant
Interval	temporary filling
Intoss	endosseus implant
Intrigue	ceramic bracket
Inzoma P990	retentive surface
Ioline	glass-ionomer cement
Ion	polycarbonate crown
Ion Ni-Chro	stainless steel crown
Ionobond	glass-ionomer cement
Ionofil-U	glass-ionomer filling cement
Ionoseal	light-cured cavity liner
Ion S	glass ionomer/cermet cement
IPS Corum	inlay/onlay, veneer ceramic
IPS Empress	ceramic-crown forming system
Irido-Platinum	wrought platinum–iridium wire
IRM	reinforced zinc oxide–eugenol cement
Isolit	gypsum pore filler
Isomolar	self-cured microfine composite
Isopast	self-cured microfine composite
Isosit SR	dimethacrylate denture teeth
ITI-Straumann	endosseus implant
Ivomat	composite inlay curing chamber

J

J-7	low-gold casting alloy
J&J Reach	toothbrush
JA	high-gold casting alloy
Jadestone	hard die stone
Japanese NiTi	nickel–titanium wire
JB	high-gold casting alloy
JC	high-gold casting alloy
JCB	medium-gold casting alloy
Jel 2, 3, 4	medium-gold casting alloys
Jelbon	Be-free, Ni-Cr bonding alloy
Jelcast	low-gold casting alloy
Jelenko O	high-gold bonding alloy
Jelspan	Be-free, Ni-Cr bonding alloy
Jelstar	palladium–silver bonding alloy

Jeltrate	impression alginate
Jeycast	gypsum-bonded investment
Jeyrock	die stone
Jeyvest	phosphate-bonded investment
JFB Alloy	cobalt–chromium casting alloy
Jico-Max	diamond bur
JP I, IA, III	medium-gold bonding alloys
JP 11, 80, 87, IV	high-gold bonding alloys
JP 5, 92	palladium–silver bonding alloys
JPW	medium-gold bonding alloy
Just White	tooth-bleaching agent

K

Kaffir D	model stone
Kaffir HXD	die stone
Kalsogen	zinc oxide–eugenol cement
Kalzinol	zinc oxide–eugenol cement
Kaoliner	ceramic fibre tape
Kelly's Paste	impression paste
Kem-Dent	inlay wax
Kemcal	model stone
Kemdent Black GP	impression compound
Kemdent Temp. Stopping	temporary filling
Kemrock	die stone
Kenbridge	high-gold casting alloy
Kent KB425	toothbrush
Kent OK, Nova, Visa	toothbrushes
Kera-Vlies	ceramic fibre tape
Kerr Endo-Post	preformed endodontic post
Kerr's Bite Reg. Paste	bite registration paste
Kerr's Compo	impression compound
Kerr's Fast Cure	self-cure acrylic
Kerr's FITT	tissue conditioner
Kerr's Impression Wax	impression wax
Kerr's Inlay	inlay wax
Kerr's Sealer	endodontic sealer
Ketac Varnish	varnish
Ketac-Bond	glass-ionomer cement
Ketac-Cem	glass-ionomer cement
Ketac-Fil	glass-ionomer filling cement
Ketac-Silver	glass-ionomer/cermet cement
Kingfisher	dentifrice
Kitty Dentafit	electrical toothbrush

Klett-O-Bond-Renfert	preshaped polymeric mesh
Kloroperka N-O	endodontic sealant
Kolynos	denture fixative
Komet	diamond bur
Kooliner	self-cure higher acrylic liner
Korecta	impression wax
Kromoglass 1, 3	glass-ionomer cements
Kromoglass 2	glass-ionomer filling cement
Kromogel	impression alginate
Kryptex	zinc silicophosphate cement
Kulzer Adhesive Bond	unfilled resin
Kulzer Adhesive Cement	dual-cure cement
Kulzer Inlay System	composite inlay system
Kurer Crown Anchor	preformed endodontic post

L

Lab Separator	separating medium
Lab-Putty	laboratory elastomer
Lab-Sil	laboratory elastomer
Laboratory 22, 33, 44	medium-gold casting alloys
Labstone	die stone
Lactona-Surgident	impression agar
Lactona-Thompson	impression agar
Lastic	impression elastomer
Lasticomp	impression elastomer
LCL 8	glass-ionomer cement
Legend	glass-ionomer filling cement
Legend	silver-free Pd bonding alloy
Legend Silver	glass-ionomer/cermet cement
Life	calcium hydroxide cement
Light-Bond	orthodontic bonding resin
Litecast B	nickel-chromium bonding alloy
Lite-Fil II	light-cured hybrid composite
LiteLine	light-cured denture reline
LP-22	heat-cure denture acrylic
Lubrofilm	surfactant
Lucitone 199	high-impact denture acrylic
Luma-Seal	light-cure fissure sealant
Lumicon Alloy	amalgam alloy
Lumicon	zinc phosphate cement
Lumifor	light-cured hybrid composite
Luralite	impression paste

Luride	fluoride gel
Luride 0.5, 1.0	fluoride tablets
Luride drops	fluoride drops
Luster-cast	gypsum-bonded investment
Lux-a-fill	light-cured hybrid composite
Luxalloy	amalgam alloy
Luxene	thermoplastic sheet
Luxene Astron Vinyl	injection-moulding acrylic
Luxon	heat-cure denture acrylic
Lynal	tissue conditioner

M

M.P.V-Delta	medium-gold bonding alloy
M.Q.	silicate cement
Macleans	dentifrice
Macleans	toothbrush
Macor-M	CAD/CAM inlay ceramic
Macromer	high-impact denture acrylic
Maestro	low-gold casting alloy
Maingold G, SG	high-gold casting alloys
Marathon	light-cured hybrid composite
Margin Repair Kit	light-cured composite paste
Mark II	machinable glass–ceramic
Maryland	type of adhesive bridge
Matchmaker	metal–ceramic porcelain
Mattibel G, R	high-gold casting alloys
Matticast R	high-gold casting alloy
Matticraft Alpha	high-gold bonding alloy
Matticraft B	palladium–silver bonding alloy
Matticraft C, H, 80	silver-free Pd bonding alloy
Matticraft E, G, JMP, S	high-gold bonding alloys
Matticraft M, Y, 45	medium-gold bonding alloys
Mattident 60	medium-gold casting alloy
Mattident G, R	high-gold casting alloys
Mattieco 25	low-gold casting alloy
Mattiflo	gold solder
Mattigold AE	high-gold casting alloy
Mattiloy	amalgam alloy
Mattiloy Plus 43	amalgam alloy
Mattinax GA, R	high-gold casting alloys
Max Pin	dentine pin
Maxibond	cobalt–chromium bonding alloy
Maxibond	orthodontic bonding resin
Maxigold	medium-gold casting alloy

Maximal	orthodontic bonding resin
Maximum Cure	
Sealant	orthodontic bonding resin
MDA	heat-cure denture acrylic
Meadway	heat-cure denture acrylic
Medicast	cobalt–chromium bonding alloy
Medinlay	high-gold casting alloy
Medior	medium-gold casting alloy
Megallium	cobalt–chromium casting alloy
Meisinger	diamond bur
Meliodent	heat-cure denture acrylic
Memory Chain	orthodontic elastic
Memosil C.D.	bite registration silicone
Mentadent P	dentifrice
Meron	glass-ionomer cement
Meta-Dent	self-cure acrylic
Meta-Fast	self-curing bonding resin
Metrocryl	
Universal	heat-cure denture acrylic
MG Newpress	injection moulding machine
Micro-Retentive	retentive mesh
Microbond Hi	
Life	high-gold bonding alloy
Microbond NP$_2$	Be-free, Ni-Cr bonding alloy
Microbond	
Porcelain	laminate veneer porcelain
Microcast MC	palladium–silver bonding alloy
Microdontic	
Pin System	dentine pin
Microfill Pontic	self-cured resin cement
Microfilm	gypsum pore filler
Microflex	flexible abrasive disc
Microjoin	self-cured resin cement
Microlok	stainless steel bracket
Microlon	heat-cure denture acrylic
Micromod	die stone
Micronium HS,	
N10	cobalt–chromium casting alloy
Microtex 84	phosphate-bonded investment
Microvest	gypsum-bonded investment
Microwhite	die stone
Midas	medium-gold casting alloy
Midigold	medium-gold casting alloy
Minacryl	
Universal	heat-cure denture acrylic
Minargent	amalgam alloy
Minerva 4	medium-gold casting alloy
Minigold	low-gold casting alloy
Miracle Mix	glass-ionomer/cermet cement

Miradapt	self-cured hybrid composite
Mirafort 4	medium-gold casting alloy
Mirage	laminate veneer porcelain
Mirage	polymeric bracket
Mirage ABC	adhesive bonding system
Mirage FLC	dual-cure cement
Mirage Bond	dentine bonding agent
Model Cement	sticky wax
Model Silicone	silicone die elastomer
Modulay	high-gold casting alloy
Modulor	medium-gold casting alloy
Moldasynt	die stone
Molloplast-b	heat-curing silicone liner
Mollosil	self-curing silicone liner
Mono-Lok	orthodontic bonding resin
Monobond S	silane bonding agent
Mooser RC Post	root canal post
Mouthguard	fluoride mouthwash
Mowrey 20/46	medium-gold casting alloy
MP Pirec	root canal post
Multibond	nickel–chromium bonding alloy
Multiform	indicating paste
Mylar	polyester matrix strip
Mynol	endodontic sealer

N

N2	endodontic sealer
Natural White	tooth bleaching agent
Naturelle Rx	silver-free Pd bonding alloy
NCM Alpha	Be-free, Ni-Cr bonding alloy
Neobond II	cobalt–chromium bonding alloy
Neocast	high-gold casting alloy
Neocolloid	impression alginate
Neotone	plasticized acrylic liner
New Era	light-cured cavity liner
New-Era	glass-ionomer cement
New-Era Silver	glass-ionomer/cermet cement
Ney	silver–palladium casting alloy
Ney Cast III	medium-gold casting alloy
Ney-Oro	high-gold casting alloy
NHP	self-cure acrylic
Ni-Ti	nickel–titanium wire
Nicrobond	phosphate-bonded investment
Nimetic Grip	self-cured resin cement
Nirabond	Be-free, Ni-Cr bonding alloy
Niranium	cobalt–chromium casting alloy
Nitinol	nickel–titanium wire
Nobelpharma	
(Brånemark)	endosseus implant

Nobil Solder	gold solder
Nobil-Ceram	Be-free, Ni-Cr bonding alloy
Nobilium	cobalt–chromium casting alloy
Noble J	high-gold bonding alloy
Nobond	separating medium
Nogenol	bite reg./impression paste
Nogenol	temporary luting cement
NoSilver	medium-gold bonding alloy
Novus	fluoroelastomeric liner
Novabond	medium-gold bonding alloy
Novabond 2	silver-free Pd bonding alloy
Novarex	cobalt–chromium bonding alloy
NPX III	nickel–chromium bonding alloy
Nu Alloy DP	amalgam alloy
Nu-Smile	tooth-bleaching agent
NuCap	calcium hydroxide cement
Nupro	polishing paste

O

Occlude	occlusion indicator
Occlusin	light-cured hybrid composite
Olympia	medium-gold bonding alloy
Olympia	othodontic elastic
Omega Alpha MS, VK	Be-free, Ni-Cr bonding alloy
Omniflex	impression elastomer
Omnigel	fluoride gel
Omnisil	impression elastomer
Opalescence	tooth-bleaching agent
Opalux	light-cured hybrid composite
OP-PO	endodontic post system
Opotow	ethoxybenzoic acid (EBA) cement
Optalloy II	amalgam alloy
Optec HSP	high-ceramic core porcelain
Optilon 399	high-impact denture acylic
Option	medium-gold bonding alloy
Optosil P	impression elastomer
Opus PCF	zinc polycarboxylate cement
Opus-Silver	glass-ionomer/cermet cement
OpusCem	glass-ionomer cement
OpusFil W	glass-ionomer filling cement
Orabase	mucous membrane dresssing
Orahesive	mucous membrane dresssing
Oral-B 10, 20, 30, 32	toothbrushes
Oral-B 35, 40, Plus	toothbrushes
Oral-B Indicator	toothbrush

Oral-B Right Angle	toothbrush
Oralin	self-cure fissure sealant
Oralin Light Curing	light-cure fissure sealant
Oralloy	amalgam alloy
Oranwash	impression elastomer
Orapol	polishing paste
Oraproph	prophylaxis paste
Organa II	laboratory hydrocolloid
Orion Delphi	medium-gold bonding alloy
Orion Libra	silver-free Pd bonding alloy
Orion Argos	palladium–silver bonding alloy
Orion	high-gold bonding alloy
Ormco	orthodontic elastomer
Ormesh	stainless steel bracket
Orocast	medium-gold casting alloy
Orplid	high-gold casting alloy
Orplid Keramik	high-gold bonding alloy
Orthalgenat	impression alginate
Ortho Gold	zinc phosphate cement
Orthocem B	glass-ionomer cement
Orthocryl	self-cure acrylic
Orthodon	die stone
Orthomite Super-Bond	orthodontic bonding resin
Orthoprint	impression alginate
Orthosit	dimethacrylate denture teeth
Osprovit	ceramic implant
Osseodent	endosseous implant
Osticon	ceramic implant
Ostilit	ceramic implant
Ostrix-B, -C, -PM	ceramic implants
Ostrix-NR	ceramic implant
Ostron 100	self-cure tray acrylic
Oxyguard	protective gel
Oxynon	soldering flux

P

P 10	self-cured hybrid composite
P 30	light-cured hybrid composite
P 50	light-cured hybrid composite
Pageant	palladium–silver bonding alloy
Paint On Colors	characterizing pigments
Pal-Bond Extra, 3	silver-free Pd bonding alloys
Paladisc LC	light-cured custom tray resin
Paladon 65	heat-cure denture acrylic
Palain Star	impression alginate
Palakav	self-cured acrylic composite

Palapress vario	self-cure acrylic
Palasiv 62	plasticized acrylic liner
Palatray	light-cured custom tray resin
Palaural	low-gold casting alloy
Palavit G LC	light-cured wax alternative
Palavit L	self-cure tray acrylic
Pallacast	low-gold casting alloy
Pallacast Wire	wrought gold alloy wire
Pallacon	low-gold casting alloy
Pallas 3, 4	low-gold casting alloys
Pallavest	phosphate-bonded investment
Palliag M, MJ, W	low-gold casting alloys
Pallium 3	low-gold casting alloy
Pallorag	low-gold casting alloy
Palloro	low-gold casting alloy
Paloy	low-gold casting alloy
Panabond 2	silver-free Pd bonding alloy
Panabond 45	medium-gold bonding alloy
Panabond Yellow	high-gold bonding alloy
Panacast 5	low-gold casting alloy
Panacast 60	medium-gold casting alloy
Panachrome	cobalt–chromium casting alloy
Panapren	impression elastomer
Panasil	impression elastomer
Panavia Ex	self-cured adhesive resin cement
Pangold	low-gold casting alloy
Pangold Keramik	palladium–silver bonding alloy
Panorama	high-copper amalgam alloy
Para-Post Plus, Unity	preformed endodontic posts
Parapin	dentine pin
Paribar	impression compound
Paste Laminate	light cured composite opaquer
Pattern Resin	self-cured wax alternative
PCR-Pin	dentine pin
PDQ	die-spacing resin
Pearl Drops	dentifrice
Pekafill	light-cured hybrid composite
Pekalux	light-cured hybrid composite
Penpin	dentine pin
Per-Fit	self-curing silicone liner
Perfection	light-cured microfine composite
Perfection Paste	self-cured microfine composite
Periograf	ceramic implant
Peripac, Improved	periodontal dressings
Peripheral Seal	denture border sealant
Perm	self-cure denture acylic
Permacure VC-1	laboratory light-curing unit
Permadyne	impression elastomer
Permaflex	heat-curing silicone liner
Permagum	impression elastomer
Permite C	amalgam alloy
Permlastic	impression elastomer
Peroxyl	tooth-bleaching agent
Pertac Hybrid	light-cured hybrid composite
Pertac Universal Bond	dentine bonding agent
Petralit	zinc silicophosphate cement
PG2	silver-free Pd bonding alloy
PGX 45	medium-gold bonding alloy
Phase II	orthodontic bonding resin
Phase	impression alginate
Phasealloy	amalgam alloy
Phillips	dentifrice
Phosphacap	encapsulated zinc phosphate cement
Photac-Fil Aplicap	encapsulated light-cured glass-ionomer
Photo Bond	dual-curing dentine bonding agent
Photo-Bond Aplicap	encapsulated light-cured glass-ionomer
Pinnacle	inlay wax
Piston Jet	injection-moulding machine
Plaque Check	disclosing agent
Plastex	heat-cure denture acrylic
Plastone L	model stone
Platigo G	medium-gold casting alloy
Platigo J	high-gold casting alloy
Platinore	cobalt–chromium casting alloy
Plax	fluoride mouthwash
Pluto 2P	high-gold casting alloy
Point Two	fluoride mouthwash
Poli-Grip	denture cleanser
Polofil, Molar	light-cured hybrid composites
Poly F Plus	zinc polycarboxylate cement
Polyan	injection-moulding acrylic
Polyapress	acrylic injection moulder
Polycap	self-cured conventional composite
Polycast	phosphate-bonded investment
Polyliner 40	heat-cured silicone liner
Polyroqq	model resin
Pontallor 3, 4	low-gold casting alloys
Porcast	high-gold bonding alloy
Porcelite	light-cured resin cement

Porcelite Dual Cure	dual-cured resin cement
Porcelite Primer	porcelain repair system
PorceLock	ceramic etchant
Pors-on 4	palladium–silver bonding alloy
Pour-N-Cure	self-cure acrylic
Power Chain	orthodontic elastomer
Precedent	glass-ionomer cement
Precious Pin	dentine pin
Precise	impression elastomer
Prema	abrasive/acid bleaching agent
Premier	diamond bur
Premium	high-gold bonding alloy
President	impression elastomer
Pressure Relief Cream	occlusion and fit indicator
Prima Rock	hard die stone
Prisma AP.H	light-cured hybrid composite
Prisma AP.H Inlay System	composite inlay system
Prisma Ceraprime	porcelain repair system
Prisma-Fil	light-cured hybrid composite
Prisma Gloss	abrasive paste
Prisma-Shield	light-cure fissure sealant
Prisma TP.H.	light-cured hybrid composite
Prisma Universal Bond	dentine bonding agent
Prisma U.B. 2, 3	dentine bonding agents
Prisma VLC Dycal	light-cured calcium hydroxide cement
Pro-Wax	surfactant
Procal	calcium hydroxide cement
Procera	wrought titanium crown
Proco-Sol	endodontic sealer
Profile	self-cured hybrid composite
Profisil	laboratory elastomer
Prolite II, 3	laboratory light-curing units
Proplast	polymer–ceramic implant
Propylor	endodontic sealant
Prosthodent VL-2	composite core paste
Protect	dentifrice
Protect	dentine isolation material
Protect	fluoride gel
Protect Liner	light-cured microfine composite
Protemp II	temporary C & B resin
Protexoflex	thermoplastic sheet
Protocol	palladium–silver bonding alloy
Protor	high-gold casting alloy

Provicol	temporary luting cement
Provil	impression elastomer
Provipast	temporary filling
Proxabrush	toothbrush
Proxigel	tooth-bleaching agent
Proxyl	prophylaxis paste

Q

QC 20	self-cure acrylic
Quasar	ceramic bracket
Quasar	orthodontic bonding resin
Quick Check	occlusal indicator spray
Quick Ligs	elastomeric ligature
Quick-Pour	laboratory elastomer

R

Radix Anker	preformed endodontic post
Rafluor New Age	fluoride gel
Rainbow	flexible abrasive disc
Rajah	medium-gold casting alloy
Ramitec	registration elastomer
Rapid	impression elastomer
Rapid Stone	model stone
Rapidur	die stone
RCI Reinforced	glass ionomer/cermet cement
Reach Anti-Plaque	fluoride mouthwash
Realor	low-gold casting alloy
Rebaron	self-cure acrylic
Recal	calcium hydroxide cement
Recon	tissue conditioner
Redifast	self-cure acrylic
Redifix	impression tray adhesive
Redigard	thermoplastic sheet
Redilon	heat-cure denture acrylic
Redilon DB	self-cure acrylic
Reditray	self-cured tray acrylic
Redphase P	silicone impression elastomer
Reflect	impression elastomer
Reflex	nickel–titanium wire
Refractory S	silica-bonded investment
Regel Star	amalgam alloy
Regisil	registration elastomer
Rely-a-bond	orthodontic bonding resin
Rema Star	phosphate-bonded investment
Rema Exakt	phosphate-bonded investment
Remanium CC	cobalt–chromium casting alloy
Remanium CD	cobalt–chromium bonding alloy
Remanium CS	Be-free, Ni-Cr bonding alloy

Rematitan	nickel–titanium wire		Seabond	denture fixative
Rembrandt			Sealapex	endodontic sealant
Lighten	tooth-bleaching agent		Sealite	light-cure fissure sealant
Renaissance	aesthetic foil for porcelain		Securipin	dentine pin
Reogan	calcium hydroxide paste		Sedanol	zinc oxide-eugenol cement
Replica	impression compound		Sensitive	dentifrice
Reprodent	denture border sealant		Sensodyne	dentifrice
Reprodent Hard	self-cure acrylic		Sensodyne Search	toothbrush
Reprodent Soft	plasticized acrylic liner		Sentalloy	nickel–titanium wire
Reprosil HF	impression elastomer		Sentinol	nickel–titanium wire
Resilient	self-cure core composite		Se+riton	self-cured acrylic filling
Resiment	dimethacrylate resin cement		Se+riton	self-cured acrylic cement
Resistal P	nickel–chromium bonding alloy		Se+riton	temporary C & B resin
Restobond 3	dentine bonding agent		Shiny-Brite	gypsum-bonded investment
Restolux SP2	light-cured hybrid composite		Shofu	amalgam alloy
Restolux SP4	light-cured hybrid composite		Siccoform	impression elastomer
Rex-Sil	impression elastomer		Signal	dentifrice
Rexillium III	nickel–chromium bonding alloy		Silamat	high-speed mixing machine
Rexodent RGI	glass-ionomer filling cement		Silaplast	impression elastomer
Rexprint	impression elastomer		Silar	self-cured microfine composite
RGI	glass-ionomer/cermet cement		Silasoft	impression elastomer
Rigel Star	low-copper amalgam alloy		Silibond	porcelain repair system
Right-On	orthodontic bonding resin		Silicap	encapsulated silicate cement
Rochette	adhesive bridge		Silicer	microcrack stabilizer
Rocky Mountain	orthodontic elastomer		Silicoater	surface conditioning processor
Roll-X	Be-free, Ni-Cr bonding alloy		Silicoater MD	surface treatment oven
Rotatec-Plus	surface conditioning processor		Sililink	silane bonding agent
Rubberoid	impression agar		Silistor	porcelain repair system
RX Imperial 2	high-gold bonding alloy		Silky Rock	hard die stone
Ryco-Sep	gypsum pore filler		Silskin II	soft maxillofacial polymer
			Silux Plus	light-cured microfine composite
S			Silver Pal-Bond	palladium–silver bonding alloy
S.S.White			Simpa	self-curing silicone liner
Alginate	impression alginate		Simplex Rapid	self-cure acrylic
S.S.White Paste	impression paste		Skillcast 60	medium-gold casting alloy
S-1	Be-free, Ni-Cr bonding alloy		SMG	high-gold bonding alloy
SA Primer	dentine primer		Smile	self-cured conventional com-
Saffron	medium-gold casting alloy			posite
Safix-Anker	preformed endodontic post		Smoker's	
Salivan	silver–indium casting alloy		Toothpaste	denture cleanser
Saphilox	ceramic implant		Snap	temporary C & B resin
Schein 20/20	light-cured hybrid composite		Snug	denture fixative
Scotchbond,2	dentine bonding agents		Soflex	flexible abrasive disc
Scotchbond			Soft Oryl	tissue conditioner
Multi-Purpose	multi-purpose adhesive		Softic 49	plasticized acrylic liner
Scotchprep	dentine bonding primer		Solarcast	low-gold casting alloy
Scotchprime	porcelain repair system		Soldavest	soldering investment
SDI Lojic	amalgam alloy		Solder Auro	gold solder
SDI Permite	amalgam alloy		Solila Nova	amalgam alloy

Sono-Cem	dual-cure resin cement
SP 70, 90	palladium–silver bonding alloy
Special Bond II	unfilled resin
SpectraBond	self-cured hybrid composite
Speed	nickel–titanium wire
Speed E	soldering investment
Spheralloy	amalgam alloy
Spirit	silver-free Pd bonding alloy
Sporicidin	cold disinfectant solution
SR Isosit	
Inlay/Onlay	composite inlay system
SR Isosit-N Fluid	separating medium
SR Ivocap	heat-cure denture acrylic
SR Separating	
Fluid	separating medium
Stabilo Temp	self-cure acrylic resin
Stabilok	dentine pin
Stabilor G,	
GL/NHS	medium-gold casting alloy
Stabilor NFIV	medium-gold casting alloy
Staline	ethoxybenzoic acid (EBA) cement
Standalloy	amalgam alloy
Starburst	low-copper amalgam alloy
Starburst	
Non-Gamma II	high-copper amalgam alloy
Starfire	ceramic bracket
Stat-BR	bite registration elastomer
Staybelite	endodontic sealer resin
Stellon	heat-cure denture acrylic
Stents	impression compound
Steri-Oss	endosseus implant
Steradent	denture cleanser
Sterngold 66	medium-gold casting alloy
Stick	impression tray adhesive
Sticky Post	self-cured dimethacrylate cement
Strator	low-gold casting alloy
Stripit	ceramic etchant
Sturdicast	medium-gold casting alloy
SuccessFil	endodontic obturator
Sumo	glass-ionomer cement
Sunrise	medium-gold casting alloy
Super Nitane	nickel–titanium wire
Super Oralium	low-gold casting alloy
Super Poli-Grip	denture fixative
Super Sterafix	denture fixative
Super Wernet's	denture fixative
Super-Bond	
C & B	self-cured acrylic cement

Super-Cast	nickel–chromium bonding alloy
Super-Cure	heat-cure denture acrylic
Super-Sep	gypsum pore filler
Superbond	orthodontic bonding resin
Supra-Stone	hard die stone
Supranium	cobalt–chromium bonding alloy
Supreme	impression alginate
Surflex F	impression elastomer
Surgical Simplex	self-cured acrylic cement
Surprise	metal–ceramic porcelain
Svedion	cobalt–chromium casting alloy
Sybraloy	amalgam alloy
Syntac	dentine bonding agent
Szabo YPG	high-gold bonding alloy

T

T-Lux	light-cured tray resin
Tab 2000	temporary C & B resin
Talladium No	
Bel-T	Be-free, Ni-Cr bonding alloy
Talladium	
Premium, V	nickel–chromium bonding alloys
Tau-Marin	toothbrush
TD71	self-cured acrylic composite
TDA Diamonds	diamond bur
TemDent	temporary C & B resin
Temp Bond	temporary luting cement
Temp D	zinc oxide–eugenol cement
Temper-Indicating	
Paste	heat-treatment indicator
Tempit	temporary filling
Templin	zinc oxide–eugenol cement
Tempo	tissue conditioner
Temrex	zinc oxide–eugenol cement
Tenet	zinc phosphate cement
Tenure	dentine bonding agent
Tetrapaque	light-cured composite opaquer
Tetric	light-cured hybrid composite
Tewerock	die stone
Tewesil	impression elastomer
The Force	nickel–titanium wire
Thermabond	nickel–chromium bonding alloy
Thixoflex	impression elastomer
Ti-Core	titanium–reinforced core resin
Ticon	nickel–chromium bonding alloy
Ticonium 44	nickel–chromium casting alloy
Ticonium T3	nickel–chromium bonding alloy
Ticonium	
Premium 100	nickel–chromium casting alloy

Tiffany	low-gold casting alloy
Timeline	light-cured cavity liner
Titancor	root canal post
Titanol	nickel–titanium wire
Titronic-K	root canal post
TMS Link	dentine pin
Toothguard	disclosing agent
Topaz	light-cured microfine composite
Topaz Glasses	blue-light protective glasses
Topcast	low-gold casting alloy
Topcraft	silver-free, Pd bonding alloy
Topol	dentifrice
Topstone	die stone
Totacide	cold disinfectant solution
Total	plasticized acrylic liner
Traitement SPAD	endodontic sealant
Transbond	orthodontic bonding resin
Transcend	ceramic bracket
Translux	blue-light surgery curing unit
Translux Lightbox	composite inlay curing chamber
Tray Dough	thermoplastic resin
Traylight	laboratory light box
Tresiolan	dentine isolation material
Trevalon	heat-cure denture acrylic
Trevalon Hi	high-impact denture acrylic
Tri-Flex Root Pin	preformed endodontic post
Trim	temporary C & B resin
Tripton	dentine bonding agent
Tristar	nickel–chromium bonding alloy
Tru-Fit	die-spacing resin
Tru Stone	die stone
Trucast II, III	high-gold casting alloys
TrueVitality	composite inlay system
Tubilitec	varnish
Tubli-Seal	endodontic sealer
Twinlook	dual-cure resin cement
Tytin	amalgam alloy

U

U.S.A.	diamond bur
Ufi Gel P	self-cured silicone liner
Ultra-Bond	dual-cure composite
Ultra-Pake	metal–ceramic porcelain
Ultra-Seal	light-cure fissure sealant
Ultra-Seal XT	self-cure fissure sealant
Ultracryl	self-cure acrylic
Ultradent	ceramic etchant

Ultrafil	hot injection gutta-percha
Ultrafine	impression alginate
UltraLight	orthodontic bonding resin
Ultratech	nickel–chromium bonding alloy
Ultratrim	orthodontic bonding resin
Unibond	Be-free, Ni-Cr bonding alloy
Unicryl	self-cure acrylic
Uniflux	soldering flux
Unilastic	impression elastomer
Unilot	gold solder
UniSolder	gold solder
Unitbond	nickel–chromium bonding alloy
Unosil S	impression elastomer
Until	self-cured resin cement
Utiloy	low-gold casting alloy

V

V.H.T. Investment	die ceramic
V-Bond	light-cured resin cement
Vacufilm	surfactant
Vacuformat-U	vacuum-forming unit
Valiant	amalgam alloy
Valux	light-cured hybrid composite
Van R	impression agar
Vanguard	thermoplastic sheet
VariGlass	light-cured glass-ionomer cement
Vel-Mix	die stone
Velva	preformed endodontic post
Verabond	nickel–chromium bonding alloy
Veraloy	amalgam alloy
Veriflux	soldering flux
Verilloid	impression agar
Verinor	medium-gold bonding alloy
Verone	impression elastomer
Versapor	augmentation polymer
Vertex Orthoplast	self-cure acylic
Vertex Regular, SC	self-cure acrylics
Vertex Soft	plasticized acrylic liner
Vertex Trayplast	self-cure tray acrylic
Vestogum	laboratory elastomer
Vi-Comp	cobalt–chromium bonding alloy
Victory	cobalt–chromium casting alloy
Vidur	laboratory hydrocolloid
VinaSoft	plasticized acrylic liner
Vintage Opal	metal–ceramic porcelain

Virginia Salt	retentive surface
Virilium	cobalt–chromium casting alloy
VisarSeal	light-cured unfilled resin
Viscogel	tissue conditioner
Visio Alpha, Beta	laboratory light-curing sources
Visio-Dispers	light-cured microfine composite
Visio-Fil	light-cured hybrid composite
Visio-Gem	light-cured laboratory resin
Visio-Molar	light-cured hybrid composite
Visio-Seal	light-cure fissure sealant
Vista	low-gold casting alloy
Vita	jacket crown porcelain
Vita Hi-Ceram	high-ceramic core porcelain
Vita In-Ceram	high-ceramic core porcelain
Vita K + B	self-cure acrylic
Vita Spray-On	metal–ceramic porcelain
Vita-Cerec	CAD/CAM inlay ceramic
Vita-Omega	metal–ceramic porcelain
Vita-VMK 68N	metal–ceramic porcelain
Vitadur N	laminate veneer porcelain
Vitrebond	glass-ionomer cement
Vivalloy HR	amalgam alloy
Vivostar	medium-gold bonding alloy
VPS	silicone impression elastomer

W

W.L.W.	silver–palladium casting alloy
W-B Precision	phosphate-bonded investment
Wards Wondrpak	periodontal dressing
Waxit	surfactant
Wettax	surfactant
White & Brite	tooth-bleaching agent
White Economy	low-gold casting alloy
WHW	heat-cure denture acrylic
Widarock	hard die stone
Widerit	phosphate-bonded investment
WIL-O-dont	light-cured orthodontic resin
Will-Ceram P	high-gold bonding alloy
Will-Ceram W1	palladium–silver bonding alloy
Wiptam	wrought Co-Cr-Ni wire
Wiron 88	Be-free, Ni-Cr bonding alloy
Wironit	cobalt–chromium casting alloy

Wisdom Dental Gel	dentifrice
Wisil	cobalt–chromium casting alloy
World 20	low-gold casting alloy
World 50	medium-gold casting alloy
World 75	high-gold casting alloy

X

Xantalgin select	impression alginate
Xantopren H, M	impression elastomers
Xantopren VL	impression elastomer
XR Bond	dentine bonding agent
XR Ionomer	glass-ionomer cement
XR Primer	dentine bonding primer
XRV	light-cured hybrid composite

Y

Yeti-Creation	diagnostic wax

Z

Z100	l.c. hybrid composite
Zelgan	impression alginate
Zendium	dentifrice
Zenith Alpha Base	glass-ionomer lining cement
Zenith Alpha Silver	glass-ionomer–cermet cement
Zetaplus	impression elastomer
Zeus Magic White	die stone
Zeusuperock	hard die stone
Zeusvest	phosphate-bonded investment
Zinroc	zinc oxide/eugenol cement
Zionomer	glass-ionomer cement
Zircate Prophy	prophylaxis paste
ZOE Plus	temporary luting cement
Zone	periodontal dressing

1st Impression	impression alginate
16/17 Platinized Wire	wrought gold alloy wire

Index

Self-activated (cont.)
temporary restoration, 70
transfer copings and patterns,
182
Setting pastes, endodontic, 169
Setting reactions, 3
Shape-retentive memory, nickel–
titanium, 197
Shaper file, 63, (Fig. 4.1d)
Shaping instruments, root canal, 52
Sharpening instruments, 40
Sheet casting wax, 182
Shelf life, 3
Shellac, 103, 108, 181, 183
Shimstock foil, 15
Siamese bracket, 129
Silane bonding, brackets, 129
Silane coupling agent, 79, 80, 144,
216
Silastic, 98
Silica, 1, 221
allotropes, 183
filler, in stone, 178
gel, 217
Silica-bonded investment, 184
Silicate
abrasives, 138
cement, 49,154
removal, 39
Silicification, 168
Silicon dioxide, 1
Silicon impregnation, 165
Silicon in cobalt–chromium alloys,
189
Silicone-reinforced alginate, 105
Silicone
duplicating material, 177
elastomer, 122
occlusal record, 73
impression material, 105, 174–7
maxillofacial polymers, 226
silicone putty impression, 100
Silicone rubber
impression wash, 17
polishing cups, 138
self-curing, 27
Silicone soft lining, 118
Silicones, 2
Silicophosphate cement, 141
Silk sutures, 224
Siloxane ester, 28, 168
Siloxane polymer, resilient lining,
203
Silver, 2
alloys, 190–1

cap splints, 96, 140
cyanide, 179
electroplating, 179
endodontic points, 57, 169
halides, 228
in cements, 157
in high-gold alloys, 185
in high-gold, metal–ceramic
alloys, 186
in low-gold alloys, 188
in wrought gold alloys, 197
Silver-free alloys, 74, 75
Silver–palladium alloys, 74, 75,
191
Silver–tin amalgam alloys, 146–9
Single crystal alumina brackets,
129, 225
Single viscosity polyether, 106
Sintering, 3
Smear layer, 160
Smear layer, dentine, 42
Sodium alginate, 173
bicarbonate, 14
neutralizer, 50
polish, 138
bisulphite, 206
carbonate, 205
carboxymethyl cellulose, 32, 207
chloride, 178
citrate, 28, 217
dichloroisocyanurate, 22
dodecyl benzene sulphonate, 217
dodecyl sulphate, 217
fluoride, 24, 217–19
hypochlorite, 22, 206
lauryl sulphate, 23
metaphosphate, 23
monofluorophosphate, 24, 28,
217, 219
perborate, 50
sulphate, 228
tetraborate (see Borax)
thiosulphate, 228
Soft-lining material, (Fig. 7.21)
Soft maxillofacial polymers, 226
Soft white wax, 122
Softening heat-treatment of gold
alloys, 186
Solbrig casting system, 190
Solder, silver, 127
Soldering, 123
Solders, 82, 191–2
Sonic handpiece, 54
Sonic scaler, 89
Sorbitol, 217

Space closure, 132
Spark machining, 198
Special impression tray, 64, 67, 200
light-curing unit, (Fig. 5.9)
modification, (Fig. 7.11)
Specific gravity, 9
Splints
fractured jaws, 96
mobile teeth, 94
Sponge, butterfly, 37
Spot welding, 196
Spreader, gutta-percha, 56
Solvent softening technique, 56
Springback, 124, (Fig. 8.4)
Sprinkle technique, acrylic, 109
Stabilization, 22
Stabilizing materials, 28
Stainless steel, 195–6
bands, 58
brackets, 227
clasps, 35, 115
components, 115
crown posts, 159
dentine pins, 42, 159, 197
denture base, 113
instruments, 196
post, (Fig. 5.10)
preformed crowns, 196
surgical implants, 196
sutures, 224
tape, 197
temporary crown, 69, 167
wire, 125, 196
wire loops, 96
Stannous fluoride, 24, 219
Stannous octoate, 204
Steel scaler, sharpening 87, (Fig.
6.3)
Sterilization
handpieces, 40
instruments, 136
root canal instruments, 54
Sterling silver, 190
Steroids in endodontic pastes, 169
Sticky wax, 183
Stiffness, 7
orthodontic wire, 123, (Fig. 8.2)
Stippling, acrylic, (Fig. 7.15)
Stock denture tooth, 35
Stock impression tray, 67, 173
modification, (Fig. 7.8)
Stomatitis, denture-related, 111
Stone, 122
casts, 104
die, 178